The Care of the Sick

Originally published in 1979, *The Care of the Sick* is a detailed and comprehensive exploration of the emergence of modern nursing.

Beginning with primitive and early historical nursing, the book traces the development of nursing through the ages and covers a variety of key topics, including the rise of the trained nurse; the problems faced by nursing during its development as a profession; education and working conditions; the government and nursing; the economics of nursing; and how the image of nursing has changed over time.

Extensive and thorough, *The Care of the Sick* will appeal to those with an interest in the history of nursing, the history of medicine, and social history.

T0273360

The Care of the Sick

The Emergence of Modern Nursing

By Vern L. Bullough and Bonnie Bullough

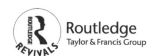

Routledge
Taylor & Francis Group

First published in 1979
by Croom Helm Ltd

This edition first published in 2020 by Routledge
2 Park Square, Milton Park, Abingdon, Oxon, OX14 4RN
and by Routledge
605 Third Avenue, New York, NY 10017

Routledge is an imprint of the Taylor & Francis Group, an informa business

Publisher's Note
The publisher has gone to great lengths to ensure the quality of this reprint but points
out that some imperfections in the original copies may be apparent.

Disclaimer
The publisher has made every effort to trace copyright holders and welcomes
correspondence from those they have been unable to contact.

A Library of Congress record exists under LCCN: 78014238

ISBN 13: 978-0-367-61133-0 (hbk)
ISBN 13: 978-1-003-10428-5 (ebk)
ISBN 13: 978-0-367-61132-3 (pbk)

The Care of the Sick

The Care of the Sick:
the Emergence of
Modern Nursing

Vern and Bonnie Bullough

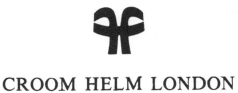

CROOM HELM LONDON

© 1979 Neale Watson Academic Publications, Inc.
Croom Helm Ltd, 2–10 St John's Road, London SW11

British Library Cataloguing in Publication Data

Bullough, Vern LeRoy
  The care of the sick.
  1. Nursing-History
  I. Title II. Bullough, Bonnie
  610.73'069'09   RT31

  ISBN 0–85664–849–3

Photo: "Nurses on Strike,"
(*Courtesy Youngstown Vindicator and Lloyd S. Jones*)

Contents

Contents

One

Primitive and Early Historical Nursing

Civilization began when cities appeared. Cities allowed men to concentrate together, to specialize, and forced them to communicate more effectively with each other. Primitive peoples in a few places especially favored by nature developed cities that sometimes grew into empires. These early civilized people, conscious of their heritage, invented writing to pass it on to future generations. The written records of these ancient civilizations, especially when supplemented by archaeological findings, allow us to reconstruct the past. It is with written records that history begins.

Nursing, however, is older than civilization. It began whenever and wherever man first began to care for the injured, the sick, the wounded. Medicine and nursing have often been represented by the same person, but at other times or in different societies there has been a distinction between the two. Paleopathologists, those specialists who study prehistorical evidences of disease (paleopathology), have found from the bone and mummy remnants of ancient man that he was afflicted with many of the same illnesses as his modern descendants. Bones found in Peru, China, England, Egypt, and elsewhere show evidence of arthritis, sinusitis, bone tumors, and osteoporosis. The tissue remains of mummies indicate that ancient man suffered from arteriosclerosis, pneumonia, pleurisy, kidney stones, gallstones, appendicitis, tuberculosis, and perhaps smallpox, as well as prolapse of the uterus and rectum. But when the medical historian tries to determine what techniques were used to treat these afflictions, he is confronted with an almost insoluble problem, since the only substantial evidence for the existence of prehistorical medical skills is that for the trepanation of the skull. Trepanned skulls have been found all over Europe in Neolithic deposits, and in Peru, Mexico, and even in the rest of North America as far north as Canada. Although historians do not agree as to why this dangerous operation was practiced so widely by the ancients, it is quite clear that it demanded attentive nursing care if the patient were to survive—and somewhat surprisingly many of them did.

Primitive Societies

Prehistoric man evidently did practice some sort of medicine, but how and under what conditions can only be conjectured, since these people have left no written records. There is, however, some indirect evidence which can amplify the character of the healing arts in the prehistoric past—the practices of modern primitive tribes. It is the primitive tribe that gives some flesh to the bones excavated from the past. Though contemporary primitives are different from the people of the distant past, they do give us a guide, in fact almost the only guide, to what may have been man's economy, society, religion, and particularly his attitudes toward the sick. Primitive peoples have been changing and making history, but at a markedly slower rate than in the more dynamic civilizations. Primitive tribes differ from each other, but it seems clear that in most of them good health was the natural state of affairs. They believe—or rather, used to believe, since primitive tribes are rapidly disappearing—that the body would remain in perfect order unless tampered with. They recognized that such things as poisons, wounds, burns, and falls would affect their health or even kill them, and that cold, heat, overstraining, too much sun, or overeating might cause some minor ailments and discomforts. In fact, they had developed a whole series of massages, potions, and other treatments to treat just such incidents. Aside from these so-called natural ills, however, most primitives believed that they suffered or died from diseases or illnesses attributable to supernatural causes. As a result the shamans or medicine men used magical or supernatural means in their cure, as well as more prosaic treatments. Most medicine men did not consider the comfort of the patient to be important in treating a disease; on the contrary, they thought that the best cure was to make the patient so uncomfortable that the evil spirit which caused disease would seek to move elsewhere. In effect the major effort was directed toward the disease and not toward the patient.

In all societies, however, the truly sick man was weak and helpless and could not fulfill the tasks that were normally expected of him. In such cases someone had to watch over the patient, nurse him, and care for him. In most primitive societies this nurse was a close female relative. At times there seems to have been an even more specialized type of nursing care. The Banyankole in Africa isolated a man with smallpox, and someone who had had the disease was chosen to look after him. There was even a set treatment for the nurse to follow. For the first few days, she fed the patient milk and hot water, encouraging him to sleep as much as possible; on the fourth day the nurse pricked the pustules with a thorn, leaving the pus to dry. On the sixth day the patient was bathed by the nurse with warm fresh water, and on the seventh day he was smeared with a white clay to absorb the pus and the peeling skin.

Other tribes gave special diets to the sick. Among the Natchez, extremely sick persons were given small quantities of coarse meal cooked in a rich broth. In some American Indian tribes, members of the patient's household prepared the concoctions prescribed by the medicine man in utensils especially set aside for the sick, but usually the sick ate what the robust and healthy did or went without. Perhaps because of this practice, patients among many primitive peoples died as often from hunger and inadequate nursing care as from the disease. The regular treatment of wounds was no treatment at all. Bleeding aroused but a casual interest, and then an incantation served as a treatment. There were exceptions, and in some primitive groups old women were called in to nurse the wounded warriors. Some of the American Indians combined pressure with a styptic to stop bleeding by filling the wound with a dry powder before bandaging it. Many South Sea Islanders tied a tourniquet made of tapa cloth tightly around the injured part. Other primitive peoples made a kind of poultice of herbs and fresh leaves which they applied to the wound.

Among some primitive people the sick or infirm were considered such a liability that they were often abandoned. Even where more humane treatment prevailed, special circumstances often demanded abandoning the seriously ill. Such cruelty and neglect occurred only where all hope of recovery had gone or in epidemics when the group needed to abandon its members in order to survive. There was also a distinction between the young and the old. An old patient might well be killed without much thought, but the sick young person would be spared. The sick and crippled were often killed out of respect and compassion, a sort of mercy killing.

We know most about primitive nursing care in the prenatal, postpartum, and postnatal periods. In some cultures the lochial period was four days; in others it was as long as forty days. The baby might be delivered in the mother-in-law's house, in the mother's house, in the women's menstrual hut, or at times in a special lying-in hut. Some primitive societies had the equivalent of a nurse-midwife, while in other groups the woman was assisted by her female relatives or by women who had had children. Every society, however, seems to have had someone to nurse the mother and care for the infant. Occasionally, it was the husband who was expected to do the nursing, as among the Kalmuks, but in most societies it was a task delegated to women, who could well be called nurses.

Among the Indians of the southeastern United States, the newborn child was washed in a stream, daubed with bear grease, and then placed in a cradle of cane softened with moss. Other Indians bathed the infant in tepid water as soon as the cord was cut, while the mother herself received a hot-water sponge bath. Usually the newborn was given a few drops of a special brew. In the Congo the mother and child were sprinkled with cold water after delivery; this supposedly revived the mother and made the baby cry. When the placenta was delivered among certain African tribes, the baby was daubed with sand and washed with tepid water, while the mother herself cut the umbilical cord. Almost every primitive society had developed a perineal binder for the mother.

Primitive man was also plagued by psychiatric problems. Mental illness in most primitive cultures was treated with considerable indulgence unless the individual was totally incapacitated or unless his bizarre behavior frightened others. The Yorubu, a central African tribe that had reached a fairly high level of sophistication before the arrival of Europeans, had a variety of psychiatric methods including some that modern psychiatrists have also found useful: rest cures, allowing the individual to act out his difficulty, and permitting him to confide in the witch doctor.

In effect it appears that primitive peoples had developed some of the procedures associated with modern nursing care including midwifery techniques, dressing wounds, the preparation of special diets, emotional support, and perhaps even isolation procedures. Unfortunately, the relation of these nursing techniques to primitive medicine is not clear. Was there an actual separation of medicine and nursing? The answer must be ambiguous—sometimes yes, sometimes no. Usually the actual care of the sick rested with the women of the community.

Ancient Egypt

Once civilization developed, changes in living habits effected changes in social structure, technology, and ideology, and these in turn affected medicine and nursing. Since this book is primarily concerned with the development of nursing in Europe and America, most attention will be given to the main sources of this civilization, namely the ancient Near East, specifically Egypt, the Hebrews, and the peoples of the Tigris-Euphrates Valley. Passing attention will also be given to the ancient Chinese and to the founders of civilization in India. Egyptian civilization, though not the oldest (this honor seems to go to the Tigris-Euphrates Valley), is the longest-lived and most stable and is discussed first.

Although the same magical, religious, and empirico-rational elements present in prehistoric and primitive societies are encountered in ancient Egypt, they are more distinct. The physician was not a medicine man or a shaman; instead there were specialization and separation of functions, with physicians, priests, and sorcerers all existing independently. Some patients would consult the physician, others the priest, and others sought healing in magical formulas. Many tried all three methods, since the Egyptians, like the primitive peoples, did not accept illness and death as natural or inevitable. They thought that life, once it had begun, should be indefinitely prolonged. If no untoward accident intervened, why should life cease? Man, therefore, did not die, someone or something assassinated him. The murderer often belonged to this world and could be easily identified: another man, an animal, an inanimate object, a stone detached from the mountain, a tree falling upon a traveler and crushing him. Often, however, the assailant was invisible and only revealed itself by the malignity of its attacks: it was a god, a spirit, the soul of a dead man that entered a living person or threw itself upon him with irresistible violence. But once in possession, the vile influence wreaked havoc. It broke bones, sucked out the marrow, drank the blood, gnawed the intestines or the heart, and devoured the flesh. The invalid perished as the destruction continued, and death speedily ensued, unless the evil genius could be driven out before it had committed irreparable damage.

Whoever treated a sick person had, therefore, two very important duties to perform. He must first discover the nature of the spirit in possession and, if possible, its name, and then attack it, drive it out, or even destroy it. This took powerful magic. But his work was not ended, for he must then use medicine to contend with the disorders that the strange being had produced in the body. This could be done by following a strict regime. The cure-workers, therefore, were divided into various categories. Some inclined toward sorcery and had faith in formulas and talismans; others extolled the use of drugs and medicines. But most of the practitioners did not bind themselves exclusively to either but distinguished between the cases where they could use natural methods and those in which magic was sovereign. The most famous Egyptian medical practitioner was the legendary Imhotep, who has also been given the credit for building the first pyramid.

Healing appeared as the successful result of a contest between invisible beings of good and evil. Therapeutic methods were based upon rituals of worship, sacrifice, and purification. Although the medical literature of Egypt that has come down to us is not large, it is rich enough for most medical historians to contend that even though all physicians used incantations or prayers at some time, there were many who treated their patients primarily with methods that we consider rational.

Herodotus, the Greek historian, implied that Egypt in its later period was a land of specialists with physicians for "the eyes, others of the head, others of the teeth, others of the belly, others of obscure diseases."[1] Aside from chance comments such as these by later Greeks, our knowledge of Egyptian medicine and nursing is based upon archaeological materials including tomb paintings, carvings in the temples, and certain papyri—that is, books written on material made from the stems of papyrus plants. The two most important papyri are the *Edwin Smith Surgical Papyrus*,[2] dealing with surgery, and the *Ebers Papyrus*,[3] which is a kind of medical textbook. There are other papyri—the *Berlin, Hearst, London, Kahun,* and two lesser *Berlin* papyri dealing with medicine—but they are neither so detailed nor so rational as the first two. (A papyrus is named after the man who first acquired it or after the place where the manuscript is kept.) There are more incantations in the *Ebers* than in the *Smith Papyrus*, perhaps because one is surgical and the other medical, but both of them approach a case more or less scientifically: (1) the provisionary diagnosis is made; (2) instructions are then given on how to examine the patient and what diagnostic signs to look for; (3) the diagnosis and the prognosis of the case are described; (4) necessary therapeutic measures are outlined, such as manipulation, drugs, and magic formulas or prayers.

Egyptian temples were often healing temples, with many people traveling long distances to be cured by their favorite divinities. Many of these temples had a "house of life" attached which was a sort of training school for physicians and medical attendants, an indication that the patients might have received what then passed for professional medical care. In the healing temples the sick and the afflicted, sterile women desiring children, and patients of every kind would spend the night, or sometimes many days and nights, in an attempt to obtain healing or comfort from the gods. The priests would look after them, pray with them, use incantations, and sometimes alleviate their troubles with practical remedies such as baths. Certainly the long rest in the temple, the appearance of significant dreams, or the bathing ritual could often have a therapeutic effect on the patient and perhaps might even lead him to believe that he was cured. The priests in these temples performed many nursing duties; in fact, some writers have called them nursing priests.

That there were specialists, or at least individuals, outside the temple who carried out nursing duties, we know because workers on some jobs were excused from work to nurse their fellow laborers. It seems natural to suppose that someone knew about first aid and elementary nursing techniques, that they liked this kind of work and were put to use. We know for certain that there were wet nurses, at least for the nobility, for there are several goddesses of nursing. It seems that some of these were also deities of parturition, watching over the mother and children, especially the royal children. The most famous of these goddesses were Nekhbet and Uzoit.

Some of our present-day nursing techniques and duties also were known in Egypt. Taking the pulse, for example, was a common practice in Egyptian medicine. Great emphasis was placed on the heart and on the vessels that went from it to every part of the body. It was, therefore, natural for the Egyptians to evaluate a patient's general condition by the quality of the pulse. "His heart beats feebly" was an alarming symptom. The Egyptians probably did not count the pulse, since they were unaware of the circulation of the blood, but they evaluated its quality. They made frequent use of linen bandages and absorbent lint made from ravelings or bits of thread, and in injuries to the nose or outer ear they used plugs, swabs, or tampons of linen. They also used a kind of adhesive plaster to close small wounds; more serious wounds were closed by surgical stitching.

Some of the treatments in the *Edwin Smith Surgical Papyrus* indicate that daily care of the patient was expected. Whether this was done by the doctor, by the doctor's assistant, or even perhaps by a relative of the patient who might act as a nurse is not clear. For example, the basic treatment for a gaping wound in the head was to bind fresh meat upon it with two strips of linen, and then to treat it every day afterward with grease, honey, and lint until the patient recovered. Some sort of dietary treatment was also prescribed, since the statement "moor him at his mooring stakes until the injury passes by" often appears. This has usually been taken to mean that the patient should be put on his accustomed diet. What this was is not known, but an indication that such a diet might be a special sick diet is found in another prescription where a man suffering from an unidentified disease was to be given a preparation of barley every day and was to be prevented from eating anything hot. Since similar references can be found in the papyri, it is quite possible that certain diets were taken for granted without detailed instructions being given. In such cases the physician or surgeon probably told the wife or "nurse" what to feed the patient. That some sort of nursing watch was kept is also indicated by the clauses that tell the physician how long treatment should last: ". . . until thou knowest that he has reached a decisive point"—which seems to imply a rather close watch.

We also know that the Egyptians had developed various splints. One was the regular wood splint padded with linen. A second is simply called "of linen," and James Henry Breasted, the editor and translator of the *Smith Papyrus*, thought that this might be a molded splint—that is, layers of linen impregnated with glue and plaster which could be molded while soft to conform to the limb. A third type was a stiff roll of linen used apparently where a softer splint was needed, as with a fractured nasal bone.[4] They had also developed other techniques that seem to require nursing care. They had a brace of wood padded with linen for insertion into the mouth of a patient suffering with constriction of ligaments controlling the mandible (tetanus?) in order to hold the mouth open and permit feeding with liquid food. They had also devised a backrest of sorts for maintaining a patient upright in the sitting posture.

The Egyptian mother, at least the primipara, was very young. Girls usually married at the age of twelve or thirteen, and their husbands were hardly more than fifteen or sixteen. When the young woman felt the first pains of labor, she called women members of her household or friendly neighbors to assist her. She retired to a corner of the house where in anticipation she had placed statuettes of the divinities of childbirth. Royal women were often delivered in a separate house, a sort of lying-in hospital. A woman was usually delivered kneeling down, sitting on her heels with one nurse holding her back while the other knelt to receive the baby in front. Sometimes she squatted on top of two bricks or stones which left space in the center to deliver the infant. Royal children were usually turned over to a wet nurse, but most mothers nursed their own children. The newborn was wrapped in a large linen cloth but was not bandaged.

Babylonian Civilization

The great civilizations that grew up between the Tigris and Euphrates rivers did not have the political unity or continuity that was so apparent in Egypt, perhaps because they were less geographically protected. Various empires appeared in this area, which is known geographically as Mesopotamia (modern Iraq), including the Sumerian, Akkadian, Assyrian, and Babylonian. Despite this, there was a cultural unity which allows historians to speak rather loosely of a Babylonian civilization.

Medical documents from this region are far more numerous than those from Egypt. The ancient Mesopotamians wrote on clay tablets which have survived in much greater quantities than the papyri. Since the documents, however, are far less orderly, much more casual, and a great deal shorter than the Egyptian ones, it has been suggested that they were a type of notation which helped to maintain an extensive oral tradition. Although the analysis of the two longest papyri, those of Smith and Ebers, would give us the essentials of Egyptian medicine, it is impossible to do the same in Babylonian medicine because no lengthy document has survived. Another difficulty is that much of our information is based on seventh century B.C. documents from the great library of Ashurbanipal. However, medical historians believe that much of the material contained in these late tablets is of much earlier origin, dating back to the early Sumerians in many cases.

Disease in the Mesopotamian area, at least in the earlier period, was considered a great curse, a divine punishment for acts against the gods or an attack of the spirits. This aggravated the position of the sick man in society, since his illness might be a punishment for some sin. He might have stolen, killed, committed perjury or adultery, spat into a river, drunk from an impure vessel, or done something else that was sinful. For this his god or guardian spirit had abandoned him, leaving him an easy prey to the demons. He was sick and suffered and deserved it, but the worst was that his suffering made his sin apparent to all. He was branded with the odium of sin and isolated in society. His daily life was altered, and he found himself in disgrace. This concept of disease as punishment for sin is also dominant in the Old Testament. God had revealed his law; those who obeyed it piously lived in happiness, but those who transgressed were punished, with illness and suffering being the chief punishments. The logic and simplicity of the thinking are difficult to overcome. Christianity endeavored to glorify suffering but never quite succeeded. In the Middle Ages epidemics were considered visitations inflicted by God upon mankind—an attitude not unknown even today.

The problem then was, as in other, more primitive cultures, to lift the spell from the afflicted. This could be effected through the aid of a priest or by "sympathetic magic," whereby the afflicted was able to transfer the disease to something else, either animate or inanimate. This is described as "making an atonement" for the sick person, and the word in Assyrian, *kuppuru*, which describes this is the equivalent of the Hebrew *kipper* of the priestly code. To cure the afflicted, three separate types of priests developed. One was the *baru*, the seer, who specialized in divination. He knew omens and how to interpret them, for the sick and for the well. He might determine through the omens what was wrong with the patient. Next was the *ashipu*, the exorcist or incantation priest, who performed the rites required for driving an evil spirit from the body of the patient. He also did not deal with sick people exclusively, since disease was not the only consequence of sin. A third type of priest, the *asu,* was more strictly a physician than the other two because he devoted all his activities to the sick. He not only knew the charms, but also the medical properties of certain drugs and perhaps even performed operations.

Such an attitude toward illness would, if carried to its logical conclusion, make the nurse unnecessary. The patient had committed his sin; he must suffer and atone for it. Let him get right with the gods. But illness might also be caused by the curses or spells of an enemy and not by the patient's own misdeeds. This would at least make people more willing to intervene. But even without this rationalization, a wife or husband would care for a sick mate, parents who loved their children would try to nurse them to recovery, and friends might nurse other friends.

That nursing care of some sort did exist can be deduced from several documents. Polygamy was legal in Babylonia, as was divorce, but if a man took a second wife because his first wife had become sick, he was not allowed to divorce the sick wife, but instead was obliged to keep her in his house and support her as long as she lived. If she preferred to leave, he was to return her dowry to her. The sick, then, were not abandoned, but somebody had to nurse and care for them. In the incantations that were used by the priests, there are several references to activities that today are nursing duties. Baths were to be given to the patient, his body was to be massaged with butter, and his wounds were to be dressed and bandaged. That this constituted nursing care is evident. That this care might be given by a sort of lay nurse can be gathered from a letter the physician Arad-Nana wrote to a patient who had a nosebleed. In his letter Arad-Nana says that the patient's difficulty was that the bandages on his nose had not been applied by experts. They had been placed on the cartilage of the nose when they should have been placed inside the nostrils. By placing them inside, Arad-Nana says, the breathing would be hindered, but the flow of blood would cease. He then adds that he would come and teach those who applied the bandages how to do it.[5]

Some of the gods of Babylonia were also nursing deities, especially Ishtar, the mother of creation, goddess of love, fertility, childbirth, and healing. She was the kind, sympathetic mother of mankind who listened to the supplications of sinners, especially those seeking relief from pain, suffering, and disease. Some of these gods were invoked to nurse the patient and to watch over him:

> May Ishun the great overseer,
> The potent spirit of the Gods,
> Stand at his head and guard him through the night
> Unto the kindly hands of Shamash.
> Night and day may he commend him.[6]

Of course, wet nurses existed in Babylonia as they did elsewhere. They were closely regulated by the law both as to remuneration and as to punishment for their failure to fulfill their responsibilities. If a child given to the care of a nurse died and the nurse was convicted of having substituted another child in his stead, her breasts were cut off.

Biblical Nursing

The third people who contributed greatly to Western civilization were the Hebrews. Though never very numerous and without great power, they exercised influence considerably out of proportion to their numbers. Most of their genius was religious: Judaism eventually gave birth to both Christianity and Islam. The ancient Hebrews lived between the Babylonians and the Egyptians, and thus were influenced by both. Their concept of disease, as has been pointed out, was similar to that of the Babylonians: God visiting punishment upon sinners. Job in the Old Testament exemplified this. But the Jewish heritage in medicine is greater in sanitation and public health than in any concept of disease. Garbage and excreta were disposed of outside the city or camp, contagious diseases were quarantined, spitting was outlawed as unhygienic, and bodily cleanliness became a prerequisite for moral purity. Although some of these concepts were Egyptian in origin, Moses and the Hebrews were the first to codify them and present them as religious tenets.

Unlike their Egyptian and Babylonian colleagues, the priests of Israel apparently avoided actual medical practice but concentrated their efforts on the observance of health rules with regard to food, cleanliness, and quarantine. This might eventually have produced an empirical medical practitioner, free of priestly interference, or it might have left the care of the sick and the afflicted to the family, encouraging the development of practical nursing care, as indeed seems to have happened among the ancient Hebrews.

Nurses are frequently referred to in the Scriptures. Most of the references are to wet nurses, but there are others. Isaiah (60:4) states that "thy sons shall come from far, and thy daughters shall be nursed at thy side"; in Numbers (11:12) is a reference to a nursing father carrying a sucking child; another appears in Isaiah (49:23). The nurse appears at times as a combination servant, companion, and helpmate. Rebekah's nurse accompanied her when she left with Abraham's servant to meet Isaac (Genesis 24:59).

Hindu Medicine and Nursing

Early Indian medicine was regarded as an aspect of sorcery, and the physician inevitably was a man of power, possessed of magical skill. Disease came from sin, confession was part of the healing rite, and demons were fought by exorcism, spells, and hymns. Much of the information about early Hindu beliefs is derived from the vedas, the holy Sanscrit books. Of the four early vedas, the most valuable for medical purposes is the *Atharva veda* which contains a number of magical formulas as well as herbal cures. Additional information is found in the *Upavedas* or later vedas, particularly the *Ayur-veda* (Science of Life) which can be partially reconstructed from references to it in other works. Particularly valuable for our picture of ancient Indian medicine are the works of Charaka (second century A.D.) and Susruta (fourth century A.D.). Since both of these scholars were influenced by the Greeks and Persians, there is considerable scholarly debate as to how much of what they say can be taken as indicative of early Indian medicine, and how much is derived from the Greeks and Persians. Almost all modern investigators agree, however, that the ancient Indians were especially advanced in surgery, particularly rhinoplasty and skin grafting. Indian physicians not only used inspection, palpitation, and auscultation, but also smelling and tasting. Five kinds of remedies were recognized: emetics, purges, irrigations, oily enemas, and remedies that produced sneezing.

Of particular interest for any history of patient care is the importance the Indian writings gave to attendants on the sick. Susruta stated that the

> physician, the patient, the medicine, and the attendants (nurses?) are the four essential factors of a course of medical treatment. . . . That person alone is fit to nurse or to attend the bedside of a patient who is cool-headed

and pleasant in his demeanour, does not speak ill of anybody, is strong and attentive to the requirements of the sick, and strictly and indefatigably follows the instructions of the physician.[7]

Similarly, Charaka wrote that the attendant should know how drugs were prepared, be devoted to the patient, have purity of mind and body, and be intelligent or clever.[8]

These attendants, however, were not a special class of medical practitioners but rather pupils of the physician. They served their physician teacher, observed and assisted him when they could, and eventually, if they performed satisfactorily, became physicians or surgeons themselves. All such attendants were male since women were attended only by their female relatives, not by professionals. There is no mention of hospitals in the early texts, and these probably did not exist until the third or fourth centuries A.D.

The Chinese Way

Ancient Chinese medicine, like its counterparts elsewhere, was closely related to magic and demons. According to tradition, medicine had originated when the Emperor Shen Nung (about 2700 B.C.) invented drug lore and acupuncture and incorporated it into the fundamental philosophy of *yang* and *yin*. Medicine then became closely allied to philosophy. The whole universe is divided into two principles, yang (male) and yin (female). Yang is light, while yin is dark, and similarly the male and female elements are on opposite sides of the spectrum for every conceivable characteristic. When the two are in harmony, the patient is in good health; illness results when they are not. The earliest Chinese medical work, and one that was studied into the twentieth century, is the *Nei Ching*, the author of which is said to have been the Emperor Hwang-Ti (about 2600 B.C.).[9] The physician was consulted only as a last resort, and many of the secrets of good health were transmitted to the adept through religious-mystical teaching. There were specialized practitioners, such as midwives, and these women also dealt with other aspects of women's health. Actual care itself was provided by the family or servants.

Nursing in Pre-Greek Civilizations

In summary, it might be said that although the ancient peoples had not developed a specialized nurse, they were usually conscious of the need for nursing care. This is especially true among the Egyptians and the

Hindus. In Egypt specialized care was probably performed by the doctor's assistants, as it was in India, although the priests, the mother or wife, or others with a special ability for nursing might be excused from other tasks to take care of a sick or wounded friend or relative. In Israel, in Babylonia, and in China, where the medical profession had not become so specialized and where the conditions of disease were somewhat different from those in Egypt, nursing was more confined to the family or servants. There were probably no doctor's assistants or priests who did nursing, but rather the women in the home were the key figures. Wet nurses, of course, existed in all these early civilizations, and from what the Old Testament says on the subject, some of these might actually have developed into a sort of practical nurse once the child was weaned (II Samuel 4:4). Nevertheless, the nurse in these societies was developing a reputation for kindliness, if the statement in I Thessalonians (2:7) can be taken literally. Here St. Paul stated: "But we were gentle among you, even as a nurse cherisheth her children."

The Greeks

It is difficult to explain why suddenly, about 2,600 years ago, a people known as the Greeks took such important and radical steps in human thought. The advances made at that time make ancient Greek medicine much closer to modern than any other historical form of medicine. It is quite possible that modern medicine could not have existed without the precedent set by the Greeks; in fact, much of modern medical terminology is based on Greek words. The advances in medicine, science, and human thought appeared to be so great and the pace so quickened that some historians describe them as the *Greek Miracle.*

Although we may not know all the reasons for such advances, the historian must attempt at least a partial explanation. Several contributing factors appear fairly obvious. Whereas the Egyptians, the Mesopotamians, and the Hebrews had a writing of sorts, the Greeks made effective use of an alphabet with symbols for vowels also. The alphabet is believed to have originated in Phoenicia around 1200 B.C. and spread from there around the Mediterranean. The Phoenicians did not have any written symbol for the various vowels. Adoption of alphabetical writing did not, of course, initiate popular education, but it made learning much easier and probably created a wider audience than had existed before. But the Greeks, especially the Ionian Greeks who lived in Asia Minor, traded with most of the other Mediterranean peoples. These commercial contacts exposed them to the cultural achievements of the Egyptians, Mesopotamians, Phoenicians, and Cretans, and each of these civilizations contained elements that would or could contribute a new approach to science and medicine, especially if combined together. Later the European Greeks continued and expanded these contacts.

This very multiplicity and intermingling that went on in the Greek world apparently created a vigorous hybrid. A factor in this invigoration was the division of the Greeks into numerous small city-states. This extreme political fragmentation, which existed throughout Greek history and which later proved to be their undoing, at first merely prevented the development of a strong, well-organized bureaucracy of the state or of the priests, both of which had maintained such a stranglehold on thought and practice in other civilizations. Individualism and critical thought could develop to a degree unattainable in the Oriental empires.

This does not mean that religious medicine was unknown to the Greeks; Greek medicine always retained a religious orientation. The Greek physicians were not disbelievers, but they could separate their practices from their religious beliefs. In Greece also, as in other early civilizations, medicine was not yet a science working behind the closed doors of a hospital or university, unintelligible in its technical detail to the untrained layman. Surgical treatment, dietary regulation, bandaging, preparation of drugs—all were often matters of common knowledge. The educated layman was even familiar with medical theories. In late antiquity the upper classes were always well versed in medicine; medical instruction came to constitute part of a general education. People of lower standing, even if unfamiliar with theory, had developed a tradition of folk medicine. Since many of the country districts never had a resident physician, the people exchanged their experiences with their neighbors, especially with those who were well known for their wisdom in such matters. In this situation nursing and nursing techniques became widespread, and nursing became more of a science than it had been earlier.

That general knowledge of nursing and medicine was so widespread worked against the development of the professional practitioner. In *The Art*,[10] attributed to the great medical writer Hippocrates, there is a section defending the calling of the physician. The writer points out that though many people are cured of their sickness without calling on a physician, correct medical treatment without so much trial and error could be given if they did so. The general extent of this knowledge appears frequently in the earlier writings of the Greeks known to us, the two poems the *Iliad* and the *Odyssey*, attributed to Homer. These poems were apparently the product of several hands, being composed over several centuries before reaching their final form about the seventh century B.C. In the *Iliad*, which is an account of the attempts to capture Troy and rescue the beautiful Helen from her lover Paris, 140 different wounds are described, some of them superficial, some penetrating. The mortality rate averaged 77.6 percent, being highest in sword and spear thrusts, and lowest from arrow wounds. There was considerable need for nursing care, and Achilles, Patroclus, and other princes often acted as nurses. In the eleventh book, Patroclus was forced to cut out the arrow from the surgeon Machaon by himself, after which he washed the wound with water and then applied a dressing to it.

Later Patroclus himself was wounded, and Achilles nursed him. There is a *cylix* (a two-handed drinking cup much decorated by artists) in the Berlin museum showing Achilles bandaging the upper arm of Patroclus. Achilles is using a two-rolled bandage that he is trying to extend over the elbow; it is evident from the position in which he has the two tails of the bandage that he might have some difficulty when it comes to the final fastening. Homer uses several terms meaning nurse: there were wet-nurses, nurse-midwives, and nurse-maids.[11]

The early stages of Greek medicine still had some of the concepts of Egyptian, Babylonian, and Hebrew medicine. For wounds, good medical and nursing techniques were utilized; the arrow was drawn or cut out, the wound washed, soothing herbs applied, and the wound bandaged. But in sickness where no external cause was apparent, there was no thought of treatment. Here, if anywhere, an evil spirit was at work. For plague no medical treatment was possible; the solution was to find how or why men had angered the gods. The real healer of the plague, described in the first book of the *Iliad*, was the prophet who prayed for its removal, thus persuading the enraged Apollo to stop shooting the plague arrows. In this the Greeks were like primitive peoples; rational causes and empirical methods tended to be more often linked to injuries than to internal ailments.

When we turn to the rise of Greek scientific thought in the sixth, fifth, and fourth centuries B.C., we note writers dealing with medical care, the best known of whom is Hippocrates of Cos (460–379 B.C.). He is often called the "father of medicine" and is best remembered today by the Hippocratic Oath, which was probably written after his death. Very little is known about his life or his ideas. Fifty to 70 books were later attributed to him, and in the third century B.C. they were collected in Alexandria into the *Corpus Hippocraticum*. It is not known which of these books, if any, were actually written by him. Some of them are textbooks, some are monographs, and some are little more than notes, with contradictory opinions found throughout the various works. Historians believe that the writings are not the work of one man, or even one group, but are a collection of medical writings, written between 480 and 380 B.C., express-ing the ideas of several men and several schools. When these works of unknown authors were eventually gathered together in Alexandria, the name of Hippocrates was affixed to them, since even by that time he was regarded as the greatest ancient physician. But when we examine these works for mention of nurses or nursing duties, we are faced with a typical difficulty in answering many problems about the ancients. There is very little specific information about nurses of nursing. Many have concluded from this silence that the task of nursing usually fell to the women of the household. The activities of the Greek woman are rarely described for us, perhaps because they were not considered dignified enough for literary treatment. The Greeks, for all their emancipation, were unwilling to admit women to the company of men; the lives of men and women in Greece were quite distinct.

This supposition that women might handle nursing duties is given support by several references in Greek literature. Xenophon, a historian, wrote a work called *Oeconomicus*, a discussion of household management. One of the duties he describes for the wife is to see that any sick servant is cared for.[12] Though women nurses are not mentioned in the Hippocratic works, there are several allusions to bedside care which might indicate that nursing care was to be given to the sick. There are instructions that the location of the patient's bed is to be considered, that undue noise is to be avoided, that kitchen smells, especially the smell of wine, should be kept from the sick. Baths are to be given, either almost continuously or at intervals, according to the illness of the patient. At times the writers in the Hippocratic corpus indicate that baths cannot be given because the houses of the patients do not have the suitable apparatus or attendants (nursing attendants?) to manage the bath. In the *Regimen in Acute Diseases*, the patient is instructed to be quiet and silent and to do nothing himself in the bath but to leave the pouring and the rubbing to the attendants or others.[13]

While in the field, the armies also had nurses who accompanied them, although there is no evidence to suggest that they were specially trained. The same Xenophon, in his *Anabasis*, indicates that when the Greeks were away from home fighting, they retired periodically to nearby villages to nurse their wounded. When they moved on, the wounded were carried with them by selected companions.[14]

Though lay nurses existed, many of them quite able, there apparently was need at times for better-trained personnel to watch over the sick, attendants who were more medically qualified than a wife, mother, or comrade-in-arms would be. The clinical histories of the *Epidemics*, a Hippocratic work, contain fairly complex and complete accounts of the symptoms the patient experienced on different days of his illness. Not all the histories are equally informative, but the detailed accounts that appear there indicate that a trained or semitrained person had kept a very close watch on the patient.[15] If we assume that the physician was too busy to spend all his time with one patient, that, in fact, it was probably too expensive to the patient to have him do so, then it seems apparent that someone else gave the information. This required a trained eye, one quick to catch the essential, a person who could anticipate the doctor's desire for necessary information—in short, a trained nurse. It could not have been an unskilled attendant since the regime for the sick or the observations could not have been carried out by him. But we know of no trained nurses, so that someone else had to take it upon himself to be the nurse. A hint as to who would do this appears in the *Decorum* of the Hippocratic collection.

> Let one of your pupils be left in charge, to carry out instructions without unpleasantness, and to administer the treatment. Choose out those who have been already admitted into the mysteries of the art, so as to add anything necessary, and to give treatment with safety. He is there also to prevent those things escaping notice that happen in the intervals between visits. Never put a layman in charge of anything, otherwise if a mischance occurs the blame will fall on you, but achievement will bring you pride.[16]

Here we have a skilled or partially skilled attendant who could perform or, perhaps better, superintend the necessary nursing. In the latter case, the members of the patient's household, probably the women, would do the nursing. The physician would have someone upon whom he could rely to carry out his order or to report to him when necessary, thus saving him many extra visits. The pupil also had a good chance of gaining experience which was very important in an era before internship was known. The combination of nurse and medical student might be far from ideal, but it is an early recognition that a nurse should have some sort of professional training.

Bandaging techniques had also been perfected by the Greeks, and they appear to have developed some standard types. Three simple types are variations of a common spiral or figure-of-eight bandage used to bind an arm or leg or to support a limb. Of the complex bandages the so-called Hippocratic rhomb covered the top of the head, and the hemirhomb was intended for the side of the face or for a unilateral dislocation of the jaw.

In the Hippocratic work on surgery, several surgical procedures are mentioned. According to the author the necessary requisites for the surgery are the patient, the surgeon, the assistants, instruments, and lights. The lamps are to be placed most carefully to give the greatest amount of light. The instruments are enumerated, an indication perhaps that some of the attendants might have been "scrub" or "circulating" nurses. Part of their duties, however, included strongarm tactics that would be out of place in present-day nursing; in Chapter Six the writer warned the assistants that when they present the part for operation, they should hold fast the rest of the body, so that it would be steady for the surgeon.[17]

An interesting development in Greek medicine on a less scientific plane is incubation. This procedure developed in the temples of Asclepius, the god of healing, and might have been influenced by Egyptian practices. The Greek temples known as *Asclepieia*, have been more thoroughly studied than the Egyptian, and we know more about what went on. A sick person would go to the temple to sleep or brood upon his illness (incubate). In his dreams the god would appear to him and cure him or tell him how to be cured. Modern scholars used to take it for granted that the priests charged for "hospitalization," but it now appears that many of these temples accepted the poor for treatment. If the god advised a lengthy cure or remedies for which the patient could not pay, the priests did not send him away. Apparently many of the more wealthy patients had endowed the temples, so that the priests could afford to care for the poor. It seems safe to say that in a world where the poor were left to their fate by the state or by the community-at-large, where lay medicine did not make any special provisions for the needy, the Asclepieia and religious medicine were of the greatest importance for the medical welfare of the lower classes. That they performed such tasks helps to explain why so many of these same institutions were taken over by the Christian Church to be run as hospitals or poorhouses.[18]

In the temples cures might have been effected naturally or perhaps through a kind of shock. Fevers usually pass in time, eyesight occasionally does return of its own accord, and rest can do wonders for most sick people. The accounts of cures in the temples show that patients, at the instigation of the god, vomited and expelled evil matter. They dreamed they were cut open, that malignancies were removed, and that they were healed. The god appeared to them and told them to do certain things. Not only the poor and the afflicted went to the temples but also the rich who could afford medical care, often after they had been termed hopeless cases by the lay practitioner. In antiquity the physician gave up much sooner than he would today, so that many "hopeless" cases could well be cured in time at the temple. Moreover, in the temple the patient would be willing to do things that he would never have done at the request of a regular physician. He would accept painstaking diets or regimes, suffer through rigorous treatment or massage, simply because the god told him to do so. Many of these people would thus cure themselves.

The important point about the Asclepieia is that the god was willing to see dire sights, to touch unpleasant things, to welcome the afflicted. He allowed his sacred precincts to become a hospital ward; he had no aversion to the natural, and therefore nature herself cooperated. The larger shrines were administered by chief priests who supervised the work of the assistant priests and minor officials. The assistant priests conducted sacrifices for the gods, received the patients, recorded their names and homes, and, more important, directed the care of the sick. A large number of assistants were attendants for the sick; they washed them, applied ointments, talked to them, and acted generally as nurses. In these temples the snake was sacred, helpful in curing the sick. The symbol of the temple came to be a single snake wrapped around a staff, from which modern medicine gets the symbol of the caduceus. However, when the medical corps of the U.S. Army adopted its symbol, it mistakenly took a wand with two serpents around it; this was not the staff of office of the gods of medicine, but of Hermes, or Mercury, the god of business and communication.

That there were other types of hospitals in Greece seems probable. Some of the great cities had doctors in residence who were paid by the community but also received remuneration from their patients. These physicians were often in charge of a sort of city hospital where patients paid for their stay, since those who could not were turned out, although some of the physicians also had an *iatreia*, a combination consulting room and dispensary where attendants and apprentices acted as nurses.[19]

In childbirth, nurses are mentioned both as attendants and as wet nurses, as has been pointed out. In his play *The Thesmophoriazusae*, Aristophanes has a man disguised as a woman enter the temple of the women to defend one of his fellow men accused by the women of maligning them. In the temple scene he accuses the women of pretending to be pregnant and then at the last minute having the nurse substitute someone else's baby which they pass off as their own to deceive their husbands. We do know that women attendants were present at births, acting in the capacity of nurses. The mother of the philosopher Socrates was a nurse-midwife. According to the Spartan constitution as given by Plutarch, the attendants in that city bathed the newborn babies not with water but with wine which was supposed to test their hardiness. In Sparta also the nurses did not wrap the children in swaddling bands, a tight band wrapped around a newborn, but instead left their limbs free to develop. Plutarch implies that in most of Greece water was usually used to bathe the newborn, and swaddling clothes and bandages were common.

In summary, the accomplishment of the Greeks in nursing, while perhaps not so great as their contribution to medicine itself, was very important. They were the first Western group to become conscious of the need for a trained nurse. Though they met this need with apprentices and attendants rather than a separate occupational group, merely that the need was recognized is extremely important in the history of nursing. Women apparently furnished the majority of the lay nurses, but like the Egyptians, the Greeks had nursing priests and attendants. That the general knowledge of medical practices and procedures was so well developed and widespread in Greece would mean that nursing care, even in the family, was on a much higher level than it had been previously.

The Roman World

The transition from the Greek world to that of the Romans was gradual. The Romans, while developing their characteristic institutions of law and government, were dependent upon the Greeks for much of their culture. In a very real sense, Rome was a Greek cultural colony. This colonization had started with early Greek immigrants into the Italian peninsula before Rome became a power. The Romans themselves traced their mythological beginnings to Aeneas, a hero of the Trojan War, and perhaps an unconscious symbol of their Grecianized culture. These contacts increased greatly in the third century B.C. as Rome began to dominate the Mediterranean. Rome eventually ruled most of the ancient cultures discussed in this chapter—the Egyptians, the peoples of the Tigris-Euphrates Valley, the Hebrews, and the Greeks. This ultimately spread Roman and Greek culture around the Mediterranean, something that had already been started by the conquests of Alexander the Great. Greek science and Roman engineering spread throughout the ancient world. It was Greek medicine that became dominant in Rome, and it was the Roman concept of Greek medicine that was transmitted to the Middle Ages.

Before Greek medicine came to Rome, there was little or no concept of a specialized medical practitioner. Rather, a type of home nursing or doctoring was practiced that maintained itself even after the appearance of Greek medicine. In early republican Rome, the paterfamilias, the head of the family, was the medical caretaker for his family which included all of his household, family servants, domestics, relatives, and so forth. In many of the larger households these men might have delegated the actual care of the sick to a slave or freed man who had some aptitude for it, but even this was supervised by the heads of the families.

That much of this folk medicine was little more than superstition with a mixture of natural remedies is apparent from an examination of a few of the writers of this period. The most famous of these early Romans, Cato the Elder, in his only surviving work, *On Agriculture*, gave advice for the treatment and care of gout, colic, indigestion, constipation, pain in the side, and so forth. He was especially impressed with the curative effects of cabbage. Cabbage juice was to be used as a poultice on all kinds of wounds and swellings, to cleanse sores, boils, and tumors, and to be taken internally to keep one regular. He also included incantations for the cure of fractures.[20]

Much more complete in his accounts of the curative effects or medicinal properties of various plants, animals, herbs, and metals was Pliny the Elder in his *Natural History*. Pliny gave both the drug preparations and an outline on how to cure. Most of his medicine was a sort of natural medicine based on purgings, drenchings, and rubbings.[21]

That this type of medicine was not very effective was hinted at by Plutarch in his short biography of Cato. Plutarch described how Cato refused to consult the Greek physicians but continued to prescribe for himself and also continued to brag that this was why he was so healthy and lived so long. Plutarch, however, implied that this was also why Cato's wife and son died.[22]

Greek medicine, in the form of temple medicine, appeared in Rome at the beginning of the third century B.C. when a temple of Asclepius was built on an island in the Tiber River. The more scientific Hippocratic medicine had gained a foothold by the middle of that same century. Despite the suspicion of the Greek practitioner voiced by Cato and others, the Greek influence slowly penetrated into Rome. The Romans, however, developed a contempt for the actual practitioner of medicine, so that most of the practitioners remained Greek, and most of the technical medical works of the period were written in Greek.

Nonetheless, the newer concepts and practices of the Greek physician began to play an important part in the education and training of the upper-class Roman. Gradually the natural remedies of Cato and Pliny were either replaced or supplemented by the more advanced techniques of the Greeks. Greek medicine became a subject of study, if not of practice, among the educated Romans. Marcus Varro, in his book on the nine liberal arts which every Roman should know, ranked medicine as the eighth. Vitruvius, another writer on the arts, represented only by his surviving work on architecture, advised his readers to include medicine among their preparatory studies. The best medical work of this type, circulated among the educated, was that of Celsus who lived in the first century A.D. His treatise *Concerning Medicine* is a section of a six-part book; the other parts were on agriculture, military arts, rhetoric, philosophy, and jurisprudence. Only the medical work has survived. He imparted much information about the medical practices of his time, including the use of ligature and the performance of cataract operations. He was especially good on dermatological subjects, and modern dermatological nomenclature seems to reflect his interest in the subject. Because Celsus appeared to know so much about medicine, some historians have claimed him as a physician, while others maintain he translated or adapted an earlier Greek medical work. Neither of these theories can be proven. Many other historians argue that Celsus represents the best of the lay medical tradition which had begun in Greece but reached full flowering in Rome.[23]

Of course, there were able professional practitioners in Rome also, the most famous of whom is Galen, probably the greatest of Greek physicians after Hippocrates. The personal life of Galen is fairly well documented. He was born in A.D. 130 in Pergamum in Asia Minor, the site of a famous temple of Asclepius. He studied medicine and philosophy for nine years in several cities, including Alexandria in Egypt, after which he returned home to become physician to the gladiators, men who fought professionally in the arena. After four years of this, he left for Rome, where he gained great fame as a practitioner, lecturer, and experimenter, eventually becoming the personal physician of the Emperor Marcus Aurelius. He died in A.D. 201. A prolific author, he wrote at least 100 treatises, and his surviving works fill some 22 volumes. Because he was so comprehensive, later physicians were often unwilling to challenge his authority, so that perhaps his very ability hindered the further development of medicine. Under Galen, medicine became, or took steps to become, a science. He was willing to submit tradition to experience and experiment and was probably the greatest medical experimentalist before the seventeenth century.

Although the Romans, except for their Greek citizens, might not have made any real contribution to medicine, in nursing they surpassed the Greeks. This was especially true in military nursing but also in ordinary home nursing. Roman armies fought all over the Mediterranean world—far enough away from Rome, so that the wounded could not be brought home to be cared for by their wives or family; care had to be provided on the spot. The first really powerful enemy of Rome was the nearby city of Veii, which the Romans besieged from 405 to 396 B.C. when it fell. During this struggle many men were injured. Livy in his *History* recorded how the Roman consul billeted the wounded soldiers with the Romans to be nursed and cared for, and how each family apparently tried to exceed the others in their care.[24] But as Rome expanded farther afield, traveling time alone forbade a continuation of this practice, the solution being the original portable hospital. This was a series of tents arranged more or less on the corridor system. Eventually tents gave way to buildings which became permanent convalescent camps located at strategic points.

Many of these hospitals were built along the frontier of the Rhine and Danube rivers, where the remains have been excavated in modern times. These hospitals contained wards, recreation areas, baths, pharmacies, rooms for attendants, and apparently even accommodations for officials taking a rest cure. Some of them could handle as many as two hundred patients. Physicians were classified among the noncombatants in the army. Every legion had its own physician as well as auxiliary medical personnel, who probably acted as nurses. Every three legions had a hospital. These were, of course, primarily military hospitals, and they were under military control and discipline. According to Vegetius in his book *The Military Institutions of the Romans*, either the prefect of the camp or the military tribune was in charge of the hospitals. Military discipline was maintained in them; the Emperor Aurelian ordered the patients to conduct themselves quietly, and if any patient caused strife, he was to be whipped. Despite this strict discipline, the numerous male nurses or attendants took good care of the sick. Vegetius himself argued that little strife could be expected from men who had to struggle with both the enemy and illness.[25] The attendant who nursed his comrades in arms was called a *contubernalis*—literally, "tent companion," perhaps from the time when hospitals were tents. There were other nursing attendants known simply as attendants or adjutants.

Besides more or less professional nurses, each Roman soldier was expected to know a minimum amount of first aid in order to nurse his wounded companions in the field. Bandages were issued to each soldier as standard equipment. At times there were even battlefield operations. The Emperor Trajan personally treated the wounded after one heavy battle, and when the bandages ran short, he tore his own clothing to bind the wounds of his men.

Not only were there hospitals for the soldier, but there were also hospitals for some parts, at least, of the civilian population. On the large Roman estates, a detached building, or at times just a room in the large house, served as a *valetudinarium* or hospital. Columella, a Roman writer on agriculture, instructed the bailiff to watch over the sick and wounded slaves on the estates and to take them to the *valetudinarium* that they might be treated.[26] Acting as a nurse was the bailiff's wife, who was especially cautioned by Columella to watch over the ill. He warned her to keep the *valetudinarium* clean and to air the wards, so that the sick would always find the rooms orderly and healthful.[27]

Whether these *valetudinaria* were meant for people other than slaves is uncertain, but there is evidence that other patients were treated in them. This historian Tacitus indicated that aristocrats and other freemen might be confined to one, perhaps on their own estates.[28] Celsus wrote about the physicians who have charge of large hospitals (*valetudinaria*) but who cannot pay full attention to individuals and resort to a superficial diagnosis.[29] Another writer, Martial, implied that there might have been places large enough to warrant many attendants and students. In one of his *Epigrams* he stated that he was lying ill, but not feverish, until the physician Symmachus and his attendants and disciples came: "A hundred hands frosted by the North wind have pawed me: I had no fever before, Symmachus; now I have."[30] These attendants might have also acted as nurses. In the larger hospitals there were several attendants; at least the philosopher Seneca referred to slaves designated as nurses for the sick and the insane.[31] Further developments in these hospitals led to a whole host of attendants carrying out medical and nursing duties referred to in the documents as *medici, optiones, optiores, capsarii, censi,* and *accensiti*.

Co-existing with these *valetudinaria* were, of course, the temples of Asclepius, already discussed in the section on Greece, and a separate kind of hospital or dispensary, the *iatreia*, which was also Greek. This started as a waiting room or physician's office but developed into a type of private hospital. For surgical operations the patients might be confined there until they were able to be moved to their homes where their families supervised the nursing care. An actual hospital development is indicated by the Roman playwright Plautus in his comedy the *Two Menaechmuses.* In the fifth act a physician appears to remove a man who was considered mentally deranged. The physician promised to watch over his patient for at least 20 days and sent attendants to bring the patient while he went to his office to prepare for him.[32] Under the empire these *iatreia* grew larger with crews of assistants, pupils, and slaves to man them and perhaps act as nurses.[33]

There were two kinds of patients whom the ancient physicians always avoided: the near dead and the childbearing woman. The reason for the first is obvious—it was a hopeless case—but the woman was a problem of morals and modesty. In Rome, however, women were much more emancipated, and the physician as represented by Soranus of Ephesus, another Greek of about A.D. 100, finally invaded the scene of parturition. His treatises on gynecology and obstetrics are the first indication we have that the male physicians were particularly concerned with the subject, although Soranus himself wrote as if child delivery and most medical care for women would be in the hands of midwives. Soranus reported that the Germans and Scythians plunged their babies into cold water immediately after birth. Others, he reported, advised washing the newborn in brine or in wine, while still others urged a urine washing as most healthful. Soranus, himself, felt strongly that an immediate "salting" was the only correct procedure, although the midwife was to take caution to see that the eyes and mouth were not sprinkled. After sprinkling, the baby was to be bathed with lukewarm water, and the mucus cleared from the nose, the mouth, and auditory canals; then the eyes were to be treated with an injection of olive oil, the umbilical cord was to be bent double, and placed in the middle of the umbilicus; finally, the baby was to be swaddled, making sure that every part was molded to its proper shape.[34]

Whether the Roman women followed his recommendations is not known. Probably the nurse-midwife continued, as she always had, to attend to most of the deliveries, assisted by a few women companions. Galen, in one of his works, referred to the midwife and told of her procedure for measuring dilation first by the little finger, then by the others. When the dilatation had reached the proper point, the nurse-midwife had the patient get up from her bed and sit on a delivery chair, a chair with the bottom cut out, where she could bear down to expel the baby.[35] According to Galen, the newborn infant was to be taken by the nurse, powdered moderately, and wrapped in swaddling clothes. These were necessary, he argued, to protect the soft skin of the baby, which was not yet prepared for exposure. For his salting or sprinkling he recommended a simple dusting powder. The child then should receive the breast and periodic baths of pure water, or what Galen called the moist treatment—milk and baths. If the mother's milk was diseased, he recommended a change to a wet nurse.[36]

A discussion of Roman nursing and medical care would not be complete without mention of Roman public health measures. They built aqueducts, sewage systems, and bathing installations of unequaled magnificence wherever they went. A few Romans also conjectured that malarial fever was produced by small animals or insects coming out of the swamps, and Roman architects accepting this hypothesis devised building techniques to prevent these invasions.

Rome had transmitted Greek medicine throughout the Mediterranean world. The tentative recognition of the need for a professional nurse that had appeared in Greece was developed by the Romans into attendants for the sick. Medical students probably still acted in this capacity, but the Romans supplemented them with other attendants. This specialization had been aided by the development of hospitals for the soldier, the slave, the insane, and the urban poor. The attendants in these institutions, both men and women, were still supplemented by the women in the household. On the large estates, the women, especially relatives, probably bore the main burden of nursing. The modern hospital had not developed, but a good foundation had been laid for it. Nursing, even though most of the "professional nurses" were probably slaves, had strengthened its position in medical care and had begun to emerge as a separate specialty.

Two

Medieval Nursing

The Middle Ages were, as the name implies, a transition between the classical or ancient and modern civilizations. The use of the term *Middle Ages* or *medieval* now is mere convenience rather than logical or descriptive. The term was applied by writers in the Italian Renaissance (fourteenth and fifteenth centuries) who were blinded by what they considered their rediscovery of the Greek and Roman world. They forgot that the medieval period which they wished to ignore was much more advanced in many ways that the Greco-Roman world, nor did they realize that their own thinking was deeply molded by the medieval world. Historians no longer regard the Middle Ages as a period of darkness. Rather, we find that there was a more or less continuous tradition of learning, which gradually grew stronger; toward the end of the Middle Ages we find such famous names as Chaucer, Dante, Frederick II, Innocent III, and St. Thomas Aquinas. In medicine we have Lanfranc, John Arderne, Henri de Mondeville, and Guy de Chauliac, who helped to reinvigorate the medical sciences. We also have the development of the first university medical schools at Bologna, Montpellier, and Paris. It seems almost poetic justice that a general medieval survey today includes the fourteenth and fifteenth centuries, the very period in which the writers considered themselves as newly enlightened, the founders of a new age. The medieval period usually includes the years A.D. 300 to 1500, but there is no sharp division between when the Roman world leaves off and the medieval world begins, or when the medieval world ends and the modern period begins.

The medieval world is distinguished from the Greco-Roman world by the appearance of two new elements or streams of culture which helped to make a different society: the Germans and Christianity. The history of the early Middle Ages is a history of the fusing of these three streams of thought, action, and ways of life—Greco-Roman, Germanic, and Christian—into one. In nursing the most important contribution was made by Christianity. The Greco-Roman contribution has already been discussed, and it was much more important than the third element, the Germanic. During the early Middle Ages, however, much of the medical heritage of the Greeks was neglected by Western Europeans. It was rediscovered in the tenth, eleventh, and twelfth centuries through contacts with the Moslems, Jews, and Byzantine Greeks, and it was this rediscovery that gave rise to the medieval university and the powerful surgeons of the later period. The Germanic element changed the geographical focus of Western civilization. Before the Germans, the center of civilization was along the Mediterranean. During the medieval period the center of Western civilization gradually shifted northward and westward, until in our day it has largely become an Atlantic civilization.

The Germans

In trying to determine the nursing techniques of the Germans, we encounter the same difficulty as with most other preliterate societies. We know very little. Some observers commented on the Germans as they came into contact with the Romans. The most famous commentary was by the Roman historian Tacitus, who wrote toward the end of the first century A.D. In his *Germania* he emphasized the devotion of the German women to their husbands and sons. The warriors, he said, "take their wounds to mother and wife, who do not shrink from counting the hurts and demanding a sight of them: they minister to the combatants food and exhortation."[1] He also pointed out that the Germans, unlike the Romans, had few household slaves, but that most German slaves were semifree serfs bound to the land as farmers. In these circumstances the care of the husband and family fell much more heavily upon the wife or mother than it did in the Roman world.

Medically the Germans believed in the magical qualities of various incantations and herbs, as can be seen in the Anglo-Saxon leech books. *Leech* is an old English word meaning physician and was later applied to the blood-sucking worms used by many of them. These leech books are collections of magical recipes and incantations used by the physicians to cure disease.

Similar to the Germans in organization and outlook were the Norsemen or Viking invaders of Europe. They, too, recognized the need for nursing care. Like the Germans, wives and sisters, if near the battlefield, served as nurses. Haldora of Iceland, in about A.D. 1000, was reported as saying: "Come then women of my household, now that the bloody battle is over, let us hasten to the fields and bind up the wounds of the warriors, friends and foes alike."

When women were not available, the men had to nurse each other. According to the *Heimskringla* saga, King Magnus the Good of Norway fought a battle in 1043 in which his forces suffered many casualties. After the battle,

> King Magnus let bind the wounds of his men, but leeches were not so many in the host as were needed then. Then went the king to such men as seemed good to him and felt their hands; but when as he had taken and stroked the hollow of their hands, then named he twelve men who seemed to him would be the softest handed, and told them to bind up the wounds

of men, and yet none of them had bound a wound before, but all these
became the greatest of leeches.[2]

King Magnus had required two important attributes in his nurses: a
mental outlook favorable to the care of the sick or wounded and soft
hands. The Germans as a whole had recognized the need for nursing care,
but they had not developed any institutionalized nursing as had the
Romans.

Early Christianity

The greatest contribution in the Middle Ages to the development of
nursing was made by Christianity, especially through Christian charity
which was influenced by both Jewish and pagan models. In Judaism,
charity and charitable obligations had been recognized in the Talmud, the
collection of Jewish civil and canon laws not included in the Christian
Bible. This had led the Jews to organize charitable societies for supporting and clothing the poor, educating the children of the poor, nursing and
educating orphans, visiting the sick, aiding the lying-in woman, sheltering
the aged, and taking care of prisoners. Since Jewish charity was restricted
to Jews, and Judaism never expanded as Christianity did, its impact was
limited. It had, however, set an important precedent for Christianity.
Charity had not been entirely ignored by the pagans, but it remained
individual rather than social.

Christianity made charity one of the leading virtues. Jesus had set an
example of solicitude for the poor and sick that could not be entirely
ignored. Christianity then took an almost revolutionary step by making
the poor and the humble the special representatives of Jesus. Thus the
love of God, rather than the love of man, became the motivating principle
of Christian charity. This was encouraged by the conditions of the early
Christians, who were a despised sect, even at times a persecuted one which
strengthened the attachment of each member to his fellow Christian.
The result was a vast organization of religious charity which spread
throughout Christendom. Hundreds and even thousands of men and
women were inspired to sacrifice their worldly interests in order to devote
themselves to assisting their fellow man.

Christian concepts of charity were further strengthened by a strong
emphasis on the sanctity of human life. Abortion and infanticide (killing
of deformed, diseased, or unwanted children) were regarded as murder.
The bloody spectacles in the Roman arena were condemned, and even
military life was criticized, since a soldier in warfare must often kill.
Almost total pacifism can be noted in the first three centuries of the
Church, although later the ban against taking human life in battle was

restricted to the clergy. The net effect of these various campaigns of Christianity was increased reverence for human life, thus giving the nurse and the caretaker of the sick a more exalted position than they had enjoyed before.

To put ideals into practice, institutions and procedures were required. Charity was institutionalized by giving the bishop responsibility for the sick, the poor, the infirm, the widow, children, and travelers; actual care of these people was delegated to the deacons, subdeacons, and deaconesses. The Christian obligation of charity is very clear in the etymology of the word *deacon*. In classical Greek the word had implied menial service, but in the New Testament it had come to mean the noble service of doing the work of God by ministering to the needs of others.

Apparently the deacons administered to the needs of the male members of the congregation, and the deaconnesses to the women. This was probably because, as the *Catholic Encyclopedia* states,[3] there was an almost universal prevalence of baptism by immersion in the early Church, a practice that was preceded by the anointing of the whole body. One of the duties of the deacon or deaconess was to perform such anointing, making it a matter of propriety that this ceremony for women be performed by other women. Another duty of the deacons and deaconesses was the care of the sick, following the example of the deaconess Phebe, mentioned by St. Paul in his Epistle to the Romans:

> I commend unto you Phebe our sister, which is a servant [*diakonos*] of the church which is at Cenchrea:
>
> That ye receive her in the Lord, as becometh saints, and that ye assist her in whatsoever business she hath need of you: for she hath been a succourer of many, and of myself also.[4]

From a survey of church records, it appears that the office of deaconess developed mainly in the Eastern Church—that is, in the Greek-speaking part of the Roman Empire, whence the modern Orthodox Church comes—and was not common in the Western Latin-speaking part of the empire, whence the Roman Catholic Church comes. Names of several deaconesses at Constantinople in the fourth century have been preserved in a letter of St. John Chrysostom. In the sixth century, the great church of Santa Sophia in Constantinople had a staff of 60 priests, 100 deacons, 40 deaconesses, and 90 subdeacons. Gradually the deaconess became less important even in the Eastern Church, until by the eleventh century the office had almost disappeared.

More important than the deaconess in the Western Church for the care of the sick was the widow. This appears in the first Pauline epistle to Timothy:

> Let a widow be chosen of no less than threescore years of age, who hath been the wife of one husband. Having testimony for her good works:

if she have brought up children, if she have lodged strangers, if she have washed the saints' feet, if she have ministered to them that suffer tribulations, if she have diligently followed every good work.[5]

In general, however, there was considerable hostility in both the Eastern and Western Churches to women holding any kind of Church office. Their duty was to marry and to beget children. There was agreement in the West, however, that some women, namely widows and virgins, should hold positions similar to the deaconesses in the Eastern Church. More light on widows comes from a series of third- and fourth-century laws known as the *Didascalia Apostolorum* and the *Apostolic Constitutions*. These laws were professedly drawn up by the Apostles and transmitted to the Church by Clement of Rome (c. 96 A.D.). The office of widow was restricted to women over 60 (younger widows were urged to remarry), and those especially designated or appointed to the position were supposed to, among other things, watch over the sick. A widow who was chosen should be careful about her conduct, to be "meek, quiet, gentle, sincere, free from anger, not talkative; not clamorous, not hasty of speech, not given to evil-speaking, not captious, not double-tongued, not a busy-body . . . ."[6]

While technically widows were especially chosen from among other widows, and virgins publicly announced their status by taking the early equivalent of a vow, and deaconesses, where they existed, were ordained,[7] such distinctions were soon lost. Almost any woman of any age who took a vow of sexual abstinence and donned a special ecclesiastical dress came for a time to be classed as a widow. Their chief duties were to care for the sick, the poor, and travelers—duties which later devolved on nuns and lay sisters. For modern nursing the major importance, despite the confusion, of deacons, deaconesses, widows, and virgins is that a group of persons were set apart whose special duties included the care of the sick. This was a forward step in the development of nursing.

The Development of Hospitals

Probably as important to the growth of nursing as the development of these caretakers of the sick was the extension of the hospital: The Roman military hospitals were replaced by civilian ones. In early Christianity the *diakonia,* a sort of combination outpatient and welfare station managed by the deacons, served as the equivalent of a hospital. When Christianity became a legal religion at the beginning of the fourth century, the need for an institution to care for the poor became even greater. Giving further impetus to this need was the closing of the temples of Asclepius. It was to satisfy this need that the first hospitals appeared.

Supervision of the hospital, as of other charitable activity, was in the hands of the bishop. The First Ecumenical (or Church-wide) Council, at Nicaea in 325, called for the establishment of a *xendocheion* (Latin, *xendochium*), or house for strangers, in each diocese.[8] The Fourth Council, held in Carthage in 398, again stipulated that each bishop was to construct such an establishment near his dwelling. By the time of Justinian in the sixth century, we have records of numerous establishments devoted to the various charitable functions: the *xendocheion,* the *nosokomeion* (house for the sick), *gerokomeion* (house for the aged), and *ptochotropheion* (poorhouse). These different names imply a distinction between institutions that did not actually exist, since definitions were rarely drawn so narrowly. The main purpose of all such institutions was to serve the needy, and it was usually easier, safer, and cheaper to serve all of them together. As a result the *xendocheion* or *xendochium* became a convenient all-embracing establishment. By the twelfth century the term *xendochium* had disappeared in the West to be replaced by our word *hospital,* or sometimes *House of God.*[9]

Coinciding with the growth of Christianity and its establishment of hospitals was a change in Roman law which allowed such charitable institutions to develop. In earlier Roman law it had been impossible to control one's wealth beyond the grave. Wills were made and recognized, but actual execution of the will depended on the executor, which made it difficult to leave money or property to establish an institution like a hospital. Changes began in the second century A.D. when various people stipulated that a specified income from certain property should be devoted to a specific program or else the property reverted to other heirs. This gave the executor a vested interest in following the outlines of the will, so that gradually, by the sixth century, hospitals and churches were legally recognized as appropriate recipients of gifts and legacies.

These early hospitals were not for all the sick but for those who could not or would not be cared for in their own homes. Included in this group were the traveler or pilgrim, the poor and the destitute, the orphan and abandoned children, the elderly, and the plague-stricken. Persons of standing and probably the majority of medieval people were nursed in their homes by their family or servants. A *xendochium* was more like a modern nursing home than a hospital. Most of the early hospitals did not even have a physician or surgeon in attendance, so that nursing can be regarded as their chief function.

The exact date of the earliest *xendochium* has been much debated. Suffice it to say that many were founded in the fourth century after the legalization of Christianity. Some Christian hospitals might have been housed in old temples of Asclepius, while others were built or made from entirely new foundations. Helena, mother of the Emperor Constantine, who legalized Christianity, built a hospital in Constantinople. St. Basil the Great, Bishop of Caesarea in Cappadocia (d. 379), founded a hospital, and so did St. John Chrysostom when he was Patriarch of Constantinople. At Edessa, St. Ephraim (or Ephrem), who died about 373, founded one during an epidemic: ". . . he had about three hundred beds fitted up in the public porches; and here he tended those who were ill and suffering from the effects of famine, whether they were foreigners or natives of the surrounding country."[10]

Theodoret, a Church historian who became Bishop of Cyrrhus in Syria in 423, wrote about Flacilla, the wife of the Emperor Theodosius, and her attempts to relieve the sick:

> She also went about the guest chambers of the churches and ministered to the wants of the sick, herself handling pot and pans, and tasting broth, now bringing in a dish and breaking bread and offering morsels, and washing out a cup and going through all the other duties which are supposed to be proper to servants and maids.[11]

The reference to servants and maids indicates who usually watched over the sick, at least in the richer families. Nevertheless, the Empress in a sense is a prototype of many later women who, though well-to-do, interested themselves in helping to relieve the distress and discomforts of the sick.

In the hospitals in the Eastern Roman Empire were groups of attendants known as the *parabolani,* members of a minor religious order. Their chief duty was to find the needy sick and bring them into a hospital, but they also acted as a burying detail and as a bodyguard for the bishop. Public places and theaters were forbidden to them, perhaps in order to avoid the danger of contagion. The order disappeared after the fifth century, perhaps because of their involvement in the various ecclesiastical and doctrinal controversies of the period.

The Eastern Church was considerably ahead of the Western Church in the establishment of hospitals. This would be only natural, for there were many more Christians in the East and the churches were richer. But the need for such institutions came to be recognized in the West also, and probably St. Jerome, who was often an intermediary for the introduction of Eastern ideas and institutions into Rome and the West, is a key figure. In one of his letters written in A.D. 399, he tells about Fabiola, a woman who had been twice married but never happily. She then found Christianity, repented of her worldly ways, and became a devoted convert. She established a *noscocomium,* a hospital for the sick, the first according to St. Jerome in Rome:

> She was the first person to found a hospital, into which she might gather sufferers out of the streets and where she might nurse the unfortunate victims of sickness and want. Need I recount the various ailments of human beings? Need I speak of noses slit, eyes put out, feet half burnt,

hands covered with sores: Or of limbs dropsical and atrophied? Or of diseased flesh alive with worms? Often did she carry on her own shoulders persons infected with jaundice or with filth. Often too did she wash away the matter discharged from wounds which others, even though men, could not bear to look at. She gave food to her patients with her own hand, and moistened the scarce breathing lips of the dying with sips of liquid. . . .[12]

Other members of St. Jerome's group imitated Fabiola. For example, Paula and her son-in-law, Pammachius, erected hospitals in Ostia, the port city of Rome, and in the Holy Land. Popes, bishops, kings, and others soon established hospitals in the West.

Unfortunately, though real concern for the sick was becoming a part of the general mores and hospitals were developing, medicine was not keeping up with the promise it had shown under the Greeks. Greek medicine was a pagan art for which there had been no room in the early Church. Christian students of Galen had been excommunicated, so that in the Christian hospitals the care of the sick fell below earlier medical standards. Gradually, however, a reconciliation took place. When Christianity became the official religion of the Roman state, it had to compromise with necessity by taking over the cultural heritage of the past. Christians became physicians and treated patients by applying the doctrines of pagan medical writers.

Also handicapping medicine was that most of the pagan medical writing was in Greek rather than in Latin, and what passed into Western medieval Europe was only those portions of Greek medical knowledge that had been translated into Latin, a simplified version often aimed at a lay audience rather than a specialist. Thus, while nursing ideals were rising, medical knowledge was on the decline. This weakened the effectiveness of the hospitals.

Monasticism and the Care of the Sick

Further obstructing the development of hospitals in western Europe were the various invasions and wars that occurred for generations. The Germanic migrations had continued for centuries, but they were no sooner settled than the Arabs began invading the western Mediterranean and southern Europe, the Vikings or Norsemen western and northern Europe, and the Huns and Magyars eastern Europe. The net effect of all this was a decline in the number of cities. This ruralization of Europe was accentuated because the Germans who had settled in the Roman Empire were an agricultural people who saw no necessity to rebuild the declining cities. The Muslim invasions of the seventh and eighth centuries curtailed the use of the Mediterranean for commerce; and without commerce, cities could not exist. With the decline in the cities and their hospitals, care of the sick passed frequently to another Christian institution—the monastery.

In a sense monasticism was a reaction against the growing worldliness of the Church. In early Christianity, membership had set the believers apart from the rest of the world, and the threat of martyrdom had sanctified them as men and women who strove not for the things of this world, but for everlasting glory. But when Christianity became an officially recognized religion, as it did at the beginning of the fourth century, and then the only legal religion, as happened at the end of that same century, vast numbers of people became Christians, and many, if not most, lacked the high motivations of the earlier believers. In effect, as soon as Christianity became socially correct and even legally compulsory, people joined the Church for worldly reasons or under duress. Under these conditions the moral level of most Christians became little different from that of non-Christians.

There was, of course, a reaction to this. It was led by ascetics, men and women who felt that life in and of the world was hopeless, that the secular Church no longer offered sufficient guarantees against the pollutions of the world, the flesh, and the devil. These people, despairing of this world and all that it contained, withdrew into themselves and into the wilderness. They hoped that in this solitude they might prepare themselves, through mortification of the flesh, for the blessed rapture of heaven. Isolation, self-flagellation, fasting, uncleanliness, and hours of intensive prayer were characteristic of these early hermits.

One of the earliest and probably the most famous of all the anchorites (so called because they lived alone) was St. Anthony (d. 356), who withdrew into the desert of Egypt to purify his soul. More picturesque was St. Simeon Stylites (d. 459), who perched for several decades on the top of a high pillar near Antioch. At first these anchorites were completely isolated, each man occupying his own patch of wasteland, cut off from the world. As the fame of the holy hermit spread, admiring followers congregated around him, so that he was no longer alone. Establishments soon developed where the hermits lived together communally, though often they did not speak to one another. These communal establishments came to be called monasteries with rules and regulations drawn up for them. St. Basil (d. 378) wrote the first monastic rule at the end of the fourth century, leading to the development of organized monasticism.

In the West, monasticism was introduced by St. Athansius (d. 373) and spread by St. Martin of Tours (d. 397) and others. It was carried to Ireland by St. Patrick (d. 461). Gradually order was brought to the Western movement by the Benedictine rule, prepared by St. Benedict of Nursia (d. 543), a Roman noble who founded a famous monastery at Monte Cassino on the road to Naples. In his rule St. Benedict rejected flagellation and excesses of mortification. A daily routing of prayer, meditation, and work occupied his monks and most of the other Western monasteries at that time adopted this rule.

St. Benedict's rule was important in the development of nursing because it emphasized care for the sick monk:

> Before all things and above all things care must be taken of the sick so that they may be served in the very deed as Christ Himself; for He has said: "I was sick and ye visited me" and "As long as ye did it to one of these my least brethren, ye did it to me." But let the sick themselves consider that they are served for the honor of God, and not grieve their brethren who serve them by their importunity. Yet must they be patiently borne with, because from such as these is gained more abundant reward. Therefore the Abbot shall take the greatest care that they suffer no neglect.[13]

St. Benedict then laid down some minimal procedures for nursing care. Baths were to be given to the sick as often as was expedient and food as often as needed. Sick monks were also to be given meat, which was denied to most of the other monks.

Monasticism spread rather rapidly in the West, attracting many men and women. Charity, threatened by the general breakdown of the state in invasions and civil wars, was increasingly delegated to those in religious orders. St. Gregory the Great, Pope from 590 to 604, requested monks and nuns to supervise the hospitals, perhaps in order to keep them operating. Increasingly, the care of all sick, not only members of their own orders, fell into their hands.

Because monks and nuns were generally better educated than the lay population, monastic control of the hospitals was a boon to nursing. While nuns were less educated than monks. there were several convents with strong educational traditions, and many nuns, like most monks, received an education in the liberal arts, which then included some training in medicine, probably from simplified Latin versions of Hippocrates and Galen. There is some indication that during the reign of Charlemagne, at the beginning of the ninth century, all clergy under his jurisdiction were instructed in first aid. After Charlemagne's time there was a great renewal in medical studies, so that by the twelfth and thirteenth centuries most of the Greek medical knowledge had been recovered, initially through Latin translations of Arabic works.

The Arabs, a tribal people on the fringe of the Roman Empire, newly unified by the religious teachings of Muhammed, had expanded rapidly in the seventh and eighth centuries conquering Roman (or Byzantine) controlled territories in Syria, North Africa, and Spain. They had also conquered Persia and northern India. Since the Muslims were rather tolerant conquerors, accepting and incorporating much of the learning of the conquered peoples into their own culture, the Greek medical corpus was largely translated into Arabic along with Persian and Indian teachings. Soon the Arabs began to make their own contributions. Among the great writers were Rhazes, who made the first medical study of smallpox, and Avicenna, whose encyclopedia of medicine, the *Canon*, was the dominant medical textbook until the eighteenth century. Gradually Arabic versions of Greek classics as well as original Arabic interpretations began to reach Western Europe, mainly through Spain, parts of which remained under Islamic control until 1492. Gradually, as the new learning permeated medieval medicine, there was increasing specialization of medical practitioners.

Specialization occurred even in the monastery, where the sick monks were kept in the infirmary under the care of an official known as the *infirmarius*. The infirmary was usually a separate building in the monastic establishment close to the *herbarium*, where herbs for the care of the sick were grown. At Clairvaux, one of the most famous of medieval monasteries, there were three infirmaries: one for the monks, one for the lay brothers, and the *infirmarius pauperum* for the poor. Most monasteries had at least two infirmaries: one inside the walls for the monks and lay brothers and a *hospice* or infirmary near the walls for the outside community and strangers. Food and beds were usually available, and sick persons were watched over.

Medical specialists were also found in convents, as demonstrated by the well-known letters of Abelard to Heloise, the famous lovers of the twelfth century. Abelard was a great teacher, with some knowledge of medicine, who acted as tutor to Heloise; he was instrumental in founding the University of Paris. Heloise, when she realized that marriage to Abelard was impossible because of his clerical status, became abbess of the convent at Paraclete. In one of his letters to Heloise, Abelard suggests a rule for her nuns including this provision:

> The Infirmarian shall take care of the sick, and shall protect them as well from sin as from want. Whatever their sickness requires, baths, food, or anything else, is to be allowed them; for there is a well-known saying, 'the law was not made for the sick.' Meat is not to be denied them on any account, except on the sixth day of the week or on the chief vigils or the fasts of the Four Seasons of Lent. . . . There must also be a watchful nurse always present with the sick to answer their call at once when needed, and the infirmary must be equipped with everything necessary for their illness. Medicaments too must be provided according to the resources of the convent, and this can more easily be done if the sister in charge of the sick has some knowledge of medicine. Those who have a period of bleeding shall also be in her care. And there should be someone with experience of blood-letting, or it would be necessary for a man to come in amongst the women for this purpose.[14]

It has been conjectured that many older people retired to a convent or monastery because they knew that good nursing care was available there. While the religious motivation was real, many older people perhaps entered them as they would enter a nursing home today. Once inside the convent or monastery, they could then work for the salvation of their souls, while their infirmities were also tended.

Byzantine Hospitals

Toward the beginning of the twelfth century, some remarkable changes occurred in western Europe. This was partly because the disorders of the last few centuries had been brought under control: invaders were repulsed; civil wars had subsided; kings were acquiring new power by consolidating their kingdoms; in general, peace and order were being restored. Trade in the Mediterranean, which had been disrupted earlier by the Muslims, was reviving, and Latin Christian outposts were appearing in the East. The difficulties that had plagued the Church itself had been resolved under strong and able popes. Cities revived and grew rapidly. Symptomatic of these changes were the Crusades, a series of wars that attempted to eliminate Muslim control of the Holy Land. These started in 1096 and continued for several centuries, although the later Crusades were directed less against the Muslims than against the opponents of the pope.

During these Crusades, the Westerners passed through Constantinople, the capital of the Christian East, where they found an advanced culture with ideas and institutions different from their own. One such institution was the large hospital, almost forgotten in the West. Such a hospital was described at the time of the First Crusade by Anna Comnena, the daughter of the Eastern Emperor Alexius. She said that in this hospital patients could be seen

> . . . walking along, sometimes blind, sometimes lame, sometimes having some other ill, and seeing you would say it was Solomon's Porch filled with men incapacitated in their limbs. I myself have seen an old woman waited on by a young one, and a blind man led by a seeing, and a footless man using the feet not of himself, but of others, and a handless man led by the hands of other men, and children nursed by strange mothers, and paralytics served by able-bodied mortals. So the number of those who were supported was double, some being served and some servers. Thus Alexius gave attendants to each incapacitated man.[15]

From Anna's description, it is obvious that much of the nursing care was given by the patients themselves, although there were probably some servants or others who helped.

Alexius' successor, John II Comnenus, established a hospital connected with the monastery of the "Pantokrator" (Almighty). Its internal arrangement was described in some detail in the founding statutes issued by the emperor. The beds were to be allotted as follows: ten surgical, eight for acute cases and eye cases, twelve for women, twenty for lighter cases, five for emergencies, and five beds for severe fractures. Each bed had a coverlet, a mattress, a blanket, a pillow, and two extra covers for the winter. There were two chief physicians, and under them in each section were two other physicians, enabling them to serve in shifts. Each section also had three assistants, two male and two female servants, and two watchmen for the night, including a man and a woman. Attached to the hospital was a bathhouse, which was to be used by the patients at least twice a week. The servants probably did the actual nursing care.[16] The hospital has been called an example of the "most touching" of the humanitarian practices in Byzantine society.[17]

Perhaps because of Eastern influence but also because its own internal development now permitted it, similar institutions arose in the West. Institutions for the care of the sick were separated from those with other functions, and new groups developed: military orders such as the Knights Hospitalers, semimonastic orders such as the Franciscans, and regular monastic orders such as the Augustinian Sisters.

Knights Hospitalers

In the middle of the eleventh century, merchants from the Italian city of Amalfi were permitted by the Caliph of Egypt to build a church, a monastery, and a hospital for the use of pilgrims to the Holy Land. The actual founder of the hospital was a monk, Brother Gerard, who was in charge of the institution in 1099 when Jerusalem was captured by the French Crusaders during the First Crusade. The hospital order was given official recognition by the pope in 1113, and it soon took upon itself not only the care of the sick but also the defense of the Holy Land. The order was chartered as the Knights of St. John, but it was often known as the Hospitalers. Its members wore a black habit adorned with eight pointed (or Maltese) crosses. In 1187 the Muslims under Saladin recaptured Jerusalem, forcing the Hospitalers to leave the city, although they were allowed to leave ten of their number behind to care for the wounded until they were able to travel. The hospital in Jerusalem, said to hold some two thousand patients, was then converted into a lunatic asylum by the Muslims.

From Jerusalem the Hospitalers went to Syria where they established a large hospital in Acre. When Acre fell in 1291, the knights went to Cyprus, then to Rhodes, and finally to Malta, where they stayed until

1798. The activities of the order were not confined to the Holy Land, however, for hospitals under their care and supervision were either established or taken over by them throughout Europe. A great many of the hospitals, especially in eastern Germany, owed their origin to the Hospitalers or to a similar crusading order, the Teutonic Knights.

Though the ruins of the famous hospital of the Knights in Jerusalem can give us only a sketchy idea of its original extent, contemporary travelers often left accounts of this institution. Among these is one by John of Wurzburg, a German pilgrim who visited Jerusalem about the year 1160. He recorded that there were

> . . . an enormous multitude of sick people, both men and women, who are tended and restored to health daily at very great expense. When I was there I learned that the whole number of these sick people amounted to two thousand of whom sometimes in the course of one day and night more than fifty are carried out dead while many other fresh ones keep continually arriving. The same house supplies as many people outside it with victuals as it does those inside, in addition to the boundless charity which is daily bestowed upon poor people who beg their bread from door to door and do not lodge in the house, so that the whole sum of its expenses can surely never be calculated even by the managers and stewards thereof. In addition to all these moneys expended upon the sick and upon other poor people, this same house also maintains in its various castles many persons trained to all kinds of military exercises for the defense of the land of the Christians against the invasions of the Saracens.[18]

Statutes and regulations for the hospitals of the Knights give us an insight into what might be expected of the nurse-soldier. Every candidate for the order had to take the usual monastic vows of poverty, obedience, and chastity, but they also promised to be "the serf and the slave" of their lords, the sick. Originally the members, as befitted knights, had been taken from the nobility, but nonnoble members were soon allowed and were usually called sergeants or servants. Probably in most cases they did the actual nursing care, while the Knights did the fighting and administering.

Every sick person coming to the hospital had first to confess and receive the Sacrament. He was then bathed before being carried to a bed where he was to be treated as if "he were a Lord." Patients were also required to make their wills, which may indicate the lack of effective cures in the hospital. Each patient (or in some hospitals every two patients) was to have a cloak of sheepskin and boots for going to and coming from the latrines located outside the hospital. The beds of the sick were to be constructed, so that they were as long and as broad as was most conventient for repose, whatever that might mean. Each bed was to have its own coverlet and special sheet.

The hospital was divided into various wards with a brother in charge of each. He was required to visit the sick both mornings and evenings. The bed linens and other supplies were issued under his order. There was also a scribe for clerical duty. In overall charge of the hospital was the commander, who was to serve the sick cheerfully, doing his duty without grumbling or complaining. In every ward of the hospital nine sergeants were posted to wash the feet of the sick, change their linens, make the beds, feed the weak, or in general help the sick in whatever way they could. Patients were allowed to choose their own food, which was served from silver vessels.

Attached to the hospitals were physicians and surgeons, an innovation in medical care and another indication of the growth of specialization. The hospital at Jerusalem had four physicians, while the one at Rhodes had four physicians, two surgeons, and an apothecary. The physicians were supposed to examine the urine, diagnose the diseases, and administer appropriate medicines. They were required to visit the patients at least twice a day accompanied by the nurse-brother.

Convalescent patients were allowed considerable freedom if they did not make unnecessary noise. They were, however, prohibited from playing cards or dice, or from reading aloud. Perhaps they also assisted in the care and feeding of their fellow patients. No patient was permitted to disobey the orders of the physicians or surgeons, or of the prescribed regime, but all patients were to be treated with special solicitude.

The Knights introduced some important sanitary measures into their hospitals, especially the one at Rhodes. The outside latrines or trenches have already been mentioned. During epidemics a strict quarantine was enforced. All persons who had been exposed to a dreaded disease were isolated for 40 days (hence "quarantine," or 40 days). If plague was present on ships in the harbor, men were prohibited under pain of death from coming ashore. If exposure to the plague had occurred through negligence, offenders were fined 50 ducats. Generally the practice at the hospital in Rhodes, and perhaps at other knightly hospitals, was to separate patients with diseases considered incurable from other patients.

At almost the same time that the Knights were established, a similar order for women, the Sisters of the Order of Saint John of Jerusalem, appeared. They erected a hospital in Jerusalem known as Saint Mary Magdalene. They also established hospitals in some European cities but not on the scale of the Knights. Many of the knightly hospitals had sisters attached for the benefit of women patients. We know that the Knights did handle maternity cases, since the regulations of the order provided that cradles were to be made for the babies of women pilgrims born in their hospitals. The cradles were supposed to prevent the infant from being endangered by "the restlessness of its mother."

The Knights still exist but are now usually known as the Order of Malta or Knights of St. John. Their flag, a white cross on a red background, is recognized in battle as the equivalent of the Red Cross. Various offshoots of the order at present include Catholic, Protestant, and Orthodox religious branches. Especially important for its modern work is the British order of the Hospital of St. John of Jerusalem, which was refounded in the nineteenth century.

Other Religious Orders

There were also other military nursing orders, particularly the Teutonic Knights and the Knights of St. Lazarus. The Teutonic Knights date from a hospital founded by Germans in Jerusalem in 1128. The original staff of the hospital was probably connected with the Hospitalers. Pope Celestine III (1191–1198) recognized them as a separate order, but they followed the rule of the Hospitalers in their hospital policies. With the fall of Acre, the last Crusader-held city in the Holy Land, to the Muslims in 1291, the order moved to eastern Germany where by gift and conquest they acquired control of much of what was to become the kingdom of Prussia. In their military conquests most of their nursing duties were neglected or forgotten, but they did establish several hospitals in eastern Germany and western Poland. They also had women members who increasingly assumed the nursing duties, as indicated by the rule of 1280, which states that women were to do the nursing "because service to cattle and to sick persons" was better performed by women. Perhaps this statement indicates the decline of the nursing ideal among the Knights themselves as they turned to other tasks.

The third military nursing order was the Lazarists or Knights of St. Lazarus, who were originally designated to care for lepers. This dedication to Lazarus in the Middle Ages was derived from a confusion of the beggar Lazarus mentioned in St. Luke, popularly regarded as a leper, with the brother of Martha and Mary whom Jesus raised from the dead. The exact relation of the Knights to the leper hospitals has been much debated, but it is generally believed that the Knights were comparatively unimportant. The order was suppressed by Pope Innocent VIII in 1490, and its possessions went to the Hospitalers.

Along with the military orders came the development of another kind of hospital order, the mendicants. Known technically as Tertiaries or third orders, they were lay people who lived in the world—that is, outside monastery walls, but under the direction of an order or rule. They rendered services to the poor, the outcasts, the needy. In a sense they represented a rededication to the religious ideals of Jesus. The most important of these third orders were the Franciscans, the Dominicans, the Carmelites, and the Augustinians.

The crucial figure in the development of the mendicant orders was St.

Francis (1181–1226) although almost equally influential was St. Dominic (1170–1221). St. Francis, a man with an overwhelming capacity for love, was so revered that he was canonized within two years of his death. There are many stories and legends about Francis, but the most important for nursing are those which depict him visiting the lepers, cleansing their wounds, and setting an example for his disciples. In order to share the feelings of the sick, he tried to imagine that he was ill, and even begged to help those less fortunate than himself.[19] Francis urged his followers to go to leper hospitals and to wait upon the lepers, and to care for the poor, the sick, and the dying. St. Dominic, although he had a similar charismatic effect on his contemporaries, was an altogether different character. His main concern was the growth of heresy, and he became convinced that a thoroughly educated clergy and more effective institutions to care for the abandoned, the sick, the forgotten were needed to combat it. Other saints of the period such as St. Elizabeth of Hungary, a Franciscan Tertiary, and St. Catherine of Siena, a Dominican Tertiary, also emphasized the care of the sick.

Many of these orders were less concerned with nursing than with the literal imitation of Jesus. Some semimonastic orders, however, did dedicate themselves primarily to nursing duties; foremost among them was the Order of the Holy Spirit. Founded by Guy de Montpellier in the twelfth century, the order was given papal recognition by Innocent III at the beginning of the thirteenth century. The pope put the order in charge of the ancient hospital of the Holy Spirit in Rome, founded originally in the eighth century, and gave them extensive privileges which helped the order to spread rapidly. This order had both men and women members and included hundreds of hospitals under its direction. Another order devoted to nursing care was the Hospital Brothers of St. Anthony. They were founded about 1095 and were known for their care of the victims of St. Anthony's Fire or ergotism, caused by a fungus growth on rye, one of the staple grains of the Middle Ages. The order was also assigned to the care of other sick, and until its suppression in the eighteenth century, it cared for the sick in the papal household. Still another order was the Alexian Brothers, who were formed in the fourteenth century to bury the dead from plague in the Netherlands, but soon undertook other duties including the nursing of the sick. They were formed into a religious congregation in 1458. At the present time there are several hospitals operated by the Alexian Brothers in the United States. Another group known as the Gray Nuns or the Elisabetherinnen was formed into a community by Pope Martin V in 1428. They were affiliated with the Franciscans but had St. Elizabeth of Hungary as their patron saint.

Nursing orders were also found among the regular monks and nuns. Among the most famous in this group were the Augustinian Sisters at the Hôtel Dieu in Paris, one of the oldest, if not the oldest, purely nursing order. The sisters were given their rule by Pope Innocent IV (1243–1254). The director of the hospital was a canon from the cathedral chapter of Notre Dame, but a sister (probably the prioress) was next in importance. She supervised supplies, linens, and the wards. All the soiled clothes in the house were collected and sorted for wash. The major laundering was done in the river Seine every six weeks, although there was a small washing every day. In the winter the sisters apparently had to break the ice in the river to do their washing, standing in the icy river as they scrubbed. The hospital had a drug department supervised by an older sister. There was also an obstetrical division with a midwife in charge of deliveries. It has been conjectured that many of the Parisian midwives were trained in the hospital. Occasionally, sisters from the hospital did private nursing in homes, especially for families who gave money to the hospital.

Medieval Hospitals

As has been pointed out, most medieval hospitals served multiple functions: the care of the poor, the pilgrim, the traveler, the orphan, as well as of the sick. Most people who could afford servants were cared for in their home. It was considered a wifely duty to nurse a sick husband and children even if servants were available. Occasionally, there were women specialists for hire who acted as nurses, while many of the orders, especially the mendicant ones, took care of the sick in the home. Hospitals were for those who had no home or who could not care for themselves. Certain patients, however, were excluded such as lepers, the blind, and the mentally ill for whom there were special institutions. One of the first hospitals to be devoted exclusively to the care of the mentally ill was established during the thirteenth century at Gheel in Belgium, a village centered around the shrine of Saint Dymphna. According to tradition Dymphna was the daughter of a sixth-century Irish chieftain who had fled Ireland to escape an incestuous marriage. Her father pursued her and in a fit of insane rage murdered her and the priest who had advised her. A shrine arose at the site, and inevitably she became the patron saint of those afflicted with mental maladies. Patients came from far and wide to be cured through her intercession. Those who remained at the shrine for long periods were boarded out with peasants in the neighborhood, while retarded children were given work in the field. Gheel is still a center for the treatment of the mentally ill and the exceptional child.

The most numerous of the special hospitals were those for lepers, who in the eleventh and twelfth centuries, perhaps as a result of contact with the Near East during the Crusades, appeared in increasing numbers. A few such hospitals were supervised by the Knights of St. Lazarus, but the bulk were not. Leper hospitals were usually separated from the city, and any known leper was required to stay in them until death. Since leprosy has a very low level of contagion, the isolation effectively eliminated the disease in most of Europe, although at great sacrifice to the persons and families involved. Medieval law regarded a leper as a dead person, so that they were often ignored in their hospitals. Usually, the lepers nursed themselves, although there were dedicated people, such as St. Francis, who assisted them.

Regular hospitals for a time received abandoned children, although they often lacked facilities for them. If the infants were small, they were placed in the lying-in ward of the hospital where they were given to hired wet nurses who often had to nurse several infants. If the child were older, or had somehow survived the wet nurse period, other nurses took over. After age six the children were more or less on their own, although in the late Middle Ages special homes or hospitals were set up to care for abandoned children, and these special institutions gradually replaced the regular hospitals in this function.

The ordinary country hospital was a small place, usually with room for less than 25 persons. It generally cared for the poor in the area and for pilgrims or travelers. Only rarely did such hospitals admit the neighborhood sick with the exception of pregnant women. Since the hospitals were small, their personnel was also limited. Most had a master, one or two brothers, and perhaps one or two sisters. Their most important work was to tend the lands belonging to the hospital and to feed the poor, pilgrims, and the sick. Urban hospitals were much more numerous and specialized.

The beds in these hospitals varied in size, but there were usually both great beds and smaller individual beds. In the former three or four persons would sleep together. These beds were given to the pilgrims, travelers, or poor. The truly sick person had a bed of his own since this was specifically stipulated in the various laws about hospitals. If a person refused to share his bed with a designated companion, he could be turned away from the hospital. Men and women, however, were separated into different wards or rooms. The seriously ill were usually put into special wards, designated as infirmaries, so that they could be given special care. Night nurses or guards were on duty in all wards, partly to assist the patients, but also to see that if they left their beds, they were properly dressed. In the Middle Ages both men and women slept naked (but with a nightcap to prevent chills); it was the duty of the night nurse to pass clothes to persons leaving their beds. Such clothes were worn partly for modesty, but mainly to prevent undue exposure since lavatories were usually outhouses. Some hospitals, however, had a series of cisterns and sluices which allowed running water to remove sewage from the hospital.

The admission procedures at a hospital were similar to those of today. The patients' clothes were removed, itemized, washed, and stored with any valuables they might have had. The patients themselves were then bathed if their condition permitted, although this was not done for any sanitary or medical reason but in imitation of the foot washing mentioned in the Bible. Patients stayed in long halls which were to be kept clean. Accounts for the hospital in Paris show that 1,300 brooms were used every year, and that once a year, usually about Easter time, all the walls were lime-washed.

During the winter a large fire was lighted in each hall; to supplement its heat, four large iron tubs filled with burning coals were moved between the two lines of beds that stood near the wall. In the summer, temperatures were controlled by opening and closing windows, and in some cases patients had pulleys that they could manipulate themselves. Beds consisted of a mattress filled with straw and suspended on cords stretched between the four corner posts. This was then covered by a linen sheet. The pillow was made of feathers, and the patient was covered by a quilt, usually made of heavy grey cloth, but sometimes bordered with leather or fur. Although the bedding attracted vermin, it was renewed only three times a year. The sheets, however, were washed more often.

The hospital routine began at five each morning when the staff, after rising, washing, and dressing, went to the chapel for services and then extinguished the lamps in the wards. As the patients awakened, the sisters went from one to another, washing faces and hands, giving drinks, and assisting them in any way they could. Later while the beds were being made, the less sick patients were allowed to walk around. After this the floor was washed down by the servants.

By canon law, the patients in the hospital were supposed to be fed before the brothers and sisters working in the hospital, and were to eat at least as well as they did. If a person were seriously ill, the nursing staff was to feed him or her, or otherwise give assistance as needed. Most hospitals had the same meal system as the Hôtel Dieu in Paris: two main meals a day, at 11 A.M. and 6 P.M. Visitors were admitted after the evening meal.

Bread was the staple food and the bulk of the meal. When possible, meat, either fresh or salted, was served, and some particularly sick patients were given meat with almost every meal. The most common meat was mutton, although veal, lamb, and pork were provided on certain feast days. Beef was prohibitively expensive. Probably most patients had some kind of meat for four of their fourteen meals during the week. Herring, fresh or salted, and other fish were served if available. Since the food came mostly from properties attached to the hospital, patients also had fresh fruits and vegetables in season, and eggs and cheeses most of the year. Milk was seldom served. In some of the hospitals, the patients were allowed, within limits, to select their own menus, but the physicians of the period complained that the sick often chose food that was not good for their illness. In England most patients were allowed several pints of beer a day; the same was true on the Continent, although in southern Europe wine was also available.[20]

In times of crisis, however, none of the hospitals were adequate, and much of the institutional care collapsed during the Black Death, an epidemic of bubonic plague that first hit Europe in 1348–1349 and caused massive social dislocation. A large percentage of Europeans, perhaps as much as a third of the population in some areas, died during the plague. Eventually most of the governmental units dealt with the plague by removing infected patients to special hospitals on the outskirts of cities and by drafting people, often unwillingly, to serve as nurses. The nurses and their patients stayed locked up with each other until the crisis had passed.[21]

During most of the medieval period, there were very few physicians or surgeons attached to the hospitals except for those of the military orders. When a doctor was needed, he was called from the city and was reimbursed for his services. Beginning in the fourteenth century, with increased specialization, many of the regulations called for physicians or surgeons either to be attached to the hospitals or to visit them regularly. Probably these resident medical men did some prescribing or surgery, but most of the care and supervision of the patient remained in the hands of the nurse.

While many medieval hospitals were administered by the Order of the Holy Spirit, a smaller number by the Hospitalers, and still others by religious groups such as the Antonines, the great majority were more or less autonomous without any contact with the others. Their only unifying point was their motivating principle, with perhaps some loose connection through common interests. This caused a wide variation in hospital administration and patient care, so that no general survey can indicate what was true in any particular situation. It seems safe to say that generally nurses had to meet certain conditions. Before entering any of the orders or hospitals they had to show that they were freeborn, celibate, free of debts, and not lepers or epileptics. If they met these requirements, they then entered into a novitiate period usually lasting a year. As a novice the nurse learned both the care and service of the sick, and the various obligatory religious duties. If the novitiate was completed success-fully, the would-be nurse was then subject to approval by the chapter. If accepted, the nurse assumed the religious habit and took the three vows of poverty, obedience, and chastity. But before a nurse could be formally recognized as a member of the order, the bishop examined him or her, in part to make sure that the number of people in the nursing orders was kept within limits. This was a deliberate policy to prevent hospitals from becoming monasteries or convents by having too many brothers or sisters.

The conduct of the nurses was carefully regulated by statute. They were to observe silence; they were not to pamper themselves; they were to accept without recrimination the food set before them; and they were not to sleep naked, but to wear nightgowns. This last requirement might have been enacted to enable the nurses to aid the sick at any time of the night if the need arose. Since most nurses belonged to an order, much of their time was occupied with religious duties. Canon law, however, warned them never to forget that their primary duty was to the sick. Generally the hospital brothers and sisters met at chapel at least three times a day, although some institutions required more frequent attendance.

In certain cases relatives were admitted into the hospitals to help nurse their loved ones. These "lay" nurses did not take a vow or enter an order, but they had to promise to honor and revere the rules and regulations of the hospital. Donors or people who gave part of their property to the hospital were also admitted to the hospitals even though they were not ill. In most hospitals they formed a distinct group, separate from the attendants and the ordinary sick, receiving special lodging, food, and care. This special treatment often became a source of much discord, but the practice continued, perhaps because it helped the hospitals to finance the care of the poor.

Many women went beyond simple nursing duties to assume much of the responsibility which we associate with the modern nurse practitioner or general practitioner. Almost all medieval midwifery was done by women, as was much of the actual diagnosis and care of other women. Women who went beyond simple nursing duties were often called "leech" or "la Lèche," or "sage femme," wise woman.

The wife was, however, still the chief nurse. Her importance was emphasized by a fifteenth-century sermon of St. Bernardine of Siena. He urged men to marry even though some men might say:

> "What need have I to take a wife? I have no labor; I have no children to break my sleep at night; I have the less expense by far. Why should I undertake this Travail? If I fall ill, my servants will care for me better than she would." This thou sayest, and I say the contrary: for a woman careth better for her husband than any other in the world.[22]

The same Anna Comnena who described the hospital at Constantinople has given us a picture of her father's last illness. He was attended by physicians, but the nursing care was by his family:

> Constantly have I seen my mother [the Empress] spending the night by the Emperor, sitting behind him on the bed, holding him up in her arms, and in a measure relieving his respiration. No words can say how she labored over him day and night contriving ways for him to lie down, and to change his position, and making all sorts of mattresses. . . .[23]

As his condition worsened, feeding became more of a problem, until his daughters and wife together took up a vigil over his bed, feeding him, moving him, and doing everything they could.

Every mistress of a medieval castle, from the empress on down, had learned some sort of home nursing. She supervised the care not only of her immediate family but often of her servants and tenants as well. Who took care of sick wives? Husbands often did, but usually with assistance from servants and friends of his wife. Husbands were somewhat handicapped as nurses because they first had to support their families. Peasant workers on the medieval manor or great farm were often given sick leave, but not for illnesses in their families. The time allowed for sick leave varied from manor to manor and season to season. On one English manor a man received three weeks' sick leave most of the year, but only fifteen days during the harvest season. Other manors allowed him a year and a day, but required him to show up for plowing; while still others allowed him only a month, after which he had to report for work whether sick or not. The test of sickness was inability to leave house or bed.

In summation, then, medieval devotion to the sick was an important forward step in nursing. To assist in carrying out this ideal, medieval people developed various institutions, especially hospitals and nursing orders. The major difficulty was that even though such care was motivated by a dedication to a higher cause, no real study of the needs of the sick had been made. Nursing was mainly an empirical science devoted to relieving pain and suffering, an important aspect of nursing to be sure. But for nursing to go beyond this, it also needed scientific know-how. This only came in the modern period.

Three

Nursing in Transition

During the later Middle Ages there was a rapid increase in the population and in the number of cities. This was the result of an increase in trade, especially international trade between the East and the West, the development of business techniques such as double-entry bookkeeping, the rise of banks, the appearance of a stable currency, and the rise of national monarchies. Industries such as textiles and leather working expanded, and new industries appeared. The size of the middle class increased; at the same time the average person became much more materialistic than during the early Middle Ages. In some ways this new urban life resembled the city-state idea of the Romans and the Greeks, and many of the intellectual leaders of the community looked to the classics for ideals or motivations. The period between 1500 and 1800 is one of change marked by terms such as the Renaissance, the Reformation, the Age of Reason, the Enlightenment, and the Age of Revolutions.

Changes that had been evolving in the later Middle Ages increased in tempo and multiplied almost explosively. Revolutionary developments took place, including the discovery of a whole new part of the world by Columbus and other explorers, the change from an earth-centered universe to the sun-centered universe of Copernicus, and the theory of the universal workings of gravitation from Sir Isaac Newton. Late in the medieval period, printing had been invented along with new paper-making techniques, putting much more emphasis on the written word. Gunpowder had also been introduced, and its use was spreading widely. Indicative of the effects of these changes were the large-scale peasant revolts, the religious changes of the Reformation, struggles for the dominance of Europe and the world, and the American and French revolutions at the end of the eighteenth century.

In the arts and sciences, the period was especially creative; it is then that modern medicine began. During the later Middle Ages medicine had revived through the study of Arabic and early Greek medicine. This revival had begun in southern Italy, especially around Salerno in the tenth century, and had spread northward, until by the thirteenth century it was concentrated in the new universities and their medical schools at Paris and Montpellier in France and at Bologna in Italy. At first this education imitated the Arabic and Greek medical learning which had come into Europe from Spain, from southern Italy (where Arab and Greek influences were strong), and from Greece itself. Soon, however, Western physicians were contributing ideas of their own. Two of the most famous were Henri de Mondeville (1260–1320) and Guy de Chauliac (1300–1370).

These men advocated two different theories concerning the healing process. Mondeville opposed the Galenic idea of the necessity of suppuration or "laudable pus," and instead tried to avoid infection, advocating a nonsupperative growing together of the wound. Chauliac felt that suppuration was a necessary stage in the healing of wounds, and unfortunately, his ideas prevailed. Despite this, however, Chauliac was one of the leaders in new surgical techniques, including the use of an analgesic.

As the new university-trained physicians grew in power and prestige, they became reluctant to engage in surgery. Many people thought it was undignified to work with their hands, and since the physicians were concerned with their dignity, many groups of physicians began to restrict their members from using the knife in surgical operations. Another reason for this unwillingness to resort to surgery was that clergymen were forbidden to shed blood, and physicians were considered clerics, although only in minor orders. They were thus reluctant to do surgery or to bleed their patients, one of the necessities of medieval medicine. To counter this unwillingness, another class of medical practitioners grew up—the barber or barber-surgeon. Most of these men were empirically trained and thus lacked the theoretical knowledge of the physicians. In some areas the physicians did lecture to the barbers, but usually they were on their own. This separation of the theory of medicine from practical surgery served to handicap both fields. In Italy, however, there was not such a drastic division, for there both the physician and the surgeon were university trained. It is to Italy that we must look for the beginnings of modern medicine.

Medical Innovations

One of the fields in which the new "renaissance" occurred was art. In order to make painting more realistic, artists began applying themselves to scientific studies. These studies resulted in the development of perspective, naturalistic scenery, and most important from the medical point of view, in an understanding of the muscular structure of the human body. Much of this new learning was at first centered at Florence where the contact between the artist, physician, surgeon, and apothecary was very close, perhaps because they all belonged to the same guild or craft. The man who is perhaps the best representative of this new knowledge is Leonardo da Vinci who was competent in so many fields that he is considered one of the greatest geniuses of all time. He made a vast number of anatomical drawings obviously based on knowledge gained by dissection and intended to illustrate an anatomical textbook which was never published.

The founder of modern anatomical studies is the Flemish-born, Italian-trained Andreas Vesalius (1514–1564). In his most famous work, *De Humani Corporis Fabrica*, he corrected many of the anatomical errors that had persisted since Galen. His work was enhanced by the illustrations of his countryman, Jan Kalkar. Other famous anatomists of the period were Eustachius (1524–1574), who described the eustachian tube and other anatomical details, and Vesalius' pupil and successor, Fallopius (1523–1564), who described the female genital organs and the semicircular canal in the inner ear. The fallopian tubes are named for him because of his pioneering work in female anatomy.

Medicine was also closely allied with the humanities, and one of the results of this alliance was a long poem *Syphilis sive morbus Gallicus* (1530) by the physician-poet Girolomo Fracastoro (1478–1550). The poem, in Latin hexameters, is a classic for both its literary style and its medical concepts; it was so influential that the term "syphilis," based on the name of its mythical hero, came to be applied to the disease that was then epidemic in Europe. So virulent was the disease that many writers of the time, including Fracastoro, believed it had been newly introduced into Europe by sailors returning from Columbus' voyage to the New World. The controversy over the origins of syphilis continues today between those who believe it derived from the New World and those who deny it. Besides his poem on syphilis, Fracastoro studied other epidemics, and his most significant work was that entitled *De contagione* (1546). Here Fracastoro illustrated three means by which contagion could be spread: by simple contact between persons (as in scabies); by *fomites*, that is from the clothing or objects of an infected person; and at a distance through *seminaria*, which in many ways seems to anticipate the nineteenth-century discovery of microorganisms.

Newly developing sciences such as chemistry were also influencing medicine. Here the key figure was Philippus Aureolus Theophrastus Bombastus von Hohenheim (1493–1541), who was nicknamed Paracelsus, that is surpassing Celsus, the ancient Roman medical writer. To Paracelsus there was no greater obstacle to medical progress than tradition, and the way to practice medicine effectively was to discard most of the books and traditions, returning to the "book of nature." Since Paracelsus had a low opinion of most of his medical contemporaries and was pugnacious and dogmatic in his own views, he inevitably became involved in a great many disputes which limited his influence on his contemporaries. In the long run his attempts to use various minerals and chemical compounds for treatment were innovative. His great difficulty, however, was that in his eagerness to challenge the existing medical systems, he erected counter systems with dogmas often as damaging as those he was challenging. His writings are a strange combination of intelligent observation and mystical nonsense. His training, like that of most of his contemporaries, had been obtained in Italy, although most of his life was spent in Germany.

All of the preceding were university men. The founder of modern surgery, however, was a man of the people who could not read Latin, the learned language of the period. This was Ambroise Paré (1510–1590). The sixteenth century had many wars which, coupled with the increasing use of gunpowder, put great demands upon the surgeons. Guns at this time did not kill as effectively as the crossbow or even the long bow, but they did cause more wounds. Paré had served his apprenticeship under various barber-surgeons before serving in the French army where he became involved in the debate over whether "laudable pus" was a normal stage in the healing of wounds. When gunpowder came into widespread use, most of the wounds, because of the impurities in the ammunition, were infected from the beginning. This had led many surgeons to accept Chauliac's idea that infection was natural. Normal treatment called for the cauterizing of such wounds by pouring boiling elder oil into them. When Paré, on his first campaign, ran out of elder oil, he dressed wounds with a salve concocted from egg yolk, attar of roses, and turpentine. He slept that night with an uneasy conscience, fearing that he might have harmed the man more than he had helped, but the next day he found that those treated with boiled oil had high fevers and their wounds were inflamed and painful, while those treated with his salve had little pain, no swelling, and no inflammation. From that time forth, he refused to cauterize wounds. He continued to experiment in treating injuries, always seeking out people who were said to know different treatments. From this he found what worked or not.

The culminating development in this period was the explanation of the circulation of the blood by the English physician, William Harvey (1578–1657), who had studied in Italy and was greatly influenced by Italian medicine. Harvey was intrigued by movement in the human body. Upon his return to England, he investigated further. What is the pulse? Obviously, it was an expression of the movement of the blood. But Galen's theory could not explain it. Galen had taught that ingested food was elaborated in the liver to become blood, that from here blood permeated the body conveyed by the vessels in a mysterious to-and-fro movement: flowing into the right side of the heart, then passing through pores into the left side of the heart, and then pursuing its way through the organism. This answer was unsatisfactory to Harvey. By 1616 he thought he had discovered the real answer, but held off publication until he was certain. Finally, in 1628 he published his work explaining the circulation of the blood throughout the body. He stated that the blood flowed from the left side of the heart through arteries into all parts of the organism, making its way through gaps in the tissues into the veins, and then was conveyed by them to the right atrium of the heart. His simple explanation helped tie physiology and anatomy very closely together. Despite opposition, his theory gradually gained ground. It was finally confirmed by Malpighi (1628–1694), who observed capillary circulation through the newly invented microscope. As a result of these discoveries, Galen and the old classicists began to lose influence, while medical science made some progress in understanding the workings of the human body.

Religious Changes

Nursing, however, was less affected by any of the new discoveries in medicine as it was by the rise of Protestantism. In the later Middle Ages, a number of religious reformers had challenged not only traditional beliefs, but Church organizations and institutions, particularly the papacy. Some of these, such as John Wycliffe (1330–1384) in England and John Huss (1372–1415) in Bohemia (modern Czechoslovakia), were declared heretics, and Huss was burned at the stake. Many groups such as the Waldensians and the spiritual Franciscans, a heretical breakoff from the Franciscan order, went underground, while others such as the Albigensians in southern France were wiped out by a series of Crusades. Religious unrest and dissatisfaction mounted, despite efforts to contain it, until it crystallized under a number of sixteenth-century leaders, the most famous of whom is Martin Luther (1483–1546). Other reformers include Ulrich Zwingli (1484–1531) in Switzerland, John Calvin (1509–1564) in France and in Geneva, Thomas Cranmer (1489–1556) in England, John Knox (1513–1572) in Scotland, Thomas Münzer (1490–1525) and Menno Simmons (1496–1561) in Germany, Michael Servetus (1511–1553) in Spain and in France, and Faustus Socinus (1539–1604), first in Italy, then in Poland and Hungary. The list of religious leaders and reformers could be extended, but these are among the most significant. The effect was to divide Western Europe into Catholic and Protestant camps, while Protestanism itself was split into competing sects of Lutherans, Episcopalians (Anglicans), Presbyterians, Evangelicals, Anabaptists (several varieties), Unitarians, and others.

Although the Protestant leaders often disagreed among themselves, they almost unanimously decried the conventual or monastic career, emphasizing instead life in the secular world. Inevitably, the first effects of Protestantism were to set back nursing, since various monastic affiliated institutions, including hospitals and schools, were closed, and numerous orders, including nursing orders, were dissolved.

Even in Catholic countries, monarchs, desirous of increasing their revenue, took the opportunity to close many monasteries and seized the endowments for themselves. Those monastic hospitals that did survive were often later destroyed or devastated during the religious wars of the sixteenth and seventeenth centuries. As a result some writers have called this period the "dark ages" of nursing. Though this is an exaggeration, nursing and the institutional care of the sick suffered a serious setback. In England, where there had been some 450 charitable foundations before the Reformation, most of them either schools or hospitals, only a few survived the reign of Henry VIII. An even more radical effect of the Protestant movement on nursing, both in Catholic and in Protestant countries, was the removal of most male nurses. Almost all the Catholic nursing orders organized after 1500 were for women, while in Protestant countries nursing increasingly became a woman's calling.

Religious leaders were aware of the lack of adequate nursing care. Luther urged the state to care for the sick and proposed that each town set up something similar to the modern Community Chest to raise funds. In other Protestant areas nurse visitors for the poor were established. The Anabaptists, under the leadership of such groups as the Mennonites, reestablished the position of Deaconess. The Mennonite Confession urged that "honorable old widows be ordained and chosen as servants [deacons], who besides the almoners, are to visit, comfort, and take care of the poor, the weak, the afflicted, and the needy, as also to visit, comfort, and take care of the widows and orphans." [1]

Calvin established an order of deacons in Geneva to minister to the sick and needy and also founded a charity hospital. The city of Amsterdam was divided into districts which were to be visited by nurse-deaconesses, usually elderly women, who tended the sick and helpless. The Moravians also revived the deaconess system in order to nurse the sick. Most such efforts, however, were only temporary, and the institutions for the sick increasingly relied upon hired assistants who had little skill and, perhaps because they were so underpaid, little interest in helping the sick.

The Catholics attempted to preserve some of their nursing orders by making certain that they meet newly enacted standards for order and discipline. The Council of Trent (1545–1563), in which Catholicism enacted a number of reforms to strengthen itself in the battle against Protestantism, reinforced episcopal control over hospitals in order to give more direct supervision. New orders such as the Brothers of St. John of God (or Brothers of Mercy) were founded. This order originated in 1538 through the efforts of the Portuguese John Ciudad (1495–1550), better known as John the Good. St. Charles Borromeo (1538–1584) gave practical effect to the attempts at hospital reform by founding and endowing a hospital at Milan. He required periodic reports from the hospital directors to insure that the hospital was as efficiently managed as possible. Several other hospitals were founded by him as was a nursing order, the Sisters of St. Charles of Nancy (or Sisters of St. Charles Borromeo), to carry on his work.

In England, after Henry VIII had closed most of the monastic hospitals, it was found that the sick of London were deprived of the aid given to them by the religious hospitals. As a result the mayor, aldermen, and citizens petitioned the king in 1538 to reopen at least some of the hospitals, arguing that this was an absolute necessity for "the ayde and comforte of the poor, sykke, blynde, aged and impotent persones beying not able to helpe themselffs nor havyng any place certeyn wheryn they may be lodged cherysshed, and refresshed tyll they be cured and holpen of theyre dyseases and syknesse." [2] Henry VIII eventually did endow some hospitals—namely, St. Bartholomew's and St. Thomas'. The Hospital of Bethlehem was also established as a home for the mentally ill.

St. Bartholomew's Hospital

There are fairly complete records for St. Bartholomew's Hospital from the sixteenth to the eighteenth centuries and to a lesser extent for St. Thomas' which indicate many of the changes in nursing during this period. When St. Bartholomew's was refounded, the charter provided for a matron and twelve additional women to make beds, "wash and attend upon the said poor men and women there." These women were to receive their board and room plus some 40 shillings or two pounds a year for their duties. The matron received three pounds, five shillings, and eight pence. The thirteen women slept together in a single large room. All told, they cared for about 100 patients. It was customary to call these attendants "sisters," a carry-over from the monastic tradition. Gradually, as the staff increased, the term *sister* came to mean the person in charge of a ward; those under her were called *nurses*.

In 1552 and again in 1557, the duties of the matron were defined. The good woman was to receive all sick and diseased persons who were sent to the hospital by the almoners, keeping a record of them. Inventory was to be taken quarterly by her. She was to count beds, bolsters, mattresses, blankets, coverlets, sheets, shirts, hose, and other materials. She was to make certain that the sisters assisted the sick, made the beds, supervised the wards, and washed and purged the patients' dirty clothes and linen. It was also her duty to see that each sister kept herself neat and clean. She had to watch that the sisters did not leave their room for the men's ward after 7 P.M. in the winter or 9 P.M. in the summer, unless there was a real emergency on the floor. She was never to allow the sisters to be idle. If they were not occupied with the sick, they were to spin or do other work. The matron was also to perform some nursing duties; these included inspections two or three times during the night to see that the children and other patients were covered and that the hospital was functioning in an orderly fashion. [3]

The sisters of the hospital were to obey the matron, who was to be regarded as their "chief governess and ruler." It was their duty faithfully and charitably to serve and help the sick by feeding them, talking to them, and easing their burdens. Nurses were cautioned to avoid scolding, swearing, or drunkenness, and were exhorted to be virtuous, loving, and diligent. They were also to spin, sew, mend sheets and shirts, and do the laundry. That the nurses did a lot of spinning is indicated by the records of the hospital. In May 1550, the sisters at St. Bartholomew's delivered twenty-one pairs of sheets to the matron which they had made from cloth they had spun and woven. In July 1566, eleven pairs of woolen sheets and seven flaxen sheets were given to the matron. Such lists continue to appear on the records for a long time afterward.[4]

The first list of sisters at St. Bartholomew's dates from March 1553. A Mrs. Rose Fyssher (sometimes spelled Fysher) was the matron, the first of some 28 women to serve in that capacity until the office of matron was changed to that of superintendent of nurses in 1878. The sisters included Elizabeth Clark, Jone Goodyere, Alys Wright, Elizabeth Trewillian, Kateryn Marshall, Alys Yonglive, Sybyll Jelly, Marget Edyman, Jone Cantrelle, Eve Williams, Johan Lamporte, and another person labeled "the foole." This might have been a feebleminded woman who was kept to amuse the sisters. There was evidently considerable turnover because a few years later only Mrs. Fyssher, the "foole," and four of the original sisters were left. The others had either died or moved on, but at any rate they had been replaced.[5]

From its refounding St. Bartholomew's had an outpatient ward with a nurse assigned there. There were also surgeons, pharmacists, and later even physicians. Surgeons were required either to dress the wounds of the injured and surgical cases at least three times a week or to stand by while someone else, perhaps the sisters, did. Physicians in 1591 were to write in a book the names of the patients and the medicines required for them, perhaps the beginning of the modern order book or the chart.

As the population of London grew, so did the hospital staff. Some of the new additions might not have equaled the caliber of the earlier sisters, for there are many instances of reprimands in the various hospital records. Complaints were brought against one sister because she did not come to her ward before 9 A.M., and when she did arrive, she scolded the patients. In 1648 one Jane Baker was dismissed for abusing the patients. She was also accused of charging them a penny for washing their shifts. Elizabeth Whitty was rebuked for entertaining men at night in the wards, even going so far as to let them play cards. Three sisters were dismissed in 1656 for disturbing the patients by their fighting, while another sister who charged patients extra for chairs and stools also lost her position. To diminish some of these abuses, the officials of St. Bartholomew's in 1653 stipulated that no sister was to be employed in the future without some previous trial as to her fitness in washing clothes or other such nursing tasks.[6]

Generally, however, despite the preceding examples, the patients were well cared for. That the matrons and sisters of the London hospitals remained in the city during the height of the plague, when most of the physicians fled, indicates high devotion to duty. There were, of course, always some who neglected their duties, and these were the ones who were mentioned in the hospital registers. To curb the abuses of these few nurses, regulations were passed. The first attempt at state regulation of nurses in the British Isles came from the Irish Parliament in 1715. This ordinance stipulated that nurses who did not conduct themselves well were to be committed to a house of correction for three months at hard labor, as well as whipped publicly through the streets on a market day between 11 A.M. and 12 noon.[7]

Qualifications for Nurses

There were some attempts to draw up a set of qualifications for nurses or sisters. One of the, if not the, first English physicians to attempt this was Thomas Fuller (1654–1734). He recognized that it was impossible for any one nurse to meet all his requirements, but the more closely she approached them, the better she would be. According to him a nurse should be

1. Of middle age, fit and able to go through with the necessary Fatigue of her Undertaking.
2. Healthy, especially free from Vapours, and Cough.
3. A good Watcher, that can hold sitting up the whole Course of the Sickness.
4. Quick of Hearing, and always ready at the first Call.
5. Quiet and Still, so as to talk low, and but little, and tread softly.
6. Of good Sight, to observe the Pocks, their Colour, Manner and Growth, and all Alterations that may happen.
7. Handy to do every Thing the best way, without Blundering and Noise.
8. Nimble and Quick a going, coming, and doing every Thing.
9. Cleanly, to make all she dresseth acceptable.
10. Well-tempered, to humour, and please the Sick as much as she can.
11. Chearful and Pleasant; to make the best of every Thing, without being at any time Cross, Melancholy, or Timorous.
12. Constantly careful, and diligent by Night and by Day.
13. Sober and Temperate; not given to Gluttony, Drinking, or Smoaking.
14. Observant to follow the Physician's Orders duly; and not be so conceited of her own Skill, as to give her own medicines privately.
15. To have no Children, or other to come much after her.[8]

Even in the seventeenth century, a nurse could be hired as was "Lettie Pyne" because she was a widow who "hath lived well" and was an "Irish Protestant."[9] This satisfied all the requirements for St. Bartholomew's.

Generally, however, hospitals wanted nurses who were trained in the care of the sick. Usually there was competition for any vacant place. As the staff grew, a hierarchy of nursing personnel developed. Helpers and watchers were added in the seventeenth century to assist the sisters. Some of these watchers became the early predecessors of night nurses. The first night nurse mentioned at St. Bartholomew's was in 1652 when it was noted that Margaret Whitaker had been at the hospital in this capacity for some five years.[10] Gradually, many of these watchers formed a class just below the sisters, that of nurses. Advancement to sister usually came from this group. By 1678 it was ordered that nurses on the floor were to be preferred for promotion to a sistership when a vacancy existed. Other staff positions were added to help the sisters and nurses; by 1771 St. Bartholomew's had some 100 women employed to care for the patients in a graded hierarchy of matron, sisters, nurses, helpers, and watchers.[11] This tended to ensure a system of on-the-job training for the higher ranks.

Slowly, working conditions for the sisters and nurses began to improve. Sisters were given separate rooms at the end of the wards and no longer had to sleep in a common dormitory room. Their pay also increased from the original two pounds a year. In 1802 when the staff at St. Bartholomew's consisted of 31 sisters, 31 nurses, and 33 night nurses, plus various attendants, each ordinary sister received slightly more than 32 pounds a year. A sister in the operating ward received 37 pounds; sisters on the foul (or disease) wards were paid 52 pounds. The two nurses in the operating wards (about 72 operations a year were performed) received nineteen pounds; in the men's foul wards they were paid 24 pounds, but they also had no night duty; while the three sisters in the women's foul wards received seventeen pounds. The rest of the nurses received four shillings a week plus an extra sixpence for the required night duty. This with various special fees brought their pay to about seventeen pounds a year. These 90-odd women cared for 3,696 patients during the year, most of them long-term patients.[12] Blue was the standard uniform color for the sisters at St. Bartholomew's, although the shades varied from period to period. In the early nineteenth century, the nurses, as distinguished from the sisters, began to wear brown, but later changed to a striped material with a blue belt.

Roaches, bugs, and other vermin continually plagued the nurses and patients of the time. Hospital records in London and elsewhere show regular attempts to remove them, but apparently not with much success. Part of the vermin problem came from the beds filled with straw or feathers, a haven for insect life. Another source of vermin were the patients themselves; they were washed only infrequently and not very thoroughly. The first pool bath was not installed in St. Bartholomew's until the 1720's. Nurses themselves still did most of the laundering in the hospitals as they had in the medieval period.

In the sixteenth and seventeenth centuries, most patients in English hospitals were probably fed a basic mutton diet, but special diets were available when prescribed by the apothecary. A typical weekly diet for 1687 was as follows:

Sunday: 10 ounces of wheat bread
                6 ounces of boiled beef without bones
                1 1/2 pints of beef broth
                1 pint of caudled ale (a mixture of ale, eggs, gruel, sugar, and spices considered especially good for the sick)
                3 pints of beer

Monday: 10 ounces of wheat bread
                1 pint of milk pottage (a thick soup)
                6 ounces of beef
                1 1/2 pints of beef broth
                3 pints of beer

Tuesday: 10 ounces of wheat bread
                8 ounces of boiled mutton
                3 pints of mutton broth
                3 pints of beer

Wednesday: 10 ounces of bread
                4 ounces of cheese
                2 ounces of butter
                1 pint of milk pottage
                3 pints of beer

Thursday: The same allowance as Sunday plus 1 pint of rice milk

Friday: 10 ounces of wheat bread
                1 pint of sugar sops (moistened cake)
                2 ounces of cheese
                1 ounce of butter
                1 pint of water gruel (thin cereal)
                3 pints of beer

Saturday: The same allowance as Wednesday[13]

When possible both old and new cheeses were to be provided, while fresh butter was available from May to October. Patients on special milk diets received milk, bread, beer, and caudled ale on Sundays. They apparently survived.

In the eighteenth century there began to be more concern over diet, especially after a certain Dr. Radcliffe gave some money to improve it. The new diet included two ounces more bread each day and a slight increase in the meat ration. Milk pottage also appeared more frequently as a breakfast meal. Patients with spending money could buy extra bread or beer. Even into the nineteenth century, when there were further revisions in the diet, beer had a regular place. By then the diet included some 40 ounces of meat a week, but there were two meatless days.

As in the Middle Ages, hospitals continued to be occupied mainly by the poor, who could not take care of themselves, and a few travelers, or soldiers, especially those of the lower ranks.

St. Vincent de Paul

In Catholic countries the most important development in nursing was the founding of the Sisters (or Daughters) of Charity by St. Vincent de Paul (1576–1660). Saint Vincent is one of those dedicated persons who appear all too rarely in history. He perhaps can be called the founder of modern organized charity. A son of poor French peasants, Vincent demonstrated great ability as a youth, was educated for the priesthood, and was ordained in 1600. In 1605 while trying to settle a legacy that had been left to him, he was captured by pirates who sent him to Tunis, where he was a slave for two years under three different masters, the last of whom was an Italian who had converted to Islam to practice polygamy. Vincent reconverted his last master, and the two (without the Italian's wives) fled Africa for Italy where Vincent regained his freedom in 1607. Later he was appointed to important positions in France where he met the rich and the powerful but never forgot his own humble origins or his life as a slave. Instead, he used his newfound influence to help the unfortunate. His first efforts were devoted to bettering the conditions of convicts in France, especially the so-called galley slaves—prisoners who were forced to serve as rowers on French ships. As his work expanded, he formed the Congregation of Priests of the Missions—priests who maintained mission services to the convicts.

During his work he became acquainted with two noble women, Madame de la Chassaigne and Madame de Brie, who spent much of their time aiding the poor or nursing the sick. On one occasion these two women asked him to solicit his congregation for aid to a family who were ill and without food. His parishioners responded with so much food that the family soon had more than it could eat or use, much of the food being left to spoil. Vincent felt that though the impulse that had provided the charity was laudable, the distribution was not. In order to organize such charity better, he brought together a society of ladies called the Confrerie de la Charité or Confraternity of Charity, pious groups of parish women who sought to provide for the needy. These societies spread rapidly throughout France and to Poland and Italy where they remained under local parish control. These women, both married and unmarried, devoted themselves to the care of the poor and the sick. As the number of women in the society increased, he grouped them into a community under the direction of Mademoiselle Le Gras (née Louise de Marillac and canonized under her maiden name). Mademoiselle Le Gras was a recent widow who was called "Mademoiselle," the French equivalent of the English "Miss," because the prefix "Madame" was reserved for noblewomen. The ladies visited the sick in their homes and provided food and care. The sick were given as much bread as they could eat, five ounces of veal or mutton, soup, and half a bottle of wine. If the patient were very ill, the women also made sure that a nurse was available.

As the order spread, it underwent some modifications, and in Paris it attracted many upper-class and noble ladies, Ladies of Charity, who often carried out their charitable duties by sending their servants to do the actual work. To assist them, Vincent began recruiting girls from the country, the first of whom, Marguerite Nasseau, arrived in 1630. These girls, Filles de Charité, were regarded by Vincent as his "daughters," but increasingly they came to be called Sisters of Charity rather than Daughters of Charity. As their number increased, Mlle. Le Gras realized that they needed both preparation and supervision. In March 1634 she vowed to devote herself to the task. The result was the organization of the Sisters of Charity, although neither Vincent nor St. Louise de Marillac would admit that they had founded an order, preferring instead to give credit to "God."

At first the Sisters had no written rule, but merely obeyed a few regulations drawn up by St. Louise. Vincent also often discussed their duties with them, and many of those talks are still preserved. As the Sisters increased in number, more formalized rules were adopted. They were to treat the sick with respect and humility. Medicines were to be given according to the prescriptions of the physician. If the patients were extremely ill or had no one to make their bed or render other nursing services, the Sisters were to intervene and take charge. In 1638 the work done by the Sisters and Ladies of Charity was extended to the Hôtel Dieu in Paris, to assist the Augustinian Sisters there in their nursing tasks. The Sisters helped serve dinner to the sick, gave them little treats, changed the sheets, adjusted the beds, read to the patients, and generally watched over them, giving nursing care whenever possible.

Vincent, however, was opposed to the Ladies and Sisters becoming nuns, since he felt there was a real need for women who could visit with the sick in their homes, which would be difficult for a nun. The women in his orders took vows only for short periods, usually a year; they could and usually did renew their vows. Both married and unmarried women were accepted, the former with the consent of their husbands, the latter with the consent of their parents. The society soon began to take care of foundlings and to serve as contract nurses for many of the hospitals in France. Under contract nursing, the hospitals agreed to board and lodge the women in return for their care of the patients. In patient care, these nurses were under the control of the hospital, but for religious matters or discipline they were under the jurisdiction of the Mother Superior in Paris, who reserved the right to transfer or change sisters as she saw fit.

Vincent did not put any written restrictions on patient load, but he advised two Sisters sent to Arras not to take care of more than eight or ten patients at any one time. He also cautioned the Sisters to obey the physicians and to treat them with respect. Vincent's contacts with the wealthy enabled him to secure funds to endow hospitals and foundling homes all over France and even outside the country. By the time of the death of Vincent and Mlle. Le Gras, the order had some 350 Sisters with some 70 establishments in France and Poland.

Saint Vincent considered the prime duty of the Sisters to be visiting the sick in their homes. This makes them the first organized visiting nurse service. He wrote:

> . . . it is true [there were] religious [orders] and hospitals for the assistance of the sick, but before your establishment there was never a community destined to go and serve the sick in their houses. If, in some poor family, anyone fell sick, he was sent to the hospital, and this separated the husband from his wife, and the children from their parents. Until now, O my God! you had not furnished the means of going to assist them in their houses, and it seemed in a manner as if Thy adorable providence, which never fails, did not extend its watchful care over them. Why, then you, my dear sisters, did God delay in granting this assistance to them? Oh! because it was to be reserved to you. . . .[14]

The first secular nursing registry was also organized in France in the seventeenth century. Theophraste Renaudot, a graduate physician from the University of Montpellier, came to Paris as physician to Louis XIII and commissioner of the poor. Seeing that unemployment was one of the big problems of the poor, he opened an employment bureau in 1630. Dr. Renaudot soon added a nursing registry; he listed the names of the persons who were prepared to nurse the sick along with a list of Paris physicians and surgeons who were willing to give free consultations and treatment to persons sent by the bureau. This nursing registry was free to the poor and available at a small fee to the general public.[15]

Early Hospitals in the Americas

In the New World hospitals were also being founded. The first hospital in the Americas was erected sometime before 1524 by Hernando Cortes, the conquerer of Mexico. It was called the *Hospital de la Purisima Concepción*, but its name was later changed to *Jesus Nazareno*. Other hospitals were soon established, so that by 1541 hospitals had been erected in most of the major Spanish towns. The first hospital in Canada was the Hôtel Dieu at Sillery; in 1658 this was transferred to Quebec. The Hôtel Dieu was founded by the Duchess d'Aiguillon in 1635, but it was not until 1639 that three Augustinian Sisters of Mercy sailed for Canada to staff it. They soon had more patients than they could handle. Almost contemporary with the Hôtel Dieu in Sillery was the Hôtel Dieu at Montreal started in 1644 by Mlle. Jeanne Mance (1606–1673), who became so interested in Canada by reading about it that she decided to make mercy work there her life mission. She arrived in Quebec in 1641 but went on to Montreal the next year. She cared for the sick from the first, although her hospital was not completed until 1644. She was a lay woman herself, but she was soon assisted by three nursing sisters of the order of St. Joseph de la Fleche. The first hospital in the continental United States was erected in Manhattan in 1658 for the reception of sick soldiers and Negro slaves. In 1717 a hospital for infectious diseases was built at Boston. A charter was granted to the Pennsylvania Hospital in 1751, and the cornerstone was laid in 1755, but the structure was not completed until 1805. The first hospital in the United States established by a private gift was the Charity Hospital at New Orleans. A sailor, Jean Louis, left the money.

Women and Nursing

Most nursing and care of the sick, however, was still carried on at home by the women of the household. Every daughter was taught by her mother or, in some cases, by her governess special formulas for making salves and lotions as well as how to care for the sick or injured. Information of this kind was handed down from generation to generation as women's trade secrets. For simple illnesses there were specific remedies. Mint was used for colic, parsley for toothache, St. John's wort for aching joints, and pounded snails were used to make poultices. Even if a physician were summoned, the nursing fell upon the women of the household. Home nursing probably increased the chances of recovery, since the hospitals, with a lack of aseptic techniques, linen shortages, and other difficulties, were not the most healthy places. On large estates some tenants might be summoned to help nurse in an emergency. In rural areas it was considered the duty of the mistress of the manor to oversee the nursing care of the tenants.

Usually a sick person at home would be put into a room scented with sweet herbs and hung with red curtains or valances; other red objects might also be put there since it was believed that the color red had healing and strengthening properties, especially in illnesses with fevers. Patients, who were now beginning to wear bed-clothes, were even dressed in red garments with red nightcaps. Very little fresh air was allowed into the sickroom. Where the beds had curtains, as they usually did in the homes of the well-to-do, these were kept closed. Thomas Sydenham, an English physician of the late seventeenth century, felt that the greatest danger to recovery was from the overnursing that the patient received at home. He tried to force his patients out of the closed and overheated rooms into the open air by making them exercise on horseback. It might be that in many illnesses the rich were less favorably placed than the poor, who through lack of money had to let nature take its own course. Of course, the poor, lacking nourishing food or good sanitation, were much more susceptible to any plague that might sweep their area.

Women took their nursing duties seriously, and a woman who did not nurse her husband, friends, or relatives was socially ostracized. The English poet Sir Philip Sidney had an aunt who had an altercation with her husband shortly before he became ill and died. He would not let her approach his sickbed. Malicious gossip had it that she had deliberately ignored nursing her husband. The poor woman even wrote to Queen Elizabeth trying to explain that she was not negligent.[16] Diaries of women of the period often have notes about dressing a poor boy's leg or nursing a servant, a husband, or neighbor.

When the women in the household were ill, or if many people in a parish were affected, those who were well attempted to nurse the others. Shortly after the Pilgrims landed at Plymouth, only six or seven persons in the company were strong enough to be up and around. Those who were well hazarded their health and lives in attending to the sick. According to William Bradford, the Pilgrim leader and historian, these able-bodied persons brought wood for the sick,

> ... made them fires, drest them meat, made their beads, washed their lothsome cloaths, cloathed & uncloathed them; in a word did all ye homly & necessarie offices for them which dainty & quesie stomacks cannot endure to hear named; and all this willingly & cherfully, without any grudging in ye least.[17]

Colonial diaries frequently mention various illnesses and the care of them. The following extract is from the diary of Mary Stockly, who visited Virginia in the early nineteenth century. What she says probably applies to an earlier age as well. During her visit most of the people in the area fell ill (probably from malaria) and could not help one another.

> I too was extremely ill but I knew the situation of the family. I know not what we should have done had not Providence directed an old woman, who had once lived in Uncle Charles Stockly's family, our way. I really was never more pleased to see anyone than I was to see her. I had no acquaintance with her, but I shared largely in her attentions. Cousin Ayers was in one room and I in the next, both almost distracted with headache. She came up to us and bathed our heads with vinegar and bound them up so good that we both felt as if we could hardly thank her enough. I felt greatly relieved from her good nursing. She slept in the room with me that night.[18]

There was more organized nursing service in some areas of the colonies, but how this functioned is not exactly certain. In New Amsterdam (now New York) nursing care was in the hands of *krankenbezoekers* and *ziskentroosters*. The former meant a seeker out of sick or a visitor of the sick, and the latter meant a, comforter of those who were ill, but in practice the two terms were used synonymously.

Epidemics

Before the twentieth century the major challenges to those who gave nursing care were epidemic diseases. These included all of the ordinary contagious diseases such as smallpox, typhoid, typhus, pertussis, diphtheria, measles, mumps, streptoccic infections, and the pneumonias besides the pandemics like bubonic plague, cholera, and influenza. A major pandemic of bubonic plague occured in the sixth century; starting in Egypt it took some 60 years to spread throughout the world. The fourteenth-century outbreak of plague was even more devastating. A colorful account of its arrival in Genoa in 1347 claims that it had started in the Genoese colony of Kaffa in the Crimea (present-day Feodosiya). According to the story the city was being beseiged by a Mongol Khan. When the disease broke out among the Khan's troops, he catapulted the bodies of its victims into the city to infect and weaken his opponents. The soldiers and colonists then carried it back to Genoa. Whatever its origin, plague spread panic and destruction throughout Europe in the next six years.

Bubonic plague is caused by the bacillus, *pasteurella pestis*, which is usually transmitted by the bite of a flea carried by an animal vector, most commonly the rat, *rattus rattus*. After the initial flea bite, the infection spreads through the lymph system to involve nearby lymph nodes. The nodes swell to enormous proportions and are called "bubos" from which the name bubonic plague is derived. The clinical course of the disease is short, marked by high fever, toxemia, delerium, and coma. If the primary target organ were the lungs, it was called pneumonic plague. Occasionally, a generalized septicemia developed with petechiae and hemorrhages under the skin. This gave the victim the darkened appearance which was described as the "Black Death." Before antibiotics the mortality rate from plague was between 25 and 50 percent, although in the fourteenth century, with its lack of sanitation in the newly developing urban areas, the death rate in some cities reached 90 percent. The impact on the populace was overwhelming.

The conceptualization of causality held by medieval people was mixed. They realized that the disease was in some way communicable, but they were unsure as to its mode of transmission. This uncertainty led to an avoidance of victims, a reliance on magical safeguards, and an accidental use of isolation techniques. The suspicion that shipping routes were somehow involved led Venice to adopt the practice of quarantine which had been developed earlier by the Knights Hospitalers. The slow but steady march of the disease throughout all of Europe and Asia, however, demonstrated that these measures were ineffective.[19]

Although the mortality rate during the plague of 1665–1666 was less than that during the fourteenth century, it was particularly disastrous to the poorer people, since most of the well-to-do fled the cities where the plague was at its worst. When the upper classes left, their servants often remained and in order to earn a living hired out as nurses. This was a particularly undesirable job, since the nurse had to remain in the infected house 28 days after a person died from the plague. Infected homes were literally sealed up, and no one was allowed to leave. Even under these conditions, some outstanding nursing was done by women, although there were others who were accused of murdering their patients in order to rob them. As indicated earlier the nurses in the various London hospitals remained at their posts. Though not entirely trustworthy, one of the most readable accounts of the plague is the semifactual *A Journal of the Plague Year*, by Daniel Defoe, who also wrote *Robinson Crusoe*.

Cholera, another bacterial disease, is characterized by a severe diarrhea which rapidly depletes body fluids and electrolytes. It is endemic in parts of India, but it has also been spread world-wide in three major pandemics during the nineteenth century. A major contribution to public health was made during the eighteenth century with the introduction of variolation, an inoculation with true smallpox. Lady Mary Wortley Montagu, the wife of the British ambassador in Constantinople at the beginning of the century, and Emanuel Timoni, a physician who had lived in that city, were responsible for starting this practice in England. It had been used in the East for several centuries, probably originating in India. Variolation was somewhat dangerous, and a far better and safer method was evolved by Edward Jenner (1749–1823) who, by 1798, had demonstrated that inoculation with cowpox would produce protection against smallpox. As his method, called vaccination, spread over Europe there was a decline in the incidence of this very dangerous disease.

Maternity Care

During the eighteenth century much more attention began to be paid to maternity cases; this resulted in the formation of many lying-in charities. Attention was also given to the education of midwives. In 1739 a small lying-in infirmary was started in England by Sir Richard Manningham with a school for both midwives and medical students. In 1741 the famous Dr. William Smellie began to teach midwifery in London. To give practical instruction to his pupils he attended poor women in their homes without taking a fee; his students, however, had to contribute to a fund for the care and support of these women. He made a major contribution to raising the standards of obstetrics by training some 900 medical students in midwifery as well as an almost equal number of women to be nurse-midwives. In France, training institutions for midwives had been established earlier, with the first in Paris in 1720. This Parisian institution was probably the first one in Europe.

As midwifery attained a more scientific status, special lying-in hospitals also began to appear for the first time. In England the Middlesex Hospital opened its doors to maternity cases in 1747; by 1749 the British Lying-in Hospital for Married Women had been founded; in 1750 the city of London Lying-in Hospital was established. Home deliveries began to benefit from some of the new techniques when the Lying-in Charity was founded to deliver women in their homes. The records of the Lying-in Hospitals show a progressive reduction in the maternal mortality rate. From 1749 to 1759 the death rate in Great Britain among women delivered in the hospitals averaged one in 42, among infants one in fifteen. By 1799–1800 the maternal deaths had been reduced to one in 913, and the neonatal death rate was one in 115. Part of this drop was caused by better techniques in the nursing and management of newborn infants.

It was the custom to wash the newborn baby with a decoction of red roses, to which had been added myrtle leaves and salt. Sometimes the infant was given a mouthwash of gin or some such strong drink. It was then wrapped in swaddling clothes, although its arms and feet were left free. By the eighteenth century in England, the child was left in swaddling clothes for only three months, but in France for a much longer period. Influential in removing all swaddling clothes from babies was Dr. William Cadogan, who in 1747 wrote *An Essay on the Nursing and Management of Children*; this rapidly went through some twenty editions. Unhappily, the good doctor also recommended breast feeding the baby only two or three times in 24 hours. Babies were also served a so-called baby pap— mixture of bread and milk or rice flour and arrowroot mixed with milk, especially ass's milk, which was the most highly esteemed as being more digestible than cow's milk. This was given to the baby through a "bubbly pot," made of horn or earthenware and often fitted inside with a piece of sponge to regulate the flow. If the child were not nursed, but only fed pap, Dr. Cadogan estimated its chance of survival as only one in ten.

During the eighteenth century there was also a big boom in the building of hospitals. Prior to 1710, 23 of the principal counties in England appeared to have had no general hospital, while in London the care of the sick was mainly confined to two hospitals. Only the larger cities had hospitals in most of Europe, although the Catholic countries had more in the countryside. Westminster Hospital in London was founded in 1720, Guy's in 1724, St. George's in 1733, and 154 hospitals and dispensaries were established during the next 125 years. Perhaps even more important for the care of the sick than the founding of hospitals was the development of the dispensary which enabled many more people to secure the services of a physician. Recovery was also more likely for persons treated at the dispensary.

Care of the Mentally Ill

Unfortunately, the care of the mentally defective or ill was far behind the care and treatment of the ordinary sick. Throughout most of the Middle Ages, insanity had not been regarded as an illness but as a sign of demoniacal possession. In severe cases torture or other cruel forms of punishment were used to drive out the devils. Some people were even burned at the stake. Fortunately, milder forms of aberration were treated more leniently. Often a pilgrimage was prescribed to a holy shrine which had a reputation for cures, such as that of St. Dymphna at Gheel in Belgium.

Those insane persons who were regarded as a menace to the community were generally imprisoned where no distinction was made between them and other inmates. Beginning in the seventeenth century, however, there was a movement to separate the mentally ill from other prisoners. It was at this time that Bethlehem Royal Hospital in England (better known as Bedlam) was converted into an "asylum" for the insane. The same thing happened to the monastery of Charenton just outside of Paris. Separation, though a step toward the recognition of mental illness, did not necessarily result in any better treatment for the patients. They were still chained, whipped, starved, put in stocks, or otherwise mal-treated. In Bedlam any person who paid twopence (two pennies) was allowed to wander through the wards, and these unattended visitors often teased the patients, stimulated their ravings, or tried to make them give a public exhibition. The behavior of sightseers had reached such a level in 1766 that the governors of the hospital attempted to lock the doors "on public holidays against all visitors." Conditions at Bedlam were vividly portrayed by the English artist Hogarth in "The Rake in Bedlam," one of a series of pictures, "The Rake's Progress."

Some attempts were made to ameliorate the conditions of the inhabitants of these hospitals. In 1700 they were for the first time called patients, indicating a need for nursing care, and incurable and curable wards were established in England, beginning in 1725, again giving some hope to a few patients. Generally, nursing in the mental hospitals was very poor. The first effective reforms in mental hospitals were introduced in France by Philippe Pinel (1745-1826) and in England by William Tuke (1732-1822). Pinel was appointed physician director of the Bicêtre asylum in Paris in 1793 and later of the Salpêtrière asylum. His first action was to remove the chains from the patients. He also wrote several treatises on insanity in an attempt to promote scientific and humane treatment of the mentally ill. He was aided by a tanner's apprentice, Jean-Baptiste Pussin, who was a nurse for the mentally ill at Bicêtre asylum. Pinel thought so highly of him and his wife that he brought them both with him to Salpêtrière when he was made supervisor there. Both the Pussins carefully nursed the patients. Pinel himself wrote of Madame Pussin: "I marvelled at her approach to the most disturbed patients, to see her calm them by sympathetic handling, and to make them accept nourishment which they had refused with violence from anyone else."

Tuke was not a physician but a merchant, a member of the Society of Friends (sometimes called Quakers). Because of the death of a fellow religionist in the asylum at York in England, Tuke attempted to start a new type of establishment for the treatment of the mentally ill. He established a house near York where he began admitting patients in 1796. In his "Retreat," as it was called, he laid great stress on sympathy and gentleness and attempted to keep his patients busy. He also used nurse attendants to look after his patients. These beginnings were continued into the nineteenth century when very effective reforms were made in the care of the mentally ill.

At the End of the Eighteenth Century

More important reforms, however, were effected in nursing itself. For the first time scholarly attention began to be paid to nursing. Early in the century a textbook on nursing had been published at Vienna. This was followed by Spanish, French, German, and English manuals. We have already discussed the ideas of Dr. Thomas Fuller on the ideal nurse, but they are also indicative of some of the other works. In Diderot's famous eighteenth-century *Encyclopedia*, which attempted to sum up all human knowledge, nursing was recognized as an important occupation. In the article "Infirmier" the encyclopedia stated that nursing

... is as important for humanity as its functions are low and repugnant. All persons are not adapted to it, and heads of hospitals ought to be difficult to please, for the lives of patients may depend on their choice of applicants. The nurse should be patient, mild, compassionate. She should console the sick, foresee their needs, and relieve their tedium. The domestic duties of the nurse are to light the fires in the wards and keep them going;

to carry and distribute nourishment; to accompany the surgeons and doctors on their rounds and afterwards to remove all dressings, etc.; to sweep the halls, and wards and keep the persons of the patients and their surroundings clean; to empty all vessels and change the patients' linen; to prevent noise and quarreling and disturbances; to notify the steward of everything they see which is wrong; to carry out the dead and bury them; to light the lamps in the evening and visit the sick during the night; and to watch them continually, giving them every aid which their state requires, and treating them with kindness and consideration.[20]

Reformers also attempted to discover how the sick and afflicted could be better treated. One of these was William Nolan, who in 1789 wrote *An Essay on Humanity: or a View of Abuses in Hospitals with a Plan for Correcting Them.* His descriptions of some of the nurses of the time are not pleasant, but he seemed to realize that tender, affectionate nursing care was almost as essential for the health of the patients as were the physician's prescriptions. Nolan also recommended that nurses be paid higher wages; this, in his opinion, would avoid many of the abuses in nursing.

Perhaps the most important reformer of the eighteenth century, however, was John Howard (1726–1790), English prison reformer and philanthropist, who also published his book on European hospitals in 1789. His interests in prisons perhaps dated from his personal experience as the prisoner of a privateer. In 1773 he was appointed sheriff in Bedfordshire and began an intensive investigation of prisons, which resulted in his chief work, *State of Prisons in England and Wales*, in 1779. In continuing his investigation he also became interested in the spread of disease, which led him to investigate hospitals. The following is his description of an infirmary in his *An Account of the Principal Lazarettos in Europe:*

> [It] is an old house in which are four rooms for patients. The floor of the room below was dirt, and the walls were black and filthy; it had in it three patients. In two of the rooms above, there were thirteen beds and fifteen patients, and a little dirty hay on the floor, on which they said the nurse lay. This room was very dirty, the ceiling covered with cobwebs, and in several places open to the sky. Here I saw one naked, pale object, who was under the necessity of tearing his shirt for bandages for his fractured thigh. No sheets in the house—and the blankets were very dirty. No vault: no water.—The diet is a three-penny loaf and two pints of milk; or rather, if my taste did not deceive me, of milk and water.[21]

Reformers like Nolan and Howard had revealed the need for reform, but there was as yet no program of reform. Moreover, with the number of hospitals increasing, the urgency of the problem became even more obvious. Undoubtedly, many of the nurses of the time left much to be desired, but whenever nursing was made a decent job, nurses responded by helping the patient in every way they could. Unfortunately, because there was a too frequent tendency to degrade the position of a nurse, to bring in untrained people to help save hospital expenses, to call upon women of the street in times of stress, and to pay nurses very little, nursing as a whole suffered.

These difficulties reached crisis proportions during the French Revolutionary and Napoleonic Wars (1789-1815) when fighting spread throughout the world (the War of 1812 in the United States is just one of its many phases). Survival became more important than reform, and unfortunately, in the minds of many people during and after the war, reform came to be abhorred. This was partly because the French Revolution, which had begun, or at least had appeared to begin, as a reform movement, had ended in a bloody revolution; this made all reformers suspect, an official attitude that did not disappear easily. Even in France, however, nursing reform was not particularly successful.

The problem can be understood by examining Paris, which on the eve of the Revolution had a population of about 700,000, of which 35,341 were hospitalized indigents, or about one in twenty. This number included 15,000 foundlings, 14,105 recipients of poor relief, and 6,236 patients in 48 different hospitals.[22] These 48 hospitals were served by 970 religious nurses, including 590 Sisters of Charity. There were also 58 Augustinians at the Hôtel Dieu which had 3,418 patients in 25 wards. The sisters cared for these patients with the help of some 800 servants and of convalescents in the hospital who were employed for minor tasks, but the ratio even counting these was about one assistant to four patients, far below what we now consider the minimum.[23] Religious orders had declined in eighteenth-century France, and the Augustinian sisters were no exception: only five of them had been in the order for fewer than ten years in 1789. The sisters did not agree with many of the new medical innovations, and they were particularly upset by a new young surgeon, Pierre Joseph Desault, who in 1788 tried to introduce changes in the wards. The Prioress, Sister de la Croix, protested that physicians' visits should be kept to the timetable established in 1708, that food distribution should not be interfered with, and that young interns were a nuisance in any case:

> The constant presence of the young surgeons . . . is infinitely dangerous, especially on the women's wards. . . . Since these young men have been admitted to the wards, the Hôtel-Dieu is unrecognizable; our refuges of rest, silence, and calm now echo with loud voices, threats, and sometimes ribald remarks. . . . in former times . . . a young surgeon would never have dared pass by . . . a sister without a deferential greeting; nowadays he keeps his hat on, hums a tune, and feels pleased if he hasn't mocked or insulted her. . . .[24]

She also opposed the removal of the large beds which held several patients and urged that they be reintroduced forthwith, since the single beds had cost the hospital some 922 places of shelter for the ailing poor.

Some indication of the hardships that nurses faced is indicated by the plea of the Prioress to the National Assembly in July 1790 when it was contemplating eliminating the novitiate. She argued, and probably rightly, that it would be impossible to find replacements for the religious nurses:

> Without firm, solemn and holy vows, how could nurses, and especially those at the Hôtel-Dieu, be expected to persevere in this demanding work? Nursing requires menial tasks, night watches and constant exposure to danger. Who else would be willing to breathe stale, noxious, pestilential air . . . listen to the heart-rending cries of suffering patients. Nurses must leave the sick or the dying to bury the dead . . . . One must have offered one's life in sacrifice like the religious of the Hôtel-Dieu, to take up so sad and burdensome a profession.[25]

Despite such pleas the law of November 3, 1789 forbade new vows, and all sixteen novices who had entered between November 5, 1788 and October 2, 1790 left. The remaining sisters, nonetheless, continued to nurse during the Revolution, although not until after 1800 were novices again admitted into the Order.

The problem was how to replace the sisters, and in the process, how to readjust the boundary lines between nursing and medicine. For generations the nurses had claimed that diet was their prerogative, but this was now disputed by the physicians. Hospital furniture, as the controversy over the beds indicated, was also a matter of dispute, as was fresh air, control of convalescents, and even the laundry facilities. The Revolutionary period also saw the rise of the hospital pharmacist, who tended to lessen the power of the nurse in the hospital.[26]

When the medical reformers first turned to the hospital wards, they stressed the needs of interns, students, and patients, in that order, with nurses finishing last. Doris B. Weiner, however, has argued that the Revolution effected an even more significant change in the hospital: recognition of the patient's right to medical care. She argues that for the first time the patient's right to public funds and attention was spelled out, and once it was recognized that a patient had rights, the nurse's traditional motivations of charity, her claims to the patient's gratitude and his meek compliance were no longer valid.[27]

While Professor Weiner's point is probably essential to understanding what happened to the traditional convent nurse, the rhetoric of the Revolutionaries was not always implemented. Nursing was regarded as women's work for the most part, but proper women did not work in hospitals unless religiously motivated. Women of the lower classes lacked the skill and training to assume responsibility, and there was not sufficient reimbursement for them to make nursing a gainful career. As the wounded from the battlefields were added to the normal numbers of sick, nursing became a critical need; rather than initiate any basic reforms, the Revolutionaries continued with the pre-Revolutionary system. On the one hand, they abolished the regular and secular congregations of religious orders, while simultaneously stipulating that "in hospitals and charitable institutions, the same persons as before shall continue individually to serve the poor and the sick, under the supervision of municipal administrators."[28]

Religious nurses were caught between their own commitment to the patient and a basically hostile state. Technically they no longer were under vows, but the government was willing to allow them to remain in the hospitals provided they swore a loyalty oath to the state. Large numbers of the nuns continued to nurse, but without new recruits the shortage of nurses grew. After 1793 the government recruited a number of women to nurse without giving them any training, or examining their suitability and then complained because they were undisciplined. Few of these remained nurses very long.

Despite mounting criticism, further "reform" did not occur until after 1800 when Dr. Jean-Antoine Chaptal became Minister of the Interior under Napoleon. Chaptal limited hospital admission to those referred by physicians, thus changing hospitals from all-purpose charitable institutions to institutions for the care of the sick. He reorganized the supply system of the hospitals, founded a school for midwives and a Children's Hospital, and on his own reestablished the religious nurses. By acting unofficially in an official capacity, in effect he bypassed the law which prohibited religious orders.

To start his new nursing orders, he asked a former Sister of Charity, Sister Deleau, to reestablish the order and open a novitiate in Paris. Napoleon acted as though he were unaware of this, and when no overt opposition appeared, other nursing orders were reestablished. Napoleon, however, insisted that the religious orders abandon their old social stratification which allowed only certain social classes to serve as sisters. The Augustinians, for example, had had three categories of helpers: (1) "filles dela chambre d'en haut" (upstairs maids), or women from honorable families who were socially acceptable as nuns, but whose orientation was secular, not religious; (2) "filles de la chambre d'en bas" (downstairs maids), or persons of piety, integrity, and good behavior, but not socially eligible for the novitiate; and (3) "servantes," who were lower on the scale and were subdivided into further groupings.[29]

Napoleon appointed his mother Letizia, "Madame Mère," as "General Protectress of Imperial Establishments of Welfare and Charity." Madame Mère in 1807 summoned all the French nursing orders to a congress held in her palace in Paris. During the congress Napoleon himself contributed 182,000 francs to their expenses although he remained unhappy at the religious orientation of the nurses. He made one more attempt to make them secular confraternities, but his mother opposed him. The result was a series of principles to which Napoleon reluctantly agreed. Some of the recommendations by Madame Mère were regressive. For example, the right of student nurses to communicate with authorities without informing the Superior was abolished. This is perhaps typical because the recommendations generally urged the establishment of traditional religious orders of nursing with the sisters in control, although somewhat less rigidly than before the Revolution.[30] The result was a resurgence of nursing orders, and nursing remained in France essentially a religious profession until almost the end of the nineteenth century.

Four

Nursing and the Age of Reform

Western society underwent such basic changes in the late eighteenth and early nineteenth centuries that people living about 1850 found themselves in a world radically different from that of their predecessors, and these radical changes have continued to our own day. During this period the middle classes grew much more wealthy and influential, effectively countering the power of the aristocracy in many countries, and government either responded to their needs or faced a revolution as in France. Symptomatic of the change was rapid urban growth, until today in the advanced industrial societies, the vast majority of people live in cities and their suburbs instead of on farms or in small villages or towns.

Instrumental in effecting change was a phenomenon to which the term Industrial Revolution has been applied. This had begun in the mid-eighteenth century in England, and had gradually spread to France, the Netherlands, Belgium, Germany, Sweden, and the United States, until by the mid-twentieth century it had reached much of the world. In its simplest form the Industrial Revolution was the application of machine power to processes formerly done by hand. This change had started in the textile industry in the eighteenth century but soon spread into other areas. At first machines were powered by water, but by the mid-nineteenth century, water power had been replaced by steam. With the perfection of steam power, railroads developed along with other means of locomotion, better roads were built, and communications improved.

The Industrial Revolution caused tremendous unrest. One of the first effects was a growth in unemployment. Most industry previously had been done in the household as a supplement to the meager farming income. As more and more expensive machines were developed, it became cheaper to take the worker to the machine rather than the machine to the worker; thus the factory system developed. People found that they had to move to strange places, give up their farms, and become almost entirely dependent on the new factories for their livelihood. Most of these factories were concentrated where water power was available, often away from previously heavily populated areas. The owners of the new coal mines, iron mills, and factories naturally wanted to produce as much as possible as cheaply and quickly as possible. To do this they cut as many corners as they could. One way to cut costs was to lay off their employees when orders declined; this left the ex-worker to fend for himself but without the old family farm to fall back on. It was also soon apparent that women and children could often do the work of men and at much cheaper rates; this resulted in the male head of the family being frequently unemployed and dependent on the wages of his wife or children. When it was pointed out to the owners of the new factories that this system was harmful to the family, or that it caused unrest, many of them agreed but argued that they had to meet the competition, and that if they changed their methods, they would go out of business, which would cause their employees to suffer more. There were no labor organizations or legal protections against exploitation, so that the workers were often exposed to almost every kind of abuse. Work days were long for all— men, women, and children—averaging from twelve to fourteen hours. Many companies fined their employees for very trivial offenses such as swearing, accidentally damaging a piece of material, or even for injuring themselves. As a result, many employees ended the week owing the company money. Since the factories were located in comparatively isolated areas, company towns were built to house the influx of employees. Workers could be expelled from their homes when they were unemployed or if they disagreed with company policy. Rates in the company store were often higher than elsewhere, but employees were nonetheless forced to buy there. To make matters still worse, workers were often paid off in the local grog or gin shop, so that a great many of them drank away their wages before getting home.

Reformers

Probably industrial conditions were worse in England than elsewhere in Europe. But the very degradation of the English working classes inspired reformers who continued in the tradition of John Howard. One such was Robert Owen (1771-1858), who demonstrated that a mill manager could actually treat his workers well and make money. Taking over a business that had utilized not only child labor drafted from Edinburgh and Glasgow, but also a large number of thieves and drunkards, he soon remade it into a model business which attracted pilgrims from all over Europe. He undertook every aspect of modern welfare work ranging from public health, temperance, and education, to social security. He achieved all this while making a handsome profit for the mill owners. While some of his later experiments such as New Harmony in Indiana were unsuccessful, he did reveal alternatives to the existing system.

Another reformer was Anthony Ashley Cooper, the seventh Earl of Shaftesbury (1801-1885), who was much more involved in politics than Owen. He felt that the state should and could enact legislation to regulate working conditions in the factories—such as the length of the working day for women and children. The first steps in this direction had already been taken before Shaftesbury's time when in 1802 child labor was limited to twelve hours a day without night work. Unfortunately this legislation applied only to cotton mills and was not well enforced even there. In 1833 Shaftesbury had this limitation extended to all textile mills and limited the working hours of children under thirteen to 48 hours a week with no more than nine in any one day. Youths between thirteen and eighteen were not to be employed for more than 60 hours a week. This, of course, was just a beginning, but it eventually led to the abolition of child labor, bettered the working conditions of women, and indirectly helped the workingmen themselves.

The philosophical leader of English reform was John Stuart Mill (1806–1873), who argued that liberty must consider the "greatest happiness of the greatest number" in a qualitative sense. His arguments carried much weight, in part because the reformers had been handicapped by their hesitancy to curb liberty; when liberty was defined as more than the freedom to do as one wants, then reform was somewhat easier. Mill argued that man must be allowed to develop his natural capacities and talents; thus he championed popular education, emancipation of women, trade union organization, the cooperative movement, and similar reforms. Other reformers urged the abolition of slavery, extension of the suffrage, religious toleration, reform of Parliament, and, most important for nursing, better and more humane care of the sick and wounded.

Aiding and abetting the reformers in the nineteenth century was a reinvigoration of religion, both Christianity and Judaism. For both Catholicism and Protestantism, the nineteenth century was a high point, while the Orthodox faith began to emerge from the domination imposed upon it by the Ottoman Turks. Within Catholicism more orders and congregations were founded than in any previous century. More than 100 of these orders had as their primary purpose nursing the sick, care of orphans, and teaching. The Society of St. Vincent de Paul was organized as a lay society to aid the poor and the sick. Protestantism meanwhile became less nationalistic and more interested in charity. Social action movements arose which paralleled the growth of the Catholic religious orders. New sects like the Salvation Army helped the urban underprivileged. Judaism, mainly as a result of the French Revolution, emerged from the ghettos of Europe, and Jews were granted full citizenship in most countries. As Jews mingled with other people, they also built charitable institutions for the care of the poor, the sick, the deaf, the blind, orphans, and the aged, which more than matched the establishments of the other religious groups.

Nursing Reformers

At the beginning of the nineteenth century, however, Protestantism was behind Catholicism in its emphasis on the care of the sick. The

Catholic Church through its nursing orders had an organized nursing care, even if it might not have met present-day standards. New Catholic orders had been founded in the British Isles in the nineteenth century, including the Sisters of Mercy (founded by Catherine McAuley, 1787–1841) and the Irish Sisters of Charity founded by Mary Aikenhead (Sister Mary Augustine 1787–1858). English Protestants conscious of their deficiency, were tremendously impressed by the Catholic nursing orders, and many agitated for Protestant equivalents. Dr. Robert Gooch (1784–1830) popularized the idea of a Protestant nursing order in several magazine articles in the 1820's, urging the formation of Protestant Sisters of Charity who would have enough education to recognize diseases, give remedies, and help relieve the sufferings of the poor.[1] The poet Robert Southey (1774–1843)[2] and some of his friends actually undertook to organize an institution for the training of nurses, but the scheme failed after only two years.

The first effective reform of nursing in Protestant circles came not in England, however, but in Germany where much the same agitation had occurred. In Protestant areas on the Continent, the deaconess movement had been reestablished, and it was from the revival of this ancient Christian office that nursing reform entered Germany. One of the leaders in reinvigorating the deaconess movement was Amelia Wilhelmina Sieveking (1794–1859), who helped nurse victims of the cholera epidemic in her native Hamburg in 1831. Recognizing the need for improved nursing, she began in 1832, with twelve other women, a Protestant Sisters of Mercy.[3] Her movement was soon overshadowed by the work of Pastor Theodore Fliedner (1800–1864), who was appointed the pastor of a small Protestant congregation in the town of Kaiserswerth in 1822.

Kaiserswerth was suffering severe unemployment because the textile mill on which most of the community depended had gone bankrupt. To assist his congregation Pastor Fliedner went on a fundraising expedition to England and Holland. During his tour he learned about Mennonite deaconesses in Holland and was impressed by the various prison reform movements in England. As his congregation began to recover economically, Pastor Fliedner turned his attention to the reformation of prisoners, and by 1826 he had formed the Rhenish-Westphalian Prison Association. Shortly after this he married Friederike Munster (1806–1842), and together they opened a home for recently discharged convicts in Kaiserswerth in 1833. The impetus for the home was given by the sudden appearance of a former woman convict whom the Fliedners had befriended. The Fliedners had no place for the girl, so she lived for a time in their children's playhouse. It was from this beginning that the immense Kaiserswerth system grew.

Almost from the first the two Fliedners had recognized the lack of facilities for the sick, especially the sick poor. Pastor Fliedner felt that although hospitals might be wonderful buildings on the outside, even the rudiments of good nursing care were missing within. To remedy this he felt that women should take a more active part in the charity work of the Church. He wrote to several of his fellow ministers who had richer congregations, asking for their opinion. Most of them agreed with him, but none was willing to assume the burden, so the Pastor and Friederike decided to handle the situation as best they could. Soon after this decision the largest and finest house in Kaiserswerth was offered for sale, and Fliedner contracted to buy it in April 1836, even though he had to launch a special fundraising campaign to pay for it. The Fliedners wanted to organize an order of deaconesses to care for the sick; but before this could be accomplished, patients began to arrive. The sick were nursed temporarily by two volunteers until the first deaconess, Sister Gertrude Reichardt, began her work on October 20, 1836.[4]

Sister Gertrude, who had had considerable experience as a nurse, had been invited to Kaiserswerth by the Fliedners to establish nursing on a sound basis. By the end of the first year, six other women had been accepted as deaconesses. Friederike Fliedner herself superintended the Order. Nurse deaconesses were instructed in both medicine and pharmacy by qualified physicians or pharmacists, so that the sisters knew something about their work. Mrs. Fliedner was opposed to rigid rules; she felt that the attitude of the nurse was more important than any rule. It was her remarkable leadership that assured the success of the undertaking, for in addition to helping her husband in all his tasks, she acted as "mother" to the deaconesses, ran her own home, and gave birth to nine children. Her notes on the Fliedner system, made shortly before she died in 1842, give a good idea of the nursing practices of the order.[5] Mrs. Fliedner's place was taken by Caroline Bertheau (1811–1892), whom the pastor married in 1843. Since the second Mrs. Fliedner had already been superintendent of a large hospital in Hamburg, the high standards set by Friederike were continued.

Nurses at Kaiserswerth wore blue print gowns and white caps. Their workday was long and hard. They rose at 5 A.M., made beds, swept their rooms, and then went to the wards to help with the patients before breakfast. Around 6:15 A.M. they had a light breakfast, perhaps a cup of coffee, and then in line with their calling as deaconesses devoted some time to prayer. They then returned to the wards where they gave the patients their medicines and began washing and dressing them. At about 8 or 8:30 A.M., the physicians began their rounds accompanied on each ward by the ward supervisor. After this there was usually a coffee break for both patients and nurses. The nurses then fed the weaker patients, did necessary mending and darning, and other ward work until dinner which was served around noon. Dinner was followed by chapel or a brief rest, after which the deaconesses again returned to the ward. There might be another break for lessons, study, or Bible reading at 2 P.M. Afternoon medicines were given about 4 P.M. If the nurse was on a children's ward, the children would then be fed, undressed, and washed preparatory for bed. Supper was served to the nurses at 7 P.M., after which some had to return to the wards to serve until 9:30 P.M.

Each nurse took her turn in rotation as night supervisor, who had to make the rounds every hour during her tour of duty. If there were difficulties, she was to wake the sister on the ward. The Kaiserswerth hospital in the 1850's included about 100 beds, which were divided into four divisions—one for men, another for women, a third for boys over six, and the last for children including girls under seventeen and boys under six. In the men's and boys' ward, night nursing was done by male nurses, also trained in the Kaiserswerth school. The sisters were not allowed to enter the male wards after 8 P.M., nor did they sleep on these wards at night. This was the job of the male watchers, who never became an integral part of the movement.

A woman who wished to enter the Order had to serve a probationary period of one to three years. The probationary sister received no money for the first six months but did get her food and lodging; after this initial period she also received a small allowance. If the probationer were successful, she was then consecrated as a deaconess in a church ceremony. She promised to serve for five years in this capacity on a very small allowance sufficient to keep her in clothing, since board, lodging, and even some of her clothes were furnished by the hospital. Under special circumstances, such as family difficulties, marriage, or other similar matters, the deaconess could leave before her term was completed. Deaconesses who became sick or old in the service of the hospital were cared for by the foundation.[6]

Other Protestant Nursing Orders

The reputation of Kaiserswerth soon spread. Other churches and hospitals began calling Pastor Fliedner, and he cheerfully answered their call. The King of Prussia wanted a deaconess house in Berlin, so Fliedner went there. Anxious to break down some of the restrictions imposed on them and thinking that the deaconess movement was an effective way to do so, women from all over Europe visited Kaiserswerth to study or observe. Among them was the English social reformer Elizabeth Gurney Fry (1780–1845), who had earlier made a reputation for her work in prisons. In fact, it was Mrs. Fry's work in prisons that had motivated Pastor Fliedner to begin his work at Kaiserswerth. A member of the Society of Friends, Mrs. Fry had very early been impressed by conditions in English prisons. Even after her marriage to Joseph Fry and the birth of several children, she could not forget what she had seen. She became an ordained minister in the Society of Friends and by 1813 had begun work among the prisoners. Her work was soon extended to include a haven for homeless wanderers, relief of the poor, and finally, in 1840 after a visit to Kaiserswerth, nursing. She established an Institute of Nursing in London to train women to care for the sick in their own homes. Besides the influence of Pastor Fliedner, she had also been approached by Dr. Gooch, the advocate of Protestant nursing orders, who had felt that she might be the woman to realize his suggestion. By the time her Institute was organized, she was in such ill health that her daughters and her sister directed most of the activities.

At first the women called themselves Protestant Sisters of Charity, but religious bigotry was very strong in England, especially against Catholics, and many people thought this was an attempt at Protestant nuns. The name was later changed to *nursing sisters*. Mrs. Fry selected women for the order, after which they trained for a short period at Guy's Hospital in London. They then devoted themselves to nursing, for which they were paid an annual stipend of twenty pounds sterling. The Institute paid their salary and acted as a registry for nurses. The money for their pay came from donations to the Institute and contributions from satisfied patients. While serving as nurses, the women lived in a home maintained by the Institute where they were rigidly supervised. Each sister wore "a neat and becoming" uniform consisting of a print dress, a voluminous apron, and a plain muslin cap. When on the street, she wore a gray dress, long black cloak, and black bonnet with no trimmings except for a black veil. After three years of service their pay was raised to 23 pounds. That they accepted pay led to considerable criticism. Other people criticized the "sisters" because their work was considered too limited, but nonetheless they were a beginning. Since they did little work in the hospital, they did not really affect hospital nursing, but perhaps they can still be called the first trained nurses in England.[7]

While Mrs. Fry was beginning her Institute, there was considerable agitation within the Church of England itself to revive the various sisterhoods which had disappeared at the Reformation. Leaders of such a movement within the Anglican Church were known as the Oxford group, the members of which emphasized the continuity of the English church from ancient Christianity. Some of them, such as John Henry Cardinal Newman, eventually converted to the Roman Catholic Church, but the majority remained Anglicans and established the High Church movement. One result of the agitation was the formation in March 1845 of the Park Village Community in London to minister to the poor. This was the first Anglican sisterhood. Among its chief organizers was Dr. Edward Bouvrie Pusey (1800–1882), the leader of the Oxford movement. While the sisterhood did not train nurses, their duties included visiting the sick in their homes and in the hospitals. The members were called Sisters of Mercy. A second group was started in 1848 under the direction of Priscilla Lydia Sellon (1821–1876), who founded a community at Devon. This order was also called Sisters of Mercy, although they were popularly known as the Sellonites. Several members of this Order accompanied Florence Nightingale to the Crimea. Since Dr. Pusey was also instrumental in the formation of this Order, it was perhaps natural for the two communities to merge in 1866.[8]

The first purely nursing order in the Anglican Church was the Community of St. John's House organized in 1848. This order, set up at a meeting of Anglican Church dignitaries in July 1848, proposed to give instruction and training to members of the Church of England who would act as nurses and visitors to the sick and poor. To do this a Training Institution for Nurses was formed. Women eighteen years of age or older who were literate were eligible for nurses' training. After admission the woman served a two-year training period in hospitals affiliated with the order, first at St. George's and Westminster, but later at King's College Hospital. If a girl completed her training satisfactorily, she could become a nurse. In special cases women could be admitted to the rank of nurse without the probationary training. There was also a third class of members, called *sisters*—those women who helped contribute to the support of the order besides attending the sick and poor.[9]

After the Crimean War the probationary period was cut to three months with a nine-month apprenticeship as assistant nurse. The various Anglican sisterhoods received encouragement by church officials as long as vows were only taken for specified periods. This difference in vows is perhaps the chief distinguishing characteristic between Anglican sisterhoods and Catholic nuns.

Nurses in Nineteenth-Century England

The motivation of the nun, the deaconess, or the sister was primarily religious. Before nursing could be fully accepted as a worthy occupation, however, the importance of secular nurses had to be recognized. This was a difficult task in part because of the hospital system itself, but perhaps chiefly because of the position of women in the nineteenth century. Though women worked, it was not considered proper for respectable women to have careers or even to be educated. Most colleges refused to admit women, and few women ever went beyond grammar school. The exceptions usually attended a training school for proper young women where they learned to curtsy gracefully, play the piano and sing and draw. They usually knew little or nothing about science, philosophy, or social problems. Women were regarded as inferior creatures who somehow had finer sensibilities. They were unable to learn as much as men, but that was because they were more moral, made of finer fabric, or because their prime duty was to be mothers. It was only through the guise of religious motivation that many strong-willed young women were able to gain some independence.

As a result, secular nursing in most hospitals was carried on by women of what were called *the lower classes.* These were women who had to work—the unmarried, widows, those whose husbands were unemployed, etc. No "respectable" woman, however, would stoop to such tasks; a lady might be a governess or teacher in socially acceptable families, but even these jobs were suspect. Since nursing was done by the lower classes, it had no prestige. Nurses in most hospitals were required to live there, and they usually had to be up at night to attend to their patients. They received very meager salaries plus board and room, although in some hospitals they did not even receive board. Nurses were not only required to make poultices, wash the patients and make them comfortable, but they were regarded as housemaids as well. The average day of the secular nurse began at 6 A.M. and did not end until 8 P.M., or later if there were emergencies. If she served as a night nurse, her shift started at 8 P.M. and lasted to 6 A.M.; the night nurses also had to remain on the wards and assist in cleaning the ward and getting it in order until 11 A.M. Most of them had acquired a fair amount of nursing knowledge, since a new nurse began by working in various positions under the direction of the matron. Sisters were usually chosen from the nurses, and matrons from the sisters; this method ensured that the existing nursing techniques were common knowledge. The long hours, low pay, and general public attitude toward nursing discouraged many women from entering nursing; and given their choice most of the nurses would have preferred domestic duty to nursing, because, though it paid slightly less, servants usually received both better board and room than nurses and used clothes from their employers. The domestic also usually had less night work.

Even those women who might have wanted to enter nursing rather than domestic service found themselves competing with the inmates of the workhouse, the English equivalent of the American home for the indigent. Since workhouses were usually run by the same people who operated the hospitals, the boards tried to save money by using paupers as nurses; most women paupers who were forced to give nursing care had neither the experience nor the desire to be good nurses; some of them saw nothing wrong with stealing food from the patients. The widespread use of paupers as nurses served to lower even further the popular image of the nurse. Charles Dickens, in his novel *Martin Chuzzlewit*, gave what he considered to be "a fair representation of the hired attendant on the poor in sickness." His typical nurse was Sairey Gamp and her colleague Betsy Prig; both were sloppy, careless, gabby old women whose fondest hopes were to get nursing service in a family where one member after another came down with the same disease. When Mrs. Gamp relieved Mrs. Prig, Dickens had her give the following report:

> "The pickled salmon . . . is quite delicious. I can partick'ler recommend it. Don't have nothink to say to the cold meat, for it tastes of the stable. The drinks is all good. . . . The physic and them things is on the drawers and mankleshelf. . . . He took his last slime draught at seven. The easy-chair an't soft enough. You'll want his piller." [10]

Obviously, Dickens had a tendency to exaggerate, but even he perhaps recognized some motivating ideal in Sairey Gamp when he had her exclaim: "What a blessed thing it is to make sick people happy in their bed, and never mind one's self as long as one can do a service."

While the various reformers tried to rouse the public from its indifference to nursing standards, most of the influential people still remained indifferent, perhaps because hospitals as a whole were for the poor, for soldiers, or for victims of epidemic disease. Even home nurses such as Sairey Gamp usually attended only the lower classes; people in the upper levels of society had their own servants to nurse them, and the evils that existed, did not affect them personally. Most of those concerned with nursing had religious motivations; their approach was to organize religious orders. Such orders could and did do valuable work, but the number of women who felt called upon to enter such nursing orders was never sufficient for all those who needed care. Many of the women who entered these orders were also less concerned with real nursing duties than with "visiting" the sick—talking, reading, and in general cheering up the patient—duties that any lady could perform without losing status; these are certainly important, but they are not the only nursing tasks. In addition to the religious orders, a strong, well-organized secular nursing service was needed.

To establish secular nursing not only was it necessary to convince hospital administrators and physicians that good nursing care was important, the public had also to be convinced;[11] more importantly, women themselves had to believe that nursing was a vital and important job worthy of their talents, and that there was nothing disgraceful in becoming a nurse. Two forces helped effect the necessary changes: scientific advances in medicine and the various wars of the nineteenth century which took women to the battlefield. In the process, for better or for worse, the nurse came to be associated with the figure of Florence Nightingale.

Florence Nightingale

As Cecil Woodham-Smith, one of her biographers indicated, it was rather unusual to call a girl Florence when she was born May 12, 1820. The name was chosen because Florence was the city of her birth. Her sister, Parthenope, born a year earlier, received her name from the Greek name of her birthplace, Naples. The two girls had been born while their parents, William Edward and Fannie Nightingale, were traveling on the Continent. The Nightingales were a well-to-do English family, and Florence was given almost every benefit that money could provide. Edward Nightingale, however, was determined that his daughters, unlike the overwhelming majority of women of the day, were to be well educated. Since he felt that no governess could educate them, he assumed this task himself and hired a governess only to teach them music and drawing. He taught his daughters Greek, Latin, German, French, Italian, history, and philosophy, all on a rather formidable timetable. This background made Florence one of the best-educated women in Europe, although she felt herself somewhat weak in mathematics.[12]

While the two Nightingale girls were growing up, their life was rigidly circumscribed. They, like other girls of their social class, were not to see, hear, or speak of certain things. Since so much was forbidden to women, they expended much of their emotions on commonplace or trivial things. A delayed letter could necessitate smelling salts or even the sickbed. Women prided themselves on being martyrs to their excessive sensibility, and "delicacy" was nearly universal. All the Nightingale women were considered to be delicate, although Florence's mother lived to be ninety-two, her sister, seventy-five, and Florence, ninety. Women in their social class were supposed to devote themselves to society, entertainment, and other such pursuits. On this point, however, Florence rebelled. She was attractive, enjoyed dancing, parties, beaux, but she also wanted to do something of value. This was a rather daring attitude when women were not only socially but legally handicapped from having an independent life, and when both convention and public opinion would be against her. But while Florence had ideas well in advance of her time, in many ways she was also affected by her environment and by our standards would be considered abnormally sensitive, overemotional, and probably prone to exaggeration.

Her decision to do something, to be somebody, was reinforced by what she considered a special call from God. In a private note she wrote: "On February 7, 1837, God spoke to me and called me to His service"— she was then not quite seventeen. The voice did not specify how she was to be called, but it probably helped strengthen her conviction that she was different. Later she underwent three similar experiences: in 1853 when she was taking a hospital post, before going to the Crimea in 1854, and in 1861 after the death of one of her closest friends and co-workers.

Outwardly at least, her first call did not affect her. She soon left on a European tour which she enjoyed immensely. On her return home, however, her determination not to spend her life "faddling, twaddling," or making "endless tweedlings of nosegays in jugs" got her into trouble with her mother. The struggle increased as her mother insisted that Florence should settle down and get married. Florence turned down one suitor. Apparently she felt that she was destined to help the miserable and helpless but was not sure how, for in 1842 she asked some friends what "can an individual do towards lifting the load of suffering from the helpless and miserable?" The friends, Chevalier Bunsen, the Prussian Ambassador to England, and his wife, told her about the work of Pastor Fliedner at Kaiserswerth. Later (sometime in the spring of 1844) after considerable brooding, she concluded that her vocation lay in hospitals among the sick. The American philanthropist Samuel Gridley Howe and his wife Julia Ward Howe (later celebrated for her "Battle Hymn of the Republic") were visiting the Nightingales, and she consulted with them. Howe urged her to "go forward"—to act on her inspiration, for he found nothing unladylike or unbecoming in it. He did add that her calling was somewhat unusual, and in England whatever was "unusual is thought to be unsuitable."

Unwilling to face her mother about her vocation, she contented herself with nursing relatives. While doing this, she made a rather startling discovery—that just being a woman did not guarantee being a good nurse. She came to realize that tenderness, sympathy, goodness, and patience were fine, but that without knowledge and skill, in other words, training, the would-be nurse was helpless. To receive such training she tried to persuade her family to allow her to learn nursing at the nearby Salisbury Infirmary; this caused her mother to have hysterics, and Nightingale herself took to bed. Unable to learn nursing through apprenticeship, she tried to learn what she could from books. She studied hospital reports, sanitary reports, books on public health, and the yearbook of the Kaiserswerth Institutions sent to her by Chevalier Bunsen. She soon had a greater understanding of hospitals and the care of the sick than almost any of her contemporaries, male or female.

From 1844 to 1851 Nightingale, her mother, and sister quarrelled over her determination to be a nurse. She bided her time, feeling hopelessly frustrated, but even more determined. Finally in 1851, over the opposition of her family, she decided to visit Kaiserswerth. Although later in life Nightingale described the nursing at Kaiserswerth as "nil" and the hygiene as "horrible," the initial visit opened up a vast potential for her.[13] After her return to England, she was even more determined to be a nurse. Her mother and sister objected so violently that she thought her plans were endangering her sister's life. But she persevered and was finally allowed to go to Paris to study with the Sisters of Charity, but she was there only a short time before she was requested to come home to take care of her dying grandmother. Still the dutiful daughter, she returned.

Shortly after her grandmother died, the Institution for the Care of Sick Gentlewomen in Distressed Circumstances, also known as the Harley Street Nursing Home, found itself in difficulties. The women in charge of the hospital asked Nightingale to take over the superintendency. Despite the opposition of her mother and sister, she agreed, and, surprisingly, once the decision was made her mother and sister accepted the inevitable. In August 1853, she began her duties. Her ideas were near revolutionary. Bells were installed for the patients to ring, lifts were installed to bring food to the floors, so that nurses would not have to leave their wards, and all religious requirements for admission were abolished. Her committee had almost balked at this last change, but Nightingale insisted. Under her direction nursing care so improved that her patients were reported as worshipping her. But she was by no means satisfied. She felt that there were great deficiencies in this and other hospitals, and she wanted to reform them. One of the greatest deficiencies was the lack of trained nurses; better nursing in one hospital, however, was not enough because this just created a demand for better nurses in other hospitals, a demand that could not be met with existing training methods.[14] In order to begin to solve this problem, she negotiated for the post of superintendent of nurses at the newly reorganized and rebuilt King's College Hospital in London. Before the negotiations proceeded very far, however, the CrimeanWar began. In March 1854 England and France had declared war on Russia; by September the allied armies had landed in the Crimea.

The Crimean War

The Crimean War is a history of blunders and mistakes. No real preparation had been made for supplying the army in the Crimea. In the first battles there were no bandages, splints, chloroform, or other drugs; the wounded lay on the ground or in the straw mixed with manure in the farmyards; amputations were performed without anesthetics with the victims sitting or lying on tubs or on old doors, and surgeons caught without candles or lamps did much of their work by moonlight. In such circumstances cholera wreaked havoc. The disasters of the cholera epidemic along with the lack of supplies produced almost total disorganization in the British Army. In order to handle the casualties, the Turkish government turned over to the British the enormous barracks at Scutari across the straits from Constantinople. As the list of casualties rose, the artillery barracks were converted into a hospital, but no one bothered to clean the buildings, which were bare, filthy, and dilapidated. No hospital equipment was available to put in the barracks, but the wounded and sick were sent there anyway. They were put on the floor and wrapped in blankets saturated with blood; no food was given to them because there was no kitchen; no one could attend to their wounds because there was a shortage of surgeons; many of the wounded lay without even a drink of water all night because there were no cups or buckets to bring water.

Such disasters were not new for European armies. The British Army had endured much worse in almost every previous campaign during the preceding two centuries. During the Napoleonic Wars whole armies had been lost because of sickness and neglect. But these earlier losses and horrors had been unknown to the English public. The disasters and incompetence of Scutari, however, became immediately infamous because one of the first war correspondents in history, William Howard Russell of the London *Times*, had accompanied the army. In dispatch after dispatch Russell described the lack of care for the wounded and the horrible suffering they had to undergo; an England made conscious by various social reformers was first surprised, then hurt, bewildered, and indignant. Newspapers demanded to know why the sick lacked adequate care. They compared the work of the French Sisters of Charity in the Crimea with the complete absence of nursing services for English soldiers.

Criticism of the government threatened to bring its downfall in Parliament. The Secretary of War, Sidney Herbert, was an old friend of Florence Nightingale's; in desperation he wrote to her on October 15 asking her to go to Scutari in command of a group of nurses with the government's sanction and at its expense. Even before hearing from Herbert, Nightingale had arranged to sail for Constantinople with a party of nurses. She had written to the Herberts about her plan, and the two letters apparently crossed. Her private expedition was now official; her commission provided for her to go to Scutari as the superintendent of all the nurses in Turkey. She began organizing her expedition immediately in order to leave by October 21. This left her four days to recruit her nurses, find equipment and uniforms and arrange transportation. She arbitrarily limited the number of nurses to 40 because she felt personally unable to control any more than that.

The announcement of her appointment caused a sensation, for she was the first woman ever to serve in such a capacity.[15] Her mother and sister forgot their previous opposition to her plans and were ecstatic; but she had little time for them. While there were many volunteers for the Crimea, there were only a few whom Nightingale would accept. Wages were set at almost double the prevailing rate in London hospitals. Each nurse was to receive from twelve to fourteen shillings a week plus board, lodging, and uniform. After three months' service this was to be raised, and after a year each nurse was to receive at least eighteen shillings. Her standards were exacting and, all told, only fourteen secular nurses passed her inspection. An additional 24 nurses came from various religious orders, including ten Roman Catholic nuns whom her friend Archbishop, later Cardinal, Manning, allowed to come under her direct supervision, a singular demonstration of both her influence and the crisis which the British believed they faced. The Sellonite Sisters sent eight nurses, and St. John's House sent six. The Protestant Institution for Nursing refused to send any nurses under the conditions demanded by Nightingale. The secular nurses were not particularly respected by some observers, and one reported that their only religious affiliation would be to the cult of Bacchus, if this god of alcoholics could be revived. Unable to find the 40 nurses she had hoped for, she sailed with 38.

From the beginning there was considerable dissension among the group, in part because of Nightingale's dictatorial methods, but since no would-be rival had her political backing, she remained in more or less absolute control. One of the early grounds for contention was the uniforms. While nuns and sisters wore their own habits, the secular nurses wore a gray tweed dress, a gray worsted jacket, a plain white cap, a short woolen cloak, and a holland scarf with the words *Scutari Hospital* embroidered in red. The uniforms were regarded as rather unattractive by the nurses, and to make matters worse they fit poorly. In the period before ready-made clothes were avilable, dresses were individually tailored, and the process involved any number of fittings. In the rush to complete the uniforms, there was no time for fittings; the nurses were allowed to do alterations themselves, but many remained unhappy. Some indication of Nightingale's power was her control of a special fund raised by readers of the London *Times* to spend as she would. This fund helped her to outfit her expedition and to bring much needed supplies and equipment to Scutari.

By November 3 the party had reached Constantinople, and the women set out for Scutari almost at once. When they arrived, they found that the chaos and confusion pictured by the newspapers had not been exaggerated. Many officers refused to take responsibility for their wounded or sick men; they told Nightingale that she would "spoil the brutes" if she assisted patients who were only "animals," "blackguards," or "scum." Medical authorities were outraged by what they considered her unreasonable demands for clean bedding, hot soup, hospital clothing, or other such "preposterous luxuries." Even before she arrived, the doctors at Scutari had been upset about her appointment, mainly because she was a woman. They felt understaffed and overworked, and the last thing they needed was a society lady and her pack of nurses. At first they either ignored her or adopted an attitude of outward submission in deference to her powerful political backing; many of them, however, tried to hamstring her whenever or wherever they could.

Nightingale soon realized that she could accomplish little without the confidence of the doctors; after first offering her nurses and supplies to the doctors and being rejected, she reverted to a traditional female role: sitting back and waiting for the males to request her assistance. She made her nurses sort linen and provisions, or do other busy work, but gave strict orders for them to leave the patients alone. This tactic irritated many of her nurses, and they rebelled when they saw the men suffering, but Nightingale refused to countermand her orders. Nurses were there to assist the surgeons, not run the hospitals.

Her first entry into the hospital itself was through the kitchen, the place where the medical men least resented her influence. At Scutari, before her arrival, the only utensils for cooking were some thirteen Turkish kettles holding 450 pints each. There was but one kitchen, and tea was made in the same kettles in which meat had just been boiled; water was in such short supply that the kettles were not even washed. Meat for the patients was issued by wards. Each ward steward put a distinguishing mark on his ward's meat—a red rag, an old nail, old surgical scissors, or a piece of uniform—and threw it into the pot. Though meat might be thrown in at different times, it was all removed together. Since there were no implements for stirring, some of the meat was fairly well cooked while some was still quite raw. Orderlies on the various wards did not always give even these inadequate meals to their patients, but were known to eat it all themselves. One nurse reported that an orderly ate eight dinners at one sitting. Shortly after her arrival, Nightingale began to cook extras from her own supplies and with her own equipment, which meals the doctors allowed her to give to certain patients. Within a week her kitchen had become what we would now call a diet kitchen, and for five months she was the only source of food for the invalids.

On November 9 the whole hospital opened up to her as a result of the almost total collapse of the British Army in the Crimea from exposure, scurvy, starvation, dysentery, and Russian defensive action. As winter set in, the hospital at Scutari was overrun with patients. In desperation, the doctors were forced to turn to her and her nurses, in fact to anyone who was willing to help; the women responded to the tragic situation with speed and determination. There were more than 1,000 men suffering from acute diarrhea when the nurses were allowed on the floors, but there were only twenty chamber pots in the whole hospital. Moreover, the privies were useless, so overflowing that the men had to wade through slime on the ward floors. To make matters worse, the drinking supply for the hospital came from wells which were contaminated by proximity to the privies. On top of all this, a hurricane struck the area, destroying many of the supplies. The harassed doctors had to ask her help.

Nightingale first forced the cleaning of the lavatories. She somehow got 200 hard brushes and began to scrub the hospital. She then insisted that the slop tubs be emptied regularly. She had no power to command the orderlies, but through pleading, begging, cajoling, and even refusing to move, she managed to get their assistance. Once the hospital was clean, she turned her attention to the laundry. She rented a house outside the barracks and put the camp followers and wives of the soldiers to work washing linens, clothes, and other necessities. These women had been living around the barracks in very bad circumstances, and this not only gave them something to do, but it also made the nurses feel better about their presence. To get hot water for laundering, she purchased boilers from her special funds. When the doctors said a thing was impossible, she usually proceeded to do it. Because of her determination, her willingness, and her ability to get supplies, she was soon purveying the whole hospital. She supplied shirts, socks, drawers, nightcaps, slippers, plates, cups, forks, knives, and spoons; she procured trays, tables, clocks, operating tables, towels, soap, and screens. She referred to herself jocularly as a "general dealer." She managed to repair and equip the wards, clean the bedding, and greet the wounded with great cheerfulness.

These initial efforts rapidly spread her reputation throughout the whole Crimean army; she still felt, however, that she had yet to prove the value of women as nurses. The surgeons remained suspicious of the women, while many of the nurses under her were upset at her unwillingness to utilize them effectively as nurses, since many knew much more about the bed care of the sick than did the surgeons themselves. They often wanted to supplement the doctor, give a different diet, or do something that he had not ordered. Nightingale insisted, however, that the nurses do nothing not authorized by the medical men. Some of her nurses, in attempts to circumvent her, wrote letters to influential relatives back home, making certain that they would be published in the newspapers. One nurse, Sister Elizabeth, even forced an investigation into the activities of Nightingale; but she herself was made to resign when her charges were declared to be exaggerated.

There was also much religious controversy among the nurses, especially after December 1854, when another party of nurses was sent out by Sidney Herbert. Nightingale was very upset, probably unjustly, that these nurses had been sent without her request, and the rivalry between the leaders of the second expedition and herself caused further difficulty. The nuns in this second group were unwilling to subordinate themselves to Nightingale; nor were the "ladies" who felt that much of nursing was beneath them. Religious bigotry was very strong in England, and the arrival of additional nuns and sisters revived rumors of a popish plot in Scutari. It was even claimed that wounded soldiers were forced to confess before they received nursing care. Such rumors were, of course, untrue, but it made Nightingale's task more difficult. The leader of the second expedition, Mary Stanley, was described by Nightingale as an unstable figure. Mary Stanley had a similar opinion of Nightingale. Eventually, the rivalry between the two women led authorities to give Stanley a separate hospital to control.

Despite her difficulties and her own high-handed methods, Florence Nightingale's prestige continued to grow. She concerned herself not only with the nursing duties in the hospital but also with the general welfare of the soldiers. She established a lying-in hospital for the wives of the soldiers. By appealing directly to Queen Victoria, she got sick pay for the soldiers while they were in the hospital. But still casualties mounted. In January 1855, there were 12,000 men in the hospital and only 11,000 taking part in the battle for Sebastopol. In the opinion of most authorities, if Nightingale and her nurses had not been at Scutari during the winter of 1854–1855, the whole hospital system would have collapsed. The soldiers knew what she was doing and loved her. The people in England almost worshipped her, but she still had to fight tooth and nail with the medical authorities at Scutari. She had a dayroom equipped for convalescent patients; she began classes in mathematics, reading, and other subjects; in effect, she established a much more favorable atmosphere for recovery. Unfortunately, almost everything she did made the medical authorities look worse. Some of her burdens were relaxed with the arrival of Alexis Soyer, a world-famous chef, who came out at his own expense to reorganize military cooking. His effect on the army diet was in the long run perhaps as lasting as Nightingale's on nursing. With better food, better nursing, and a conscientious interest in their plight, the morale of the soldiers improved tremendously.[16]

The Nightingale Legend and Changes in Nursing

A legend began growing up about Florence Nightingale. She became a modern Joan of Arc. Popular biographies were written about her; she was the "lady of the lamp," probably one of the most-written-about women in history. In the process, nursing emerged as a valuable and honorable profession. Florence Nightingale and her nurses almost alone emerged from the Crimean War with a shining reputation. To honor her work a committee was formed in November 1855; they established a general fund which she was to use at her discretion—the so-called Nightingale Fund. Many of the troops subscribed; almost all England contributed. The only opposition came from the army surgeons, who were conspicuous by their absence as contributors. At the same time as this demonstration of public support, her struggle to establish her authority in the Crimea had been won. But the war was almost over. In April 1856, peace was proclaimed; by July the last patient had left the barracks hospitals, and her task was ended. On July 28 she embarked from Constantinople for England. All England began planning mass demonstrations for her when she landed. The people wanted passionately to honor her, but she, the unwilling heroine, slipped into England with scarcely anyone knowing of her arrival, surprising even her family.

Nursing, however, could never be the same after the Crimean War. The popular image of the nurse had been transformed. Sairey Gamp was no longer the typical nurse; it was Florence Nightingale, the lady of the lamp. No longer would a nurse be typified as a tipsy, promiscuous menial servant. Instead, the nurse now had to bear the image of Florence Nightingale—strong yet compassionate, controlled in the face of suffering, seeking only to relieve the distress of her fellow man. Also transformed in the process was the British soldier; this transformation had also been wrought by Nightingale. Through her support his image changed from that of a drunken brute, the scum of the earth, to a symbol of courage, loyalty, and endurance. His officers could no longer afford to overlook him. Florence Nightingale wanted to make certain that both images were preserved.

It was to this dual purpose that she dedicated the rest of her life. She was haunted by the mortality of the Crimean disaster. Seventy-three percent of the army had been lost in six months from disease alone. She wanted to do something about this; as a popular figure she knew she could reach the public. But she felt that by playing on her name, she would irritate and antagonize the old guard in the medical profession, who were already so suspicious of her. To avoid this she deliberately sought obscurity. After her return from the Crimea she never made a public appearance, never attended a public function, never issued a public statement. Within a few years most people assumed she was dead. But she was not; she was working hard. She convinced Queen Victoria of the necessity for reform, but for either of these two women to be successful in army reform they had to work through Parliament. Florence relied on her old friend Sidney Herbert as well as on other members of Parliament. Talking about the need for reform was not enough; she also had to have concrete evidence.

In order to support her arguments for reform, she turned to the newly developing field of statistics. By 1857 she had written a lengthy report on hospitals in war entitled *Notes on Matters Affecting the Health, Efficiency, and Hospital Administration of the British Army.*[17] The nearly 1,000 closely printed pages of the report were crammed with figures, facts, tables, and statistical comparisons. In much of the report she was doing the work of a trailblazer. In preparing it she worked to the point of exhaustion, but she still kept pushing herself. She felt she had to give her Parliamentary friends the facts and figures with which they could argue for reform. Her studies showed that even in peacetime the living conditions in the barracks of the British Army were so bad that the mortality rate in the peacetime army was double that of the civilian population—even though soldiers were chosen for their physical well-being.

Even while working for army reform, Nightingale continued her interest in nursing.[18] In 1859 she wrote a little book, the most popular of all her works, *Notes on Nursing*,[19] designed for the average housewife. In its time it caused a mild sensation by emphasizing the role of good nursing care in assuring a speedy recovery. She also pointed out the need for the nurse to relieve the "apprehension, uncertainty, fear" which every patient suffers. Women were advised to put flowers in the sickroom, or better yet to make sure that the sickroom had a view, and to attend to other such minor matters that make the bedridden person feel better. In that same year she also published *Notes on Hospitals*,[20] designed to show that hospitals, through better construction, better management, and improved sanitation, could help cure the sick.

The Nightingale School

Shortly after *Notes on Nursing* was published, she utilized the Nightingale Fund, which had grown to over 45,000 pounds, to start a training school at St. Thomas' Hospital.[21] Her reason for choosing St. Thomas' was that its matron, Mrs. S. E. Wardroper, was the only woman in any existing London hospital whom Nightingale trusted to manage her school.[22] Wardroper and Nightingale converted the resident medical officer to their plan, although there was considerable opposition among the doctors on the staff who felt that trained nurses might trespass on their authority. Opposition to the nursing school was led by the senior consulting surgeon at St. Thomas' who was also president of the College of Surgeons. Eventually, however, the prestige and persistence of Nightingale triumphed, and the school was established.

The initial response to advertisements seeking applicants to the training school in May 1860 was discouraging. When the school opened on July 9, 1860, there were only fifteen candidates. The training period was to last one year. Students, who were called probationers, lived in a "nurses' home," a concept originated by Nightingale herself. Each probationer had a bedroom to herself; there was a common sitting room, while the sister in charge had a bedroom and a sitting room of her own. Probationers wore a brown uniform with a white apron and white cap. Board, lodging, washing, and uniforms were provided. In addition each probationer was given ten pounds for her personal expenses during training.

Despite the publicity given the school, it actually made no sharp break with the traditions established by the earlier nineteenth-century training programs. Apprenticeship remained the basic educational strategy, supplemented by lectures from members of the medical staff and ward sisters. Probationers kept notebooks which they submitted periodically, and they had to pass both written and oral examinations. Every month a report was made out on each of them by Mrs. Wardroper. She graded them on punctuality, quietness, trustworthiness, personal neatness, cleanliness, ward management, and technical effectiveness.[23]

In keeping with Nightingale's own beliefs, the school emphasized good character or morality more than the cognitive aspects of education. No pupil was admitted without a certificate of good character, and constraints were built into the system to monitor the students once they were admitted. The nurses' home was basic to this protective system. Probationers were forbidden to leave the home unless they went in pairs and their mission had been determined in advance to be a wholesome one. On and off duty, they were watched closely by the matron and sisters to ensure they did not succumb to the temptations of the world. Discipline for those who strayed was strict. For example, flirtation was punished by instant dismissal. Nightingale believed that this strong emphasis on morality was a crucial aspect in her life-long struggle to raise "nursing from the sink."[24]

The school was also tied to the British class system, since students were admitted either as nurse probationers or special probationers. The special group were of higher social origins; they paid for their board and room and were in turn given more medical lectures. The lower-level nurse probationers, on the other hand, were paid a small stipend. The regular probationers signed a contract to work for three years for a nominal fee after they finished the probationary year, while the special probationers were required to stay only two years.[25]

An important characteristic of the St. Thomas' school, and one not achieved by most non-English schools, was its relative autonomy. Both the school and the hospital nursing service were organized under the matron. This meant that the nursing service and educational hierarchy were independent of the medical staff in selecting, retaining, and disciplining students and nurses, although they were under physician supervision for patient care.[26]

Other Nightingale Reforms

Nightingale's hopes for effectively reorganizing the British Army medical services suffered a disastrous blow with the death of her close friend and advocate, Sidney Herbert in 1861. She, however, continued to press for reform. The first real recognition of her efforts for better army medical services came from the United States during the Civil War. The Union consulted her for help in organizing hospitals and in caring for the sick or wounded. She sent evidence to the United States to back up her suggestions, which received wide publicity and had much influence. Following her recommendations, the Union forces appointed a sanitary commission and provided for the inspection of camps. Women were also utilized as nurses. Unfortunately, she had no channel of communication with the Confederacy, although she wanted very much to help them also.

By the end of the American Civil War, her own health had so collapsed that she retired to her bed where she remained for the last 50 years of her life. While the nature of her illness is not clear, she did consider herself ill and used her illness to extract work from her friends. She not only continued to work for reforming and reconstructing the army medical services, but also became a member of the Royal Sanitary Commission on the Health of the Army in India. Though never able to visit India, she nonetheless became an expert on the country. Through numerous studies and reports and voluminous correspondence, she researched and criticized the medical and nursing facilities in India. She found that military hospitals in India were inferior in construction and comfort to barracks; often the hospitals were mere sheds. In these hospitals patients were washed and nursed by ward coolies hired at four rupees a month. These servant-nurses were not soldiers and did not have any sense of dedication, so that they often fled from epidemics or any real danger. When a soldier became critically ill, one of his comrades from the regiment was delegated to nurse him, but this too often took the form of beating the coolie for not giving better nursing care. She found that there was only one tub and basin per 100 men in a hospital. Patients were washed, therefore, by pouring water over them from a tin pot.

The British hospitals in India made no effective provision for convalescents, and even nearly recovered patients had to spend all their time in bed. Gangrene and erysipelas were widespread. Many soldiers preferred to conceal their illness rather than enter a hospital where such conditions prevailed. Never one to shirk a task, Nightingale decided that improving these conditions required nothing less than raising the whole sanitary level of India. One task for her always led to another. Her work in military hospitals had led her to civilian hospitals; sanitary work for troops in India led her to work for the health and welfare of the Indians themselves. None of her reforms were accomplished without much opposition, which was sometimes able to modify or even nullify her work, but still she persevered.

Because she wanted to do so much, Florence Nightingale often despaired that any real reform would be accomplished. This feeling drove her to renewed effort. To have more time for her work, she deliberately cut herself off from most of her friends, keeping only a few intimate contacts. She often worked day and night, utilizing her illness as an excuse to avoid doing what she did not want to do, which left her time and energy to accomplish what she felt she must. By 1868 a sanitary department had been organized in India; some of her other ideas were gradually being adopted in the British Army, and her nursing school was producing trained nurses.

The Visiting Nurse

While engaged in these many tasks, she also helped establish the visiting or district nurse. The chief mover in this reform was William Rathbone (1819–1902), a Liverpool Unitarian merchant-shipowner, from a family with strong philanthropic and liberalistic traditions. His attention was directed to the inadequacy of home nursing in Liverpool, which led him to found in 1859 a district nursing service with one trained nurse. A single nurse soon proved so insufficient that he decided to establish, at his own expense, a corps of nurses trained to nurse the sick poor in their own homes. He naturally turned to Florence Nightingale for help, assistance, and advice. According to Rathbone she gave his scheme as much consideration as "if she herself was going to be superintendent." She concluded that the only satisfactory solution was to train more nurses for the task. Repeatedly, her answer to a problem was more training for nurses. She suggested to Rathbone that he approach the Royal Liverpool Infirmary for assistance in opening a training school, guaranteeing in turn that a fixed percentage of the nurses trained would remain in the Infirmary. As a result, in 1860, at his own expense, he established a Training School and Home for Nurses in cooperation with the Infirmary.[27]

But Rathbone decided that this was still not enough. Once aroused, he investigated the nursing situation further. He found that the workhouse infirmaries in Liverpool and elsewhere were literally filled with sick people who had no real nursing care. What nursing there was, was done by able-bodied paupers, many of whom were drunken prostitutes. In fact, the situation was so bad that in the Liverpool Workhouse Infirmary a policeman patrolled some of the wards to keep order. In 1864 Rathbone suggested that a staff of trained nurses and a matron be sent to the workhouse. He was strongly seconded by Nightingale. The two reformers were aided by the publicity attending a death in the workhouse from gross neglect. Shortly after this, twelve nurses and their matron, Agnes Jones (1832–1868), arrived at Liverpool to begin a nursing experiment financed by Rathbone. At the same time a general investigation of all workhouses in England was begun, largely through the influence of Rathbone and Nightingale. The eyes of England were in a sense upon the Liverpool experiment as a demonstration of what could be done.

Fortunately, Agnes Jones proved an effective superintendent. Like

Nightingale, she had come from a well-to-do family and, inspired by the example of Nightingale, had trained first at Kaiserswerth, then at the Nightingale School at St. Thomas'.[28] Despite almost impossible difficulties (so many, in fact, that Nightingale called it "Scutari over again"), the Liverpool experiment succeeded. Wards were increasingly opened to the nurses when it was found that not only was the condition of the sick improving through the use of trained nurses, but even more important to the economy-minded governors, the new system cost less than the old. Fortified by this success the two reformers continued to press for a thorough reform. Finally even the conservative British Medical Association was aroused after *Lancet*, its official publication, appointed a commission which urged reform along lines already suggested by Rathbone and Nightingale.

By 1867 reform of the workhouse system had been accomplished.[29] Although it was not as thoroughgoing as Rathbone and Nightingale would have liked, it was a beginning. Lunatics were separated from the physically sick; the poor and the healthy separated from the ill and the bedridden. Nurses and matrons were paid. Moreover, the Liverpool district nursing service was growing so rapidly that by 1867 Liverpool had eighteen districts. Other reforms started by Nightingale were beginning to spread, but the main difficulty in furthering nursing reform was no longer the opposition of administrators, but rather the shortage of trained nurses. Even the Nightingale School itself had failed to meet the standards in nursing training set by Nightingale, so that under her direction it was reorganized in 1871. Examination standards were raised, and more study was required. She became more influential in the administration of the school; every girl who now trained there became personally known to her, and once a girl became a Nightingale nurse, it was difficult to escape her influence. She corresponded with many of them.

As more of her reforms were realized, she became less demanding, less frenzied, more willing to compromise. She also found herself less able to concentrate and was forced at times to turn down opportunities to extend the fields for trained nurses. In 1874 William Rathbone asked her to help organize district nursing in London, but she refused. She did write a very influential pamphlet, *Suggestions for Improving the Nursing Service for the Sick Poor*, which Rathbone used to advantage. In accordance with her suggestions he also founded the Metropolitan Nursing Association.[30]

Nursing Opposition to Florence Nightingale

By 1887 many of the hospitals in England and Scotland had superintendents or matrons who had trained at the Nightingale School.

Parties of Nightingale nurses had gone to the United States, Australia, Canada, India, Ceylon, Germany, and Sweden. Training schools on the Nightingale model had been set up in Britain and in other countries, while much of the direction of the district nursing was based on her concepts. Perhaps a sign of her vast success was that nursing itself was becoming so independent that other leaders had arisen in the profession to challenge her leadership. In 1886 a group of nurses proposed the creation of an independent body of examiners, separate from all training schools, to certify nurses. Any nurse satisfying the examining board would be entitled to have her name placed on a registry of nurses: she would be a registered nurse.

Such a board, it was argued, would ensure a standard of excellence in nursing, so that the public would be protected against employing nurses who were incompetent or disreputable. Surprisingly, Nightingale opposed the proposal. She argued that nursing was still too young and disorganized for such an organization, and that qualifying a nurse by examination ignored the character training which she considered as important as the technical skill. Despite her opposition the unofficial British Nurses' Association, led by their patron Princess Christian, daughter of Queen Victoria, continued to apply for official recognition. Unwilling to concede defeat, Nightingale fought them with every weapon at her command; through her efforts the British Board of Trade refused to register the British Nurses' Association as a public company. The Association refused to be put off, however, and petitioned the Queen herself for a royal charter, which was granted in 1893. In the royal charter the word "register" was removed, and the Royal British Nurses' Association had only the right to the "maintenance of a list of persons who may have applied to have their names entered" as nurses. This, despite Nightingale's opposition, was a long-term gain for nursing. While the standards of the association were probably lower at first than those of the nurses from the Nightingale schools, it could apply a minimum uniformity to standards for nurses and facilitate the recognition of nurses.

As Nightingale grew older, her eyesight began to fail, her memory grew bad, and the curtain of old age descended. By 1901 she was blind, but honors still came to her. In 1907 the International Conference of Red Cross Societies listed her as the pioneer of the Red Cross movement. In 1910, the Jubilee year for the founding of the Nightingale Training School, there were more than 1,000 training schools in the United States alone. She was almost unconscious of the jubilee celebrations and died in August 1910. In deference to her wishes, she was not buried in Westminster Abbey, as was usual for British leaders and heroes, but instead in the family grave at East Wello, her only memorial a line on the family tombstone: "F. N. Born 1820. Died 1910." She had lived for more than 90 years.

In summary, Nightingale was a brilliant woman whose achievements in research, in reforming the British Army, and in establishing nursing schools were monumental. Her major achievement was probably establishing secular nursing as a respectable occupation for women. Her accomplishments at Scutari made her a heroine to the British populace and facilitated her accomplishments after the war. Yet even with this public power, she still found it necessary to work indirectly. Her half century of seclusion in her bedroom convinced her various male friends, including Sidney Herbert, that they should present her arguments to Parliament and wage the public fights for reform. She often claimed to be a feeble woman and protested that public struggles should be handled by great, strong men.[31] While this strategem was undoubtedly the key to her effectiveness in nineteenth-century England, it set precedents of indirection and artifice which still plague nursing. Her refusal at Scutari to allow the nurses in her party to give even basic nursing care without orders from the army surgeons was also a crucial precedent in defining nurses as subordinate to physicians in all aspects of their work, even basic nursing care in which physicians lacked expertise. Her insistence on valuing character over knowledge and skills set precedents for nursing education which have been slow to change. Florence Nightingale remains nursing's greatest leader, but the mark she left on the profession was also the source of some of its problems.

Bacteriological Revolution

Other events of the nineteenth century also contributed to the development of nursing and to the transformation of hospitals from pesthouses into institutions for the treatment of illnesses. Hospitals had already become primarily institutions for the sick, but the nosocomial infections made them so unsafe that anyone with an alternative avoided them.

One of the leading innovators in changing this situation was Ignaz Philipp Semmelweis (1818–1865), who became an assistant at the Viennese Lying-in Hospital in 1846 after studying medicine in Vienna and Budapest. Here the mortality rate from puerperal fever often reached thirty percent. Horrified by conditions in the hospital, he took a leave of absence. Upon his return he found a fellow professor dead of the blood poisoning he had contracted from a finger puncture during a postmortem examination. Semmelweis was struck by the close resemblance of symptoms from blood poisoning to those of puerperal fever. He jumped to the conclusion that his friend's death had been caused by infection from the dead body, and so were the deaths of the victims of puerperal disease, who were often examined by students returning from postmortem examinations.

His hunch was verified from the hospital statistics. In one section of the Lying-in Hospital, midwives were trained, and medical students did very little examining. In this section the mortality rate was much lower than in the ward where the physicians alone did the examination. Semmelweis immediately insisted that every doctor or student disinfect his hands with chlorine water before making an examination. Almost immediately there was a decline in the mortality rate. This simple reform ought to have been adopted everywhere at once. But opposition came from Semmelweis' colleagues, the professors of midwifery, who regarded his discovery as an indictment of their methods, since they felt it implied that they themselves had brought many women to premature graves. The struggle of Semmelweis and his followers against most of the leading gynecologists of the day become so intense that Semmelweis was denied permission to lecture at the University of Vienna. He returned to Budapest, where he died rather tragically at age 47 of the very disease that had indicated to him the cause of puerperal fever. His difficulties partly arose because he had discovered a preventive technique without discovering the cause of the disease. The American Oliver Wendell Holmes had also independently discovered the contagious nature of puerperal fever.

The fruits of Semmelweis' work only came when germs themselves were discovered by Louis Pasteur (1822–1895). His discovery was aided by the development of better microscopes. Pasteur first studied fermentation in the manufacture of alcohol. He confirmed that alcoholic fermentation was caused by the vital processes of small living creatures, yeasts. Turning from alcohol to sour milk and rancid butter, he found that here also minute living organisms participated in the process. These microorganisms he found could be killed by heat. He first applied this heat treatment (*pasteurization*) to wine, then to milk. But he was not satisfied. Where did the microbes come from? By various experiments he concluded that the germs came from the air, from water, from other humans or animals, from the ground. In other words there were swarms of minute unicellular living creatures, bacteria, and other microorganisms, some of which were harmless and some of which were not, everywhere. He turned to various diseases, first to silkworm infection, then chicken cholera, splenic fever (anthrax), and others. For each of these he managed to find an answer. For anthrax he found that isolated cultures several weeks old were much weaker and produced a milder form of the disease which would still give immunity. The process was similar to vaccination as an immunization against smallpox and was now applied to other diseases. Above all he found a remedy for a particularly horrifying illness— rabies. After prolonged and laborious experiments, he produced a vaccine by drying the spinal cords of animals infected with rabies. When this was injected into victims who had been bitten by rabid animals, it could produce an immunity before the dreaded and fatal attack of rabies set in.

Pasteur's practical achievements soon produced direct results in other fields, mainly through the work of Robert Koch (1843–1910). Koch served as a physician in a small German town where there were periodic epidemics of splenic fever. He studied the disease and verified earlier work that had indicated that animal victims of the disease had rodlike organisms in their blood. He also found that another researcher had been able to transmit the disease to healthy animals by the inoculation of blood from diseased animals. This made it extremely probable that the bacillus actually caused splenic fever, but how could it be transmitted? Koch kept a stock of mice infected with the disease, examined their blood repeatedly under the microscope, and discovered that the bacilli in question grew into long threads, propagating themselves by transverse fission, and forming spores. These spores retained their virulence for years, so that if they reached an animal body through its food or the air, they could grow into bacteria. Contagion, Koch had shown, was not caused by mysterious substances but by microorganisms.

Koch detailed his work in a paper in 1876, making him the first to describe the life cycle of a contagious organism. As his research continued, Koch found that a particular bacillus always caused a particular disease. He then concluded that infectious disorders were caused by specific organisms. Following Koch's work, almost immediately Neisser discovered the gonococcus as the cause of gonorrhea; Ebert and Gaffky discovered the typhoid bacillus, Hansen the cause of leprosy, and Laveran that of malaria. Koch himself continued to experiment until, by 1882, he had isolated the tuberculosis bacillus, proving that tuberculosis was not a nutritional deficiency, as was then believed, but an infectious disease. The cholera bacillus was discovered in 1883, and the diphtheria, tetanus, and pneumonia organisms in 1884. Weichselbaum later discovered the meningococcus; this was followed by the discovery of the bubonic plague bacillus, and of many others.

With the changing concept of disease, the accidental discoveries of Semmelweis and Holmes could no longer be ignored. The application of these discoveries helped surgery to advance tremendously. Before the late nineteenth century there were two main handicaps to surgical operations. They were so extremely painful that the surgeon had to act swiftly, and operations had to be very short. Also mortality, especially from wound infection, was extremely high. Usually operations were attempted only as a last resort. There had been many earlier attempts to secure a generalized loss of sensation or even a local numbing, but most of the results had been unsatisfactory. The first breakthrough came with nitrous oxide or laughing gas, which the American dentist Horace Wells (1815–1857) first used for an operation in 1844. It caused complete anesthesia, but only for very brief periods. Next came the discovery of ether as an anesthetic by an American dentist and physician William Morton (1819–1868), who in 1846 gave a public demonstration in Boston. Another American, Crawford W. Long (1815–1878) of Dansville, Georgia, had used ether as early as 1842, but this was unknown for many years, so that Morton is usually given credit for the discovery. Sir James Young Simpson (1811–1870) of Edinburgh introduced the use of ether into Europe, and in 1847 pioneered the use of chloroform in obstetrical and surgical cases.

With one obstacle out of the way, the surgeon could now attack infection. The man who overcame this difficulty was Sir Joseph Lister (1827–1912). As professor of surgery in Glasgow, he was struck by the difference in the mortality rates between cases of simple and of compound fractures. He asked himself what could be the difference between an open and closed wound to cause this? Obviously, the answer to such a simple question was that the open wound communicated with the air. Pasteur had already shown that bacteria was present everywhere in the air; thus it was logical that bacteria would enter the wound from the air. Lister experimented with disinfectants—especially carbolic acid—and his results, which he began publishing in 1867, were astounding. He soon extended the use of carbolic acid to all fields of surgery, establishing what he felt was the "antiseptic" principle. Despite his results, medical people were slow to accept his techniques; gradually, however, they were adopted in most of the Western world. Others improved upon his techniques by boiling instruments, washing and disinfecting the hands, using rubber gloves, and sterilizing linen.

By the 1870's the foundations of modern nursing had been laid and with it the foundation of the modern hospital—the key to modern medicine. Nursing was ready to go forward.

Five

The Rise of the Trained Nurse

Nursing reform within any country is influenced both by what has been done in other countries and by independent reform movements within the country itself. Florence Nightingale, for example, had studied the nursing done by various Catholic orders and by the Kaiserswerth deaconesses, but her reforms depended to a great extent on an English tradition of long standing. In the United States, where ties with England had always been close, the English example was influential, but there was also an independent reform movement.

Almost all the leading early American cities had almshouses which included infirmaries for the sick and poor. Some, such as Philadelphia and New York, had voluntary hospitals, but most nursing care was at a very low level. In the almshouses most of the care was given by other inmates; in the hospitals, nursing was classed with scrubbing floors; no special training was needed, and none was sought. Often, in fact, the nurses were prisoners serving their time in the hospital wards. Although various reformers decried the lack of adequate medical care, methodical attendance on the sick was probably undertaken only by the Catholic religious orders until well into the nineteenth century.

One of the earliest attempts at better nursing care was made at the New York Hospital in 1798 when attendants were given a series of lectures on various aspects of sick care. Another early attempt was made by Dr. Joseph Warrington of Philadelphia, who in 1839 helped found the Nurse Society of Philadelphia, modeled on Elizabeth Fry's movement in England. Prospective nurses were given lectures by Dr. Warrington, who also demonstrated his concepts on a manikin. After attending six cases under his direction, the women received a certificate entitling them to serve as home nurses. The society continued to give training in home nursing throughout the nineteenth century, but not until 1897 was the course extended to a full year.[1]

Particularly influential in forming American concepts was the work of Mother Elizabeth Ann Bayley Seton (1774–1821), the first native-born American to be canonized a Roman Catholic saint. After her conversion to Catholicism, she organized the St. Joseph's Sisterhood at Emmitsburgh, Maryland, in 1809. The Order soon adopted the rule of the Sisters of Charity of St. Vincent de Paul, and a union with the French society was effected in 1850.[2] Another Catholic Order, the Sisters of Mercy, reached the United States in 1843 and, through the efforts of Mary Xavier

Warde, its American founder, established hospitals in Pennsylvania, Illinois, and Missouri.[3]

Protestant reformers in America, as in Europe, greatly admired the work of the Catholic nursing orders and sought to mobilize Protestant women for works of charity without establishing convents. Bishop William August Muhlenberg (1796–1877) was instrumental in forming Episcopal sisterhoods. His ideas on the subject were implemented by Anne Ayres who, after hearing him talk, decided in 1845 to devote her life to charity. At first she established a parish school for girls, but during the cholera epidemic of 1849, she and her followers worked in the emergency hospitals. A parish infirmary was established in 1853 in which the sisters, organized as the Sisterhood of the Holy Communion, worked; in 1859 they moved into the newly opened St. Luke's Hospital in New York.[4]

Sister Anne, with Muhlenberg's assistance, established the general criteria for the sisterhoods, so called because the women were to live together as sisters. Membership was renewable at the end of specific periods. Sisters were to live in the institutions in which they worked, while board, laundry, and room were to be furnished by the institution. Personal expenses were to be met by the candidate herself or by her friends, although a special fund was available for those without means. Generally, however, the women who entered the sisterhood came from the upper levels of society. The affairs of the sisterhood were to be in the hands of an elder or superintending sister, who apparently was appointed by and responsible to Muhlenberg. Candidates for the group had to serve a probationary term of six months and then be voted into membership subject to approval of the Sister Superintendent. Rules were established for hours of work and rest, food, and clothing.[5] In St. Luke's hospital, the sisters served at the upper level of nursing, while much of the actual nursing care lay in the hands of non-sisters. Every ward had a sister in charge of two day nurses and one night nurse. As a sister and as one who had had some education, she was in control of the drug closet from which she administered the prescriptions ordered by the physician. The sister also had charge of the diet of the patient, subject to some general directions from the physician in charge.[6]

The Lutheran counterpart of Muhlenberg was the Reverend William Alfred Passavant (1821–1894) who introduced the Kaiserswerth deaconess order into Pittsburgh in 1849.[7] The deaconesses in Pittsburgh soon began to serve in hospitals, the earliest of which was founded by Reverend Passavant himself.[8] Fliedner himself visited Passavant in Pittsburgh and Muhlenberg in New York.

Though the sisterhood movement led to better nursing, it labored under two handicaps. The most telling was simply the lack of sufficient recruits to the sisterhoods: as hospitals expanded in number and in scope they increasingly turned to professional secular nurses—even St. Luke's began hiring trained nurses when they were available in 1877. In fact, by 1892 the sisters had been more or less eased out of nursing, indicative of the change of nursing from a voluntary religious vocation to an emerging profession.[9] Still more of a handicap to the sisterhoods was the antagonism towards such groups by Protestants who considered them havens for secret Catholics. Many nineteenth-century Protestants feared the growing influx of Catholic immigrants into the United States, and anti-Catholicism was a major factor in American politics. Not until well into the twentieth century—some would say not until the election of John F. Kennedy as President in 1960—did the old animosities begin to erode in most of the country. So great was the anxiety among Protestants that Muhlenberg for a time dissolved the sisterhood, although it was reorganized in 1873 as the Sisterhood of St. Luke and St. John.[10]

Elizabeth Blackwell and Her Co-Workers

The most effective leadership for reform in nursing practices, however, came from women interested in the struggle for women's rights. Their interest was at least twofold: in part they wanted to see that the patient had better care, but they were also interested in widening the occupational possibilities of women. Though there were earlier forerunners of the American women's rights movement, the campaign is usually dated from the Seneca Falls (New York) Convention in 1848.[11] Here the women adopted a general platform which included a statement about women's right to enter the various professions, clearly including medicine. The medical barrier had first been broken by Elizabeth Blackwell, but only after she had applied to 29 medical schools. The circumstances of her admission into Geneva College (later absorbed into Syracuse University) indicate the barriers that women had to overcome. The faculty opposed her admission, but hated to take the responsibility for denying the request of Dr. Joseph Warrington, a powerful Philadelphia physician, who was Blackwell's patron. As a result they decided to shift the onus of rejection onto the students by having them vote on her admission, with the proviso that one negative vote would blackball her. The students, however, voted unanimously to admit her because they saw a chance not only to embarrass the faculty but also to divert themselves. When one lone man attempted to vote no, students pounced on him from all quarters, and in either mock or real fear, he changed his vote. Blackwell was admitted and arrived at the school on November 6, 1847. The contradictions of women's position in society were effectively demonstrated on the day she graduated at the head of her class (January 23, 1849) by her refusal to walk in the commencement procession because it would be unladylike. It was the custom for all women to be seated in the church before the students marched in, followed by the various male guests. Blackwell had to show that she, despite her medical degree, was still a lady, and so she entered the church with the ladies rather than the students.[12]

After her graduation she went to Europe for further study and then returned to New York only to find most of the medical doors closed to her. Her main efforts were soon concentrated on the New York Infirmary, a 40-bed hospital, which opened on May 12, 1857, and was staffed entirely by women: herself, her sister Emily, and Marie Zakrzewska. Emily, following in Elizabeth's footsteps, had started medical education at Rush College in Chicago, but after the Illinois Medical Society had censured the school for admitting a woman, she had transferred to Western Reserve which granted her a degree. Marie Zakrzewska had been the chief midwife in a Berlin hospital, and she had been encouraged by some of the physicians to study medicine. To do so, she had come to the United States but had encountered one obstacle after another; it was only when she met Elizabeth Blackwell that she was able to give up embroidering tasseled caps, the way she had supported herself, and enter Western Reserve.

The New York hospital had been a project on which Blackwell had worked for several years; she officially inaugurated it in December 1855 with an "Address on the Medical Education of Women," in which she tried to show that medicine was a work in which women had always been engaged. She received backing for her project from various American reform leaders, including William Ellery Channing and William Lloyd Garrison. Most of her male supporters emphasized the importance of Blackwell's hospital in training nurses and kept quiet about the possibilities of training future female physicians. Her charter, in fact, had granted her the right not only to care for the indigent sick but also to graduate women physicians and train nurses. The close ties of Elizabeth Blackwell with the women's rights movement is indicated by the marriages of Samuel, one of her brothers, to Antoinette Brown, America's earliest ordained women preacher, and of another brother, Henry, to Lucy Stone, who was such an ardent feminist that she insisted on preserving her maiden name as well as eliminating the word "obey" from the marriage ceremony. Susan B. Anthony, perhaps the most prominent of the early fighters for women's rights, became very upset at the marriage of these two strong-willed women because she thought that marriage would mean a loss to the suffrage cause, but marriage or lack of it did little to stop any of the Blackwells, natural or in-law, from carrying on the battle.[13]

Eight months after the Infirmary opened (May 12, 1857), the training of nurses began on a limited scale. Free courses, four months long, were given. Many of those who applied were turned away, since one of the problems was the unsuitability of many of the women who came to the Infirmary seeking training in nursing or medicine. In her diary, Elizabeth Blackwell recorded rather sadly that nursing was such an unpopular type

of work that it did not attract "the best class of women students." Part of
the difficulty was also that Blackwell felt that she could not devote as
much time to nursing as was necessary, since for her the most important
task was to show that her Infirmary, manned by women, could maintain
as high a medical standard as any all-male institution.[14]

Her work, however, bore fruit in other cities such as Philadelphia
and Boston. In attempting to establish her New York Infirmary, she or
her co-workers lectured throughout the East and inspired other women to
match their efforts. Marie Zakrzewska, for example, had spoken to a
group of Philadelphia women assembled in the parlors of Lucretia Mott
in an attempt to get funds for the hospital. She failed to get the funds,
simply because the Philadelphia women decided to organize a hospital of
their own.[15] Boston soon followed Philadelphia in attempting to make
certain that women had an opportunity to secure medical and nursing
training.

The influence of Florence Nightingale first reached American nursing
through Elizabeth Blackwell; the two had been friends before the
Crimean War, and in 1859 Blackwell had visited Nightingale again just as
she was organizing her plans for the Nightingale Training School for
Nurses at St. Thomas' Hospital. Their personalities, however, were
radically different; Miss Nightingale was much more intolerant and
demanding than Dr. Blackwell. It was perhaps for this reason that the
English movement only had one key leader—Florence Nightingale—who
attempted to keep nursing reform separate and distinct from the women's
rights movement. The United States, on the other hand, had a whole host
of leaders, many of whom were intimately and directly involved in the
struggle for women's rights. Marie Zakrzewska, for example, had left
New York during Blackwell's absence in England in order to take up a
medical post in Boston. When she found the new position at the New
England Female Medical College was not up to her standards, she
founded the New England Hospital for Women and Children in 1862 and
transferred to it the nursing school she had started in 1860. Under her
direction women gave their services in the hospital for six months in
exchange for instruction; they were then considered qualified for private
nursing service. She trained six women at the medical college, and some
30 more during the next decade. In 1872 the school was reorganized when
the hospital moved to a new building in Roxbury, Massachusetts. Five
nurses were in the first class at the new hospital, including Linda Richards
(1841–1930), who rather erroneously claimed to be America's "first
trained nurse." Certificates were given to the nurses who successfully
served a year in the hospital and attended the twelve lectures offered
during the year.[16]

After her return from England, Elizabeth Blackwell campaigned for
a real women's medical college with a four-year course, as well as nurses

trained on the Nightingale plan, which had not yet been presented to the public. She argued that even though more women had begun to study medicine, most were "imperfectly trained" and would in the long run harm not only the medical profession, but women's struggle for equality as well. Her plea for nursing training was especially well received because of the continued obstacles to women in medicine and because many of the would-be women physicians turned to nursing in which somehow or other they felt they could remain more feminine. The Women's Medical College in Philadelphia had graduated its first class of seven physicians in 1851, but the attitude of the regular medical men to this is indicated by the action of the county medical society, which in 1858 urged its members to "withhold from the faculties and graduates of the female medical college all countenance and support." This recommendation was confirmed by the Pennsylvania State Medical Society in 1859 without objection. It was not until 1871 that the Woman's Medical College secured recognition for its graduates as consultants, although in 1869 both the Philadelphia and Pennsylvania hospitals had opened their clinical lectures to women. In 1876 the national society broke the sex barrier by recognizing Sarah Hackett Stevenson as an official delegate to the American Medical Association convention held in Philadelphia.[17]

The Civil War

Because of the medical opposition to female physicians and the hesitancy of many women to become doctors, most of the women's rights supporters concentrated on nursing. In fact, the graduates of the Women's Medical College served as nurses rather than as surgeons or physicians during the Civil War. Giving some glamour to the growing recognition of nursing as a woman's profession was the publicity given Florence Nightingale. She had caught the public imagination and become an international heroine; the American poet Longfellow had turned her into a mythical heroine in his poem which included the lines:

> A lady with a lamp shall stand
> In the great history of the land,
> A noble type of good,
> Heroic womanhood.[18]

A great many women probably had a burning ambition to emulate the popular image of Nightingale, an ambition for which they had some encouragement after the appearance of her *Notes on Nursing*, which had an American edition in 1860, a few months after it first appeared in England.[19] In fact, by the Civil War, the women's rights movement and the demands that women be given the right to enter the medical professions had already laid an effective groundwork for changes in nursing. Although there was still considerable unwillingness by the male physicians to accept women in their domain, there was no real doubt that nursing was suitable for women, and that there they could do an effective job. The Civil War gave them the opportunity to prove the importance of nursing.

As soon as the Civil War broke out, both Northern and Southern women immediately volunteered their services. Ladies's Aid Societies or Soldiers' Aid Societies sprang up all over the country, the first Northern one appearing at Bridgeport, Connecticut, on April 15, 1861, the day the first volunteers were called by President Lincoln. These women offered to sew for the soldiers, to collect necessary supplies, food, clothing, blankets, and other such things, as well as to provide some means of communication between the soldiers and their distant relatives.[20] The women's rights movement was much stronger in the North than in the South, so that women were perhaps more vocal in their demands on key officials, although the Southern women were also handicapped because of the lack of any really centralized authority; as a result, there were many Southern local societies, a few state societies, but no unifying body as in the North. Perhaps the most influential of all the women's groups was started by the women of New York City on April 25, 1861, in the rooms of Elizabeth Blackwell's New York Infirmary for Women and Children. Included in the original group were the leading ladies of the New York women's rights movement and the leading society women of the city, such as the Roosevelts, the Astors, and the Schuylers. Two men, Elisha Harris, superintendent of the quarantine hospital for immigrants on Staten Island, and Henry Bellows, pastor of the First Unitarian Church of New York, were also invited by Elizabeth Blackwell. The result of this meeting was a decision to call a mass rally of New York women at Cooper Institute.[21]

The rally was held on May 3, 1861, the call having been signed by "ninety-two most respected gentlewomen." About 4,000 women gathered in the auditorium to form the Women's Central Association for Relief, headed by Dr. Valentine Mott, the dean of American medical men. Most of the other positions, however, were filled by women. One of the major objectives of the association was the training of nurses. The New York group had also thought of itself as a coordinating group for all other such women's groups in the country; their efforts led to a mission to Washington under the direction of Henry Bellows and the formation of the U.S. Sanitary Commission on June 9, 1861, the so-called fifth wheel of the Civil War.[22]

Tied closely with the nursing effort was Dorothea Dix, who had arrived in Washington in April 1861 and immediately volunteered her services to the government as coordinator of an as yet nonexisting nursing program. Dix had achieved fame for her work in improving prisons and in the founding and establishment of "insane" asylums. Since she was such a famous and influential woman, the War Department, unwilling to antagonize her, finally accepted her offer of some 100 "trained nurses." On June 10 she was granted a commission as "Superintendent of the United States Army Nurses."[23] Even before she had received her commission, however, Dix had contacted Elizabeth Blackwell, seeking her help and advice on the training of nurses. Dix's chief difficulty was the overwhelming number of women wanting to serve; few had had any experience, and some perhaps had other motives than nursing. In order to screen the deluge of volunteers, she listed the following requirements: "No woman under thirty years need apply to serve in the government hospitals. All nurses are required to be very plain looking women. Their dresses must be brown or black, with no bows, no curls, no jewelry, and no hoop skirts."[24]

Despite the dampening effects of admitting to such requirements, would-be nurses still responded. Perhaps typical of the replies was the following: "I am in possession of one of your circulars, and will comply with all your requirements. I am plain looking enough to suit you and old enough. I have no near relatives in the war, no lover there. I have never had a husband and I am not looking for one. Will you take me?"[25]

Dorothea Dix's position as superintendent of army nurses was not without its difficulties, many of which arose from her ambiguous status as a woman in a man's world. She was never empowered to enforce discipline over any army personnel, and, in fact, in October 1863, nurses were placed under the exclusive direction of medical officers, even further limiting her powers. It should also be pointed out that some of the difficulties were caused by the women themselves. Many were imbued with ideas of what a proper lady should or should not do, since woman's role in society, at least that of the "proper" woman, was extremely confining. Moreover, women had not yet learned to be nurses; they were, however, trying. When army doctors chastised them for ignoring orders, some of them became prima donnas of self-righteousness. Still, they were available, and the only alternative was to use able-bodied men, something that every good army commander was hesitant to do.[26] Male nurses were usually disabled soldiers who ceased to be nurses as soon as they were found to be able-bodied. Some of the male nurses, such as Walt Whitman (1819–1892), served unofficially. Whitman, who was regarded as too old to serve in the army, became interested in the plight of the wounded when he visited his wounded brother George. On his return to Washington, he served as an unofficial nurse to Northern and Southern soldiers in the army hospitals. He left a record of his experiences in his prose *Memoranda During the War* (1875), and in some of his poems published in *Drum-Taps* (1865) and *Sequal to Drum-Taps* (1865–1866).[27]

Louisa May Alcott (1832-1888), another of America's literary greats, served as an official nurse in the Civil War under Dorothea Dix. She left nursing when her health failed, but her experiences were preserved in her letters which were published under the title of *Hospital Sketches* (1863).[28] Both Whitman and Alcott achieved their great renown in literature. Many women, however, became famous as nurses. One of the best known was Mary Ann Bickerdyke (1817-1901), known as "Mother Bickerdyke" and as the "General in Calico." A statue in her honor was erected in Galesburg, Illinois. She had attended Oberlin College, and had studied nursing on her own, eventually establishing herself as a "botanic physician" in Galesburg. In 1861 she went to Cairo, Illinois, where the army had established a camp, and soon after to Mound City where many wounded had been gathered after the battle of Belmont. Her reports on the filth, malnutrition, and disease at the Cairo military installation led General Grant to make her organizer and chief of nursing, hospital, and welfare services for the western armies. She later made extensive and careful preparations for General Sherman's march through Georgia. Under her supervision about 300 field hospitals were built, staffed, and equipped.[29]

A military title was given to at least one woman, Captain Sally Tomkins. Before the war Tomkins had been a well-to-do, civic-minded Southern woman whose charitable activities included some volunteer nursing. In July 1861, after the first Battle of Bull Run, called First Manassas by the Confederacy, the Confederate Government realized that it lacked sufficient hospital accommodations. Appeals were made to people to open their homes, and Tomkins took charge of a 25-bed hospital in the home of a friend, Judge John Robertson, in Richmond. As the Confederacy attempted to improve its medical services, the temporary, makeshift hospitals set up for the immediate crisis were ordered closed to conserve medical supplies. Tomkins refused to close her hospital, appealed directly to President Jefferson Davis, and was allowed to keep Robertson Hospital open. To comply with regulations for government control, however, Davis appointed her a captain in the cavalry. Though she received no pay, she could issue orders and draw supplies. During the four years of the war, she took care of some 1,300 sick and wounded soldiers.[30]

As with Florence Nightingale in the Crimea, so it was with nurses in the Civil War—the male establishment did not know quite how to deal with them. Georgeanna Woolsey, one of a family of four sisters who became nurses,[31] wrote that the women nurses endured much opposition:

> Hardly a surgeon of whom I can think received or treated them with even common courtesy. Government had decided that women should be employed, and the army surgeons—unable, therefore, to close the hospitals

against them—determined to make their lives so unbearable that they should be forced in self-defence to leave.[32]

Part of the problem, however, was that the surgeons themselves were not particularly competent. Jane Stuart Woolsey, another of the Woolsey sisters, wrote that contract surgeons were themselves victims of the system:

> They had no position, small pay, and mere nominal rank. They were a temporary expedient in the first place—and who shall say what better one could have been devised for the emergency?—but the emergency went by, and the expedient was stretched into a corps of fifteen hundred men to whose hands were committed the wards of almost all General Hospitals. They served their little term, made their little experiments, and disappeared. The class was bad; it was under no bonds to be anything else; the exceptions were many and more honorable. I have known a "contract surgeon" for three months—six months—to refuse to attend a dying man, or attempt to ease his mortal agony because the patient was "no good anyhow" and the surgeon "had company." I have known one to operate on the slightly injured member and let the shattered one go, and on being "relieved" for drunkenness, begin in a neighboring hospital a fresh career of cutting off the wrong leg. . . . But I have also known contract surgeons faithful, sagacious, tenderhearted, carrying their professional skill and their professional honor into the meanest contraband hut at any hour of the day or night, spending day and night with their soldier patients, watching them, devising every manner of expedient for their relief, humoring their fancies, telling them cheerful stories, tending them like brothers and sons.[33]

Inevitably it was the incompetent surgeon who made life miserable for the nurses, fearful that his incompetency would be observed and known, although the nurses had little power to do anything about it.

The Civil War did get women into the hospitals. Some 3,200 Northern and a proportionate number of Southern women worked as nurses in the war. In the process they guaranteed that nursing would become a woman's profession, something that it has been trying to overcome in recent years. Nowhere can the equation of nursing and women be more effectively demonstrated than in the various patriotic biographies that came out during and after the war. A whole host of women earned such names as "Mother," "Sister," "Aunt," "Lady," or "Angel," if not among the troops, then in the minds of the reading public.[34] Women were beginning to break down many of the barriers erected against them, and nursing allowed them to enter the job market and yet keep within what was regarded as a traditional woman's role. The more enlightened of the medical community began to plan to utilize nurses more effectively.

S. D. Gross, president of the American Medical Association at its 1868 meeting, presented a resolution which stated that it was

> just as necessary to have well-trained, well-instructed nurses as to have intelligent and skillful physicians. . . . there ought to be, in all the principal towns and cities of the Union, institutions for the education of men and women whose duty it is to take care of the sick, and to carry out the injunctions of the medical attendant.[35]

Gross became chairman of a committee which reported in 1869 that good nursing was "half the battle in disease. . . . Thousands of human beings are daily lost by bad nursing." The report cautioned, however, that nursing was "as much of an art and a science as medicine," and that it was a mistake to suppose that "any and every individual, whether male or female, is fitted for such an occupation." Instead, every large and well-organized hospital ought to establish a training school for nurses.

> While it is not at all essential to combine religious exercises with nursing, it is believed that such a union would be eminently conducive to the welfare of the sick in all public institutions; and the Committee therefore earnestly recommend the establishment of nurses' homes, to be placed under the immediate supervision and direction of deaconesses, or lady superintendents . . . and [that] . . . district schools should be formed, and placed under the guardianship of the county medical societies in every State and Territory in the Union, the members of which should make it their business to impart . . . instruction in the art and science of nursing. . . .[36]

The medical profession had recognized the importance of nursing, but before many would be attracted, nursing itself had to change. In 1870 it was more or less standard for a nurse to have charge of about 30 patients on a ward. Day nurses served from 7 A.M. until 10 P.M., while night nurses served from 10 P.M. until 3 P.M. the following day. They were usually allowed four hours leave of absence a week, with time off for church every alternate Sunday. Included in their nursing duties, besides the care of the patient, were cleaning the fireplaces, washing the stairs, sweeping and dusting the wards, serving the patients, washing dishes, and laundering the bandages, so that they could be used again. The most important factor in changing nursing was the growing women's movement. Symbolic of this was the interest of *Godey's Lady's Book and Magazine*, a popular women's magazine, which pointed out the need for better nursing care and for a new attitude toward nursing itself.[37]

New Training Schools

Indicative of the change was the founding, within a six-month period, of three new training schools patterned on the English model.

Bellevue Hospital opened its school in May of 1873, followed in October by the Connecticut Training School in New Haven, and in November by the Boston Training School at Massachusetts General.

The Bellevue school originated through the efforts of Louisa Schuyler, one of the leaders in the U.S. Sanitary Commission and an organizer of the State Charities Aid Association. The Association was a voluntary body for the care of paupers, orphans, and the sick. One of the visiting committees, headed by Mrs. Elizabeth Hobson, visited Bellevue Hospital. The committee reported that most nursing was done by prisoners, that drunkenness was common, that fees were collected from the patients for services, and that, in general, filthy and deplorable conditions existed. They recommended establishing a nurses' training school, but the hospital commissioners and the medical board were somewhat hesitant. To overcome their reluctance, Dr. Gill Wylie, a member of the staff, voluntarily visited England to see what was being done in that country. While he was there, Hobson's group managed to raise $23,000 to establish the school. When Wylie returned, armed with advice from Nightingale and other English nursing leaders, the school began on an experimental basis in some of the hospital wards.

Sister Helen (Miss Bowden), trained in University College Hospital, London, was superintendent. At first the students considered uniforms the badge of a servant, but when Sister Helen and one of the students, Euphemia Van Renssalaer, a member of a prominent New York family, made one consisting of a blue-and-white seersucker dress, white apron, collar and cuffs, it was soon adopted. As the medical staff of the hospital became impressed with the student nurses, more wards were turned over to the control of the nursing school. As the new wards were added, Linda Richards was hired as night supervisor. It is believed that the nursing practice of recording notes about the patients' condition grew out of her practice of keeping notes for her nurses.[38]

Women were also influential in establishing the Boston Training School. They finally persuaded the hospital authorities to open the school, but it was subordinated to the needs of the hospital. No Sister Helen helped to organize the school, so that it lacked the continuity of Bellevue. Two superintendents served during the first year before Linda Richards successfully took over the job. She later also organized the training school at Boston City Hospital, although there was no standard uniform for the school until 1878. It was at Massachusetts General in 1881 that ward maids were first employed, to relieve the nurses of some of their onerous duties, so that the nurses could then devote more attention to the patients.[39]

The Connecticut Training School grew out of a report of a doctors' committee in 1872 which studied the practicability of training nurses. The result was the establishment of a training school, but as a separate entity from the hospital (as with Bellevue). When the school opened, it had three pupils; they served all day in the wards, sat up at night with the sick, cooked, and distributed the meals for patients, and occasionally heard lectures on nursing.

All three of these schools and the many which followed in the next half century, with the possible exception of a school in Waltham, Massachusetts, claimed to be based upon the Nightingale model.[40] Actually the use of the model was selective. Although some of the early training schools had funds to start,[41] none of them were endowed or even adequately financed.[42] Consequently, the hospitals expected more work from the students and felt justified in providing even less academic substance, although they often paid students minimal stipends. The model of weekly lectures at St. Thomas' was less carefully followed in the early American schools.[43] Another radical difference was that American schools did not contract for services after training; instead, the period of training was quickly lengthened to two years, and students signed contracts promising to stay the full time.[44] Those who left early were considered to have violated their contracts and were dishonorably discharged—and hence not eligible for a certificate.[45] Lectures were not ordinarily given during the second year, and in many schools students did private duty nursing in homes and surrendered their fees to the school.[46] The Illinois Training School for Nurses in 1887 was the first school to extend course work into the second year.[47]

The hospital schools in this country did not separate their students by social class or prior education, although after 1900 the academically stronger schools tended to stop the earlier wide-scale practice of paying students a stipend. Thus, there was some selective recruitment of more affluent students into the stronger schools, since poorer students needed the stipends.[48]

Probably the most controversial element of the original Nightingale model was its emphasis on the independent female nursing hierarchy under the direction of the matron, who answered to a nursing school board rather than to the hospital board in matters of educational policy. An alternate approach emphasizing physician control was used in those American schools established before 1873, and afterward was best represented by the school at Waltham, Massachusetts. Dr. Alfred Worcester, founder of the "Waltham Plan," had adapted it from a Swiss school. He argued that since nursing was a "subordinate branch of medical practice" and that since the nurse was "first, last and all the while only the doctor's assistant," only the physician could say what kind of training she should have.[49] When the Johns Hopkins Hospital School was being set up, the opposing methods of control were discussed at length. A compromise between the two alternatives was agreed upon, and the school was placed under the hospital board of trustees rather than under a separate board, but a nurse was made superintentent of the school and of the hospital nursing service.[50] This pattern preponderated in American hospitals, although eventually the nurse administrator came to be further separated from the hospital board when a physician or lay hospital administrator was made top executive. As a result the American superintendent had—and still has—considerably less authority than the British matron.

The one aspect of the Nightingale model adopted without modification in America was the strong emphasis on morality, devotion to duty, and self-sacrifice rather than on intellectual training. An 1898 survey by Jane Hodson of 325 American and Canadian nursing schools reported that candidates were selected for the schools by means of letters of recommendation, and that one of those letters usually had to be from a clergyman who could attest to the good character of the prospective student.[51]

At the end of the nineteenth century, students in most American schools started with a two-month probationary period during which they went to the wards to make beds and do other simple nursing tasks. At the end of this period, they were evaluated; if found satisfactory, they were allowed to wear the school uniform and attend lectures on applied science.[52] Ward duty always took precedence over the lectures, however, as indicated by the following passage:

> Some knowledge of Anatomy, Physiology, Materia-Medica and Hygiene being found necessary, every training school has established a theoretical course which must, however, always be incidental to the ward work, though moving as it were hand in hand with it. Training schools for nurses can thus never be ranked as strictly educational . . . and the term 'school' might be misleading, not indicating the fact that the time of the pupil nurse is largely spent in actual physical labor.[53]

The usual hours on duty were from 7 A.M. to 7 P.M. with three hours off for dinner, study, and recreation. Night nurses whose work was considered "less laborious" worked from 7 P.M. to 7 A.M. without time off.[54] Apparently, by 1898 the larger hospitals were able to keep most of the students busy because the practice of sending students to do private duty in homes, so that the schools could collect the fees, was common only in the smaller schools.[55]

Strengths of the Nursing School Movement

Immediate results of the new nursing schools were seen in patient benefits. Most observers of the time remarked on the change. For example, soon after the training school was established at Bellevue, the appearance of the wards was reported to have improved dramatically.[56] Though some of the early schools, such as the Boston Training School at Massachusetts General Hospital, had been established primarily to improve educational opportunities for women,[57] this concern soon became secondary.[58] Hospital administrators had found that establishing a nursing school not only improved conditions, but often reduced the cost of nursing, since much of the work could be justified as training. Moreover, by encouraging women in increasing numbers to enter nursing, they ensured that there would be a growing supply to meet the demand caused by the rapid growth of hospitals which reflected the changing nature of medicine. Medicine itself could adjust to the change because many of the services previously offered by physicians, were now being relegated to nurses. Growth was indeed rapid. In 1890 there were fifteen nursing schools; in 1900 there were 432, an almost 3,000 percent increase.

With the discovery of anesthesia, the bacteriological revolution initiated by Pasteur and Koch, and the work of Lister in developing antiseptic surgery, the foundations for modern medical and surgical treatment of illness had been laid. The hospital now became the chief focus of modern medicine, which would not have been feasible without nursing care of a much higher order than had been given by the untrained—and often unmotivated—nurses of the past. The medical revolution which occurred in the late nineteenth and early twentieth centuries was largely financed and facilitated by the labor of student nurses, and in America the basic reform in medical education coincided with the rise of modern nursing.

Obviously, the system did not look the same to a late nineteenth-century observer as it does to us today. Where we might see exploitation, most early nurses saw an opportunity for women to enter a useful occupation, and it was women who counted since the training school movement virtually eliminated males from nursing. In Hodson's survey of 325 schools, there were only eight general hospitals and 21 insane asylums which admitted male students.[59] While this discrimination has had serious negative consequences for the profession, it did give a monopoly to women at a time when they had few other occupational opportunities. The choices for untrained women outside of the home were virtually limited to retail clerking, factory labor, domestic service, or prostitution.[60] With some education a woman could teach or work in an office as a "typewriter," but education for most women was circumscribed, since public high schools and coeducational colleges on a broad scale are essentially twentieth-century developments. Although the women's colleges, like Smith, Barnard, and Vassar, were established simultaneously with the nursing schools, they were expensive, and their curriculums were not designed to prepare for a career.[61] Thus, despite its exploitive nature and the very real possibility of an early death from tuberculosis or other infectious disease,[62] nursing, nevertheless, offered a reasonable alternative to women of modest means who wanted an education which would equip them for a career. One of the biographers of Annie Goodrich explains her reason for entering nursing school in 1890 after her family had suffered financial setbacks:

> Annie, always an independent girl with a keen sense of responsibility, felt the need to be self-supporting. . . . She was quite honest with herself and admitted that she did not like nursing—far from it. She hated sickness and had a horror of death; nevertheless, since few vocational fields were open to women at the time she decided that entering the nursing profession was the best way to solve her problem.[63]

Thus, the system worked in many ways. The hospitals and physicians were pleased to have the service of a dedicated group of workers at such modest cost; the patients were better cared for than ever before; and nurses were afforded the opportunity to do useful work outside the home.[64] Although there were occasional shortages of candidates, the schools could manipulate admission standards to satisfy their needs for staff.[65]

The entrance of women into nursing was world-wide. The formation of the Red Cross, the growth of imperialism, the expansion of Christian (and, to a much less extent, Jewish) medical missions, all contributed to the growth of nursing. In all of these America and England were prominent, as were other Western European countries. As a result, many of the newer nursing concepts became internationally accepted.

The Red Cross

The man behind the Red Cross was Jean Henri Dunant (1828–1910) of Geneva, Switzerland. Henri (the name he used to distinguish himself from his father, Jean-Jacques Dunant) was a deeply religious Calvinist. As a teen-ager he took part in a "League of Alms," a group of young men who visited the poor of Geneva. They preached, distributed medicine, nursed the sick, and even gave them money. Dunant's Sunday afternoons were spent in the prisons of Geneva discussing religion with the inmates; Sunday evenings were centered around a group known as the Christian Union of Young People, one of the founding bodies in 1855 of the International Young Men's Christian Association. Henri would have spent his life working on such projects, but his father insisted that he be a businessman.

Through his family connections Dunant joined a banking firm which sent him to Algeria in 1853, where he conceived a rather grandiose scheme for building flour mills to grind wheat which the natives would plant. He organized a company to sell shares in this project, but it was soon floundering, and many of his friends went deeply into debt. To save what he could, he sought support from Emperor Napoleon III, a nephew of the earlier Napoleon. To improve his case, he wrote a highly laudatory biography of Napoleon III which he intended to present to the Emperor and thus win him over. With his book in hand, he set out to meet the ruler of France.

Napoleon at this time was in Italy fighting against Austria in one of the wars that eventually led to a united Italy. The war was not well planned on either side; through a series of blunders the French and their Italian allies fought the Austrians at Solferino, a small town in Lombardy, on June 24, 1859. The battle was probably the most murderous of the century: some 350,000 men fought in the one-day battle, and there were more than 40,000 casualties. The French had ambulance equipment and medical personnel to care for only 3,000 men, while the Austrians were even less prepared. In this chaos Dunant appeared en route to see Napoleon. When he saw the wounded still lying on the battlefield, he forgot about his original mission; instead, he devoted his time to caring for the casualties of the battlefield. By evening he had some 300 volunteers obeying his orders, treating Italian, French, and Austrian troops. When his resources were exhausted, he wrote to his friends in Geneva, and under the spell of Dunant's compassion and horror they dispatched volunteers. Gradually some sort of order came out of the battlefield.[66]

When his relief work was well under way, Dunant dashed off to see Napoleon III; his mission was unsuccessful, and he returned to care for the wounded. In fact, he devoted so much of his time and energy to the task that he became ill and was forced to return to Switzerland. Dunant, however, continued to be haunted by what he had seen at Solferino, especially the lack of adequate medical care for the sick, the wounded, and the dying. In order to carry his message to a larger audience, he published a book, *Un Souvenir de Solferino* (*Recollections of Solferino*), in which he painted war in all its horrors. In concluding the book he asked:

> But why have I told of all these scenes of pain and distress, and perhaps aroused painful emotions in my readers? Why have I lingered with seeming complacency over lamentable pictures, tracing their details with what may appear desperate fidelity?
>
> Would it not be possible, in time of peace and quiet, to form relief societies for the purpose of having care given to the wounded in wartime by zealous, devoted and thoroughly qualified volunteers. . . . There is need . . . for volunteer orderlies and volunteer nurses, zealous, trained and experienced, whose position would be recognized by the commanders or armies in the field, and their mission facilitated and supported.[67]

Three printings of the book were issued within four months. Dunant made sure that important persons in most of the European countries were given copies. He also made converts to his idea, the most influential being Gustave Moynier, the president of the Genevan Society for Public Benefit. Moynier threw the support of the society behind Dunant, and a conference to discuss Dunant's proposals was called at Geneva on October 26, 1863. Sixty-two delegates from sixteen nations as well as the Prussian Order of Knights Hospitalers attended. Several resolutions were passed at the conference which the delegates were to submit to their governments for approval. One of the immediate results was the founding of national relief committees, first in Prussia and then in the other German and Italian states and in Spain. Dunant himself managed to get France tentatively to accept the resolutions. When England also agreed, another conference was scheduled for Geneva in August 1864. It was at this conference that the justly renowned Geneva Convention was framed. The United States, then involved in the Civil War, only sent unofficial delegates. By 1866 twenty countries had adhered to the Geneva Convention for the Amelioration of the Fate of Wounded Soldiers of Armies in the Field. The growing body came to be known as the Red Cross from its symbol, a red cross on a white background. This was a modification of the Swiss flag, a white cross on a red background, indicative perhaps of the Swiss influence in its founding. Later, when the Muslim countries joined the International Red Cross, they adopted the Red Crescent to avoid the religious symbolism of the cross. The first effective use of the Geneva Convention was during the Austrian–Prussian War in 1866 when Prussia declared that she would employ the provisions of the Geneva Convention. Austria, which had not yet agreed to the Convention, was forced by international opinion to follow suit. Other countries soon joined, although the United States did adhere until 1882.

Once the Red Cross was successfully established, Dunant became less involved in its activities. He had gone bankrupt in 1867, partly from devoting so much time to Red Cross activities, but also because he was not a very effective businessman. When Dunant's bankruptcy became known, the Genevans in control of the Red Cross feared that this might reflect on the Red Cross itself; as a result, they pushed him into the background. While he still occasionally spoke for the Red Cross, he turned increasingly to other dreams for improving the world. He conceived of an international world library society, a society to prevent war, and others, none of which really became effective. Then for fifteen years (1875–1890) he disappeared from the international scene. His whereabouts were, of course, known to his friends and family, but it was not until toward the end of that period, when he and his family came to a financial agreement which gave him some security, that the world realized that he was still alive. In 1890 he became a patient in the deaconess hospital in the Swiss village of Heiden. He remained in Heiden the rest of his life, not even leaving it when he was awarded a share of the first Nobel Peace Prize in 1901. During his last years he was in a coma; he died in 1910.

Since the Red Cross was originally designed to alleviate the wounded in battle, it seems natural that it would have a great influence on nursing. This influence, unfortunately, was not felt very strongly in the United States or in England. In the United States the society was rather late in getting organized, and then it was as a private agency—even though it had a Congressional charter—with very limited financial backing. Under Clara Barton's leadership the Red Cross concentrated on disaster relief rather than nursing or medical care; it was not even the official body for supplying nurses in the Spanish-American War.[68] The English Red Cross suffered from some of the same handicaps, although it was organized earlier. In most of Europe, however, the Red Cross became an official, or at least a semiofficial, agency of the government with both national and international prestige behind it.

Nursing Reform in Europe and Elsewhere

The Red Cross did not attempt to impose uniform nursing practices but adopted or modified the existing nursing tradition in any particular country. In the Scandinavian countries where the Kaiserswerth movement had recently been established, the Red Cross sought to establish secular nursing groups, based to some extent on the Nightingale reforms. In Germany, where the Kaiserswerth movement was very advanced, the Red Cross established motherhouses on the Kaiserswerth model; it was not until much later that strictly secular nurses appeared, and then they had to fight the motherhouses for the control of nursing by nurses rather than religious orders.

The rise of the secular nursing movement was aided in Germany, as it was in the United States, by the various women's movements. As a result of this struggle, nursing was divided into three categories: free secular nurses, nurses in the various religious orders, and the sisterhoods of the Red Cross societies. In Switzerland, Holland, and most other Protestant countries, nursing was also shared between religious societies and free secular nursing groups, with increasing emphasis on the latter. In Russia nursing was at first done by religious orders, among them the Kaiserswerth deaconess movement, which had been introduced there early from Germany. When the Russian Red Cross was organized, however, it was given charge of the training of the nurses. Here the Red Cross schools were secularized and the title of "nurse" could only be awarded through examination.

Most Catholic countries, where nursing had long been recognized as the more or less exclusive province of the religious orders, were somewhat slower to reform their systems, perhaps because the need was not so immediately apparent. The advances in medicine, however, required better nursing care, and the nuns found that their previous methods were inadequate. They, too, turned to newer methods of training. The religious orders that usually were first affected by the new training concepts were those located in multireligious countries like the United States; here, competition with secular institutions encouraged efforts toward reform. The Sisters of Mercy in Chicago and the Sisters of St. Mary's in Brooklyn opened their own schools in 1889; by 1910 almost every active hospital order in the United States had fairly well-developed training schools. In Europe and in Latin America, however, some of the orders were more reluctant to change their old ways, perhaps because they lacked the pressures that were present in the United States.

In France, nursing reform followed the defeat of the French by the Prussians in the Franco-Prussian War (1870–1871), which demonstrated the inadequacy of much of the old French methods of nursing, which had already been under attack. Commissions from 1833 had reported on the insufficiency and bad organization of nursing in the Parisian hospitals, but little had been done. Many of the Parisian hospitals no longer used nuns as nurses, but instead paid low fees to anyone who would nurse the sick, which inevitably led the so-called nurses to exploit the patients. Finally, following the Franco-Prussian War, the Municipal Council of Paris reorganized all the city departments, including the one dealing with hospitals.

Nursing schools were opened at four Paris hospitals: the Salpêtrière, Bicêtre, Pitié, all in 1878, and in 1894 at the Lariboisière, largely through the efforts of Dr. Bourneville, a prominent neurologist, ardent republican, and free-thinker. Unfortunately, since few of the pupils in the schools were literate, it was necessary to start at the very lowest levels, and since reading and writing were not compulsory, some of the nurses failed to advance. Lectures, as in American hospitals of the time, were also given at inconvenient times, and it was often difficult for even the dedicated student to attend. Despite the inadequacy of the schools, they did overcome the opposition of many groups who had resisted any change in nursing procedures. Nuns gradually accepted the idea of education for nurses, attending the optional instruction first in civilian dress, then openly and officially in habit.[69]

Such schools could only be makeshift expedients, however. The way had been prepared for better nursing by the establishment of universal compulsory public education after the Franco-Prussian War, but French nursing needed a leader. This role fell to Dr. Anna Hamilton (1864–1936), who introduced the Nightingale system into France. Hamilton, like

Florence Nightingale, was born near Florence, Italy, of an English father and a French mother. She received a medical degree but became more concerned about her patients' care than about prescribing medicine for them. In attempting to improve this care, her interests turned increasingly to nursing. The result was a doctoral dissertation on the care of the sick in hospitals in which she criticized nursing as it then existed in France and recommended some of the reforms of Florence Nightingale.[70] She was given an opportunity to realize her ideas when she was summoned to reform the nursing in a Protestant hospital in Bordeaux. This hospital had established a short Red Cross nursing course earlier, but it was more like a nurses' aide training program than a nursing school.

Dr. Hamilton remained determined to reform French nursing; with the aid of a young Englishwoman, London-Hospital-trained Catherine Elston, she did. Other hospitals soon followed her methods, until by 1907 her program was established in Paris itself under the Director-General of the Paris Department of Public Charities. This meant the end of the service of the Augustinian Nuns as nurses at the Hôtel Dieu in January 1908 after centuries of service. The nuns, who had resisted the changes in nursing procedures, soon modified their opposition, entered training, and regained much of their nursing reputation. Once the barriers had fallen, numerous other groups, religious and political, entered the movement for better nursing care.[71]

Nightingale methods were introduced into Spain by nurses trained under Hamilton, but nursing reform was much slower there because of the position of women in Spanish society. English influence was also important in introducing nursing reform into Italy. Here Amy Turton, an Englishwoman, the Princess Strongoli, a lady-in-waiting to the Queen of Italy, and Grace Baxter from Johns Hopkins led the reform program. An English matron, Edith Cavell, was in charge of the first reformed training school in Belgium in 1907. Cavell (1865–1915) later came to be considered one of the nurse heroines of World War I when the Germans executed her during their occupation of Belgium for helping French and British soldiers to escape.[72]

In the United States the lack of affiliation between nurses and the Red Cross was remedied when Mabel T. Boardman succeeded Clara Barton as head of the Red Cross. Evidence of this change was the formation of a Red Cross Nursing Service in 1909 under the direction of Jane Arminda Delano (1862-1919), a Bellevue-trained nurse. After World War I the American Red Cross was instrumental in helping to establish or reestablish training schools in Prague, Czechoslovakia; Warsaw and Poznan in Poland; Sofia, Bulgaria; and Istanbul, Turkey. In each of these countries, the American Red Cross cooperated with the national society in extending nursing reform. From these schools grew others. The Warsaw graduates, for example, staffed the new Cracow school which was established by a Rockefeller Foundation grant in 1925.[73]

Imperialism and Nursing

While nursing reform in much of Europe and in America was being effected by forces within these countries and by the Red Cross, Western concepts of nursing were also being carried to the rest of the world. This was because Western civilization had become imperialistic: European and American power and influence were being extended over the rest of the world through conquest, trade expansion, exploitation, and other means. This movement had started with the discovery of America and the settlement of the North and South American continents. It had continued with the discovery and settlement of Australia and New Zealand, and the English conquest of India. But the movement had slowed down toward the end of the eighteenth century when the United States and Latin America had gained independence. During the late nineteenth century, however, the movement reached a new height, stimulated by the Industrial Revolution. The application of machine processes and the development of the factory systems vastly increased the production of marketable commodities. Countries that had become industrialized, first England and then others, sought new markets for their goods. Explorations in the underdeveloped areas of the world revealed a wealth of raw materials and potential customers for Western goods. The result was an exploitation of areas less-advanced industrially, an exploitation made easier because the same knowledge that had transformed production had created new military equipment and developed new war techniques. Underdeveloped areas found it practically impossible to resist European invasions.

England was in the lead in this expansion, but other states—France, Germany, the United States, Belgium, and Italy—quickly followed. Old imperialistic powers such as Spain, Portugal, and the Netherlands which had played an important part in the early expansion of Europe lost ground, although they participated to a lesser extent. Between 1870 and 1910 European domination spread over the globe, in effect also making Western civilization dominant. The entire continent of Africa was partitioned among the European powers, becoming French Africa or German Africa or British Africa. Asia and the numerous islands of the Pacific were almost completely parceled out into political dependencies or economic spheres of influence. China was divided into British, French, German, Russian, and even American spheres. The United States took over the Philippines, Hawaii, Alaska, and Puerto Rico, and extended its influence everywhere. Only Japan in Asia was able to emerge from the struggle comparatively strengthened, and she soon also began expanding in the Far East.

Imperialism was undesirable in its exploitation of subjugated peoples and increased competition among nations. The French were afraid that they would have less territory or prestige than the British; the Germans wanted their place in the sun; and Japan argued she had to expand to save herself. The result was that international tension grew apace. Unfortunately, European wars could no longer be localized because European interests were all over the globe. Eventually, also the subject peoples resented Western domination and wanted independence. This helps account for the many revolutions of the last few years and the many newly independent countries, in Africa especially.

But imperialism perhaps had some side effects which benefited the subject peoples. One of the indirect results was the introduction of Western medicine and nursing to the rest of the world. Imperialism usually required armies, and armies required medical attendants; Western physicians and nurses appeared all over the world to care for soldiers and civilians outside the fatherland. The Americans, as an aftermath of the Spanish-American War, helped establish nurse training schools in Cuba, the first of which opened in 1899.[74] Several other schools were established in Cuba by the Army and were staffed by American nurses until 1909 when Cuban nurses took over the schools. In the Philippines agitation for nursing training schools began soon after the American occupation. It was not until 1907, however, that a school was established at the Philippines Normal School. By treaty the United States was committed to provide education and medical care for the native peoples of Alaska, so that hospitals and eventually training schools were founded there also. When the United States Marines occupied Haiti in 1915, one of the results was a nurse training school under the direction of two Navy nurses.[75] They were later replaced by Red Cross nurses and eventually by Haitians. What was true for the United States was more or less true for the other imperial powers.

Many of the constituent members of the British Empire (now Commonwealth), such as Canada, New Zealand, and Australia, were themselves Western in origin. Nursing reform in these areas followed much the same pattern as in the United States and England. Most of the early hospitals in Canada were staffed by nuns and many were older than the hospitals in the United States. The distinction of introducing the first training school into the country is held by the General and Marine Hospital at St. Catherine's, Ontario. Dr. Theophilus Mack organized the school in 1874 by importing two Nightingale nurses from England. At about the same time, Montreal General Hospital was seeking advice from Nightingale to organize its own school. The school was founded in 1875, but because of the absence of a satisfactory superintendent, it was only successfully established in 1890. Toronto General took steps as early as 1877 to organize its school, but it was not opened until 1881. Catholic sisterhoods made efforts to keep up with the progress in nursing. The Sisters of St. Joseph inaugurated a school for nurses in September 1892 in Toronto. Others soon followed. By 1909 there were 70 Canadian schools for nursing, most of which had a three-year program similar to the American ones.[76]

Missionaries and Nursing

Helping to expand nursing reforms were various missionary groups. Most of Christianity's expansion has been due to widespread evangelical efforts. Missionaries had followed the early Spanish and Portuguese explorers in the Americas and elsewhere; often they were the explorers themselves. The nineteenth century witnessed a tremendous expansion of Christianity outside Europe and America led by Catholic, Protestant, and Orthodox missionaries.

Older Catholic religious orders such as the Jesuits, Franciscans, and Dominicans were supplemented by many new societies. By 1910 there were around 41,000 Catholic missionaries in Africa, Asia, and Oceania. This new wave of missionary endeavors produced the sought-after results. At the beginning of the century the Philippines, long held by Spain, were the only part of the world outside Europe and America where the Catholic Church was firmly established. There were Catholic groups in India and elsewhere, but their numbers were rapidly shrinking. By the end of the nineteenth century, however, there were millions of Catholics in India, China, and Africa, and increasing numbers in Japan and Korea.

Protestant Christianity showed much the same result. New Protestant missionary groups such as the Baptist Society for Propagating the Gospel among the Heathens, the Presbyterian and Congregationalist London Missionary Society, and the Episcopal Church Missionary Society were founded. By 1910 active Protestant missionaries totaled over 18,000, and Protestantism in one form or another won almost an equal number of converts as did Catholicism. The Orthodox Church also joined in this movement, especially the Orthodox Church of Russia. Other Orthodox Churches had just freed themselves from Turkish rule and were as yet too weak to proselytize, but they too joined when they could. By 1910 the Orthodox Church had some 15,000,000 followers in Asia. All told, Christianity was professed outside traditionally Western Christian circles by some 41,000,000 persons, most of whom were missionary converts.

Proselytizing was often carried out in underdeveloped areas through medical missions, hospitals, and nurse training schools. Protestants perhaps established more such missions than Catholics did, but both groups were active.[77] Some of these medical missionaries, like Albert Schweitzer, achieved international fame for their work. But whether famous or not, most were dedicated healers. While the establishment of training schools was usually not the primary aim of these missionaries, they did found them. The American Gordon S. Seagrave, the "Burma Surgeon" of World War II, is perhaps typical of many of these missionaries. Trained at Johns Hopkins University in the United States, he went to Burma in 1922. His first success was removing a goiter—the first time in northern Burma that a goiter had been successfully removed. This led to such a rapid increase in his surgical case load that Seagrave needed nurses to help him and to staff his hospital. Like many another missionary before him, he decided to train his own nurses. To do so, he started literally from nothing, translating or writing his own nursing texts. He turned to outside help for trained nurses to teach actual nursing procedures; when this was accomplished, the school was soon graduating nurses. Since most of them did not have the educational background of many Western nurses, there was much more repetition in instruction; but once they learned, these missionary nurses proved very satisfactory. Soon, in fact, Burmese women were running his training school.[78]

In China one of the first hospitals to establish a training school was St. Luke's in Shanghai, under the direction of both the Presbyterian and Methodist missions. Several other schools, mostly mission ones, were established between 1900 and 1909. The Rockefeller Foundation established the Peking Union Medical College in 1920, which helped set high standards for Chinese nursing. By 1937, at the time of the Japanese invasion, there were 183 training schools recognized by the Chinese Nursing Association. In Korea the Severance School was opened in 1906, the pioneer of many future schools there.[79]

The American Board of Missions sent Linda Richards to Japan in September 1885 to develop a training school. The school, affiliated with the Charity Hospital in Tokyo, graduated its first four pupils in June 1888.[80] Shortly before this the Japanese Red Cross joined the international association and began the training of nurses. Nursing in Japan, as well as in much of Asia and Africa, differed from that in Europe and America by its emphasis on the outpatient department. When the patient had to stay in the hospital, his family stayed with him, caring and cooking for him, even sleeping near him. Nurses took temperatures, but the medicines were usually administered by the patient's family on instructions from the nurse. Under this system the nurse was like a doctor's aide. The Japanese model in particular spread throughout much of the Far East with the Japanese conquests into Korea, Taiwan (Formosa), and elsewhere.

The first regular training school in India was established in 1886 in

Bombay through funds made available by the Countess of Dufferin, wife of the English Viceroy. The course offered by the school, under the direction of English nurses, was at first for one year, but it was soon extended to three years.[81] The Zenana Bible Medical Mission opened its school at Benares in 1888. The Canadian Presbyterian Mission established a training school in 1898, and the American Evangelical Lutheran Mission opened a school at Guntu in 1899. Nursing in India, however, was severely handicapped by the caste system. It was considered an "untouchable" profession, with the result that women whose background fitted them for nursing were reluctant to enter the profession.

In Africa nursing programs were instituted by the various colonial powers, by the missions, by the Red Cross, and by the numerous international bodies that were founded after World Wars I and II. In Liberia the first training school was established at Phebe Hospital in 1921 by the American Lutheran Mission. Several others soon followed, so that by the end of World War II there were four training schools, three of which were under mission auspices. Training in these schools followed the American plan. Ethiopia, which for a long time was the only independent African country besides Liberia, was even slower in getting its programs established. Not until after World War II did the Red Cross and various mission bodies open schools. Especially important was the Princess Tsahai Memorial Hospital and Nursing School established in memory of a daughter of the then emperor who had trained in England but died after her return to Ethiopia. In the Union of South Africa, the first nursing school was established in the 1880's. The first nursing registration in the British Empire was established at Cape Colony in 1891.[82]

In Latin America, most of which achieved independence in the early nineteenth century, there was a long tradition of nursing by religious groups. The European ties of these countries were with Spain or Portugal, both of which were slow to reform their own nursing systems. Women in many of the Latin American countries were not encouraged to take regular studies; and in those families where women were more emancipated, nursing was considered work for nuns or servants, not for a proper young lady. Because of these factors, nursing reform came slowly south of the Rio Grande. In a few countries—Brazil, Argentina, Chile, Uruguay, and perhaps Mexico—there were some attempts to introduce modern methods around the turn of the century. Effective reforms did not develop until after World War I, when many Latin American physicians and surgeons began to take postgraduate training in the United States. Here they encountered a different type of nurse, which they very much admired and tried to introduce into their own countries. For help they turned to the United States, especially to the Rockefeller Foundation, which set up training schools throughout Latin America and awarded postgraduate fellowships in the United States or Canada. The Red Cross helped found schools in a few countries, while Catholic orders in Brazil, Colombia, Mexico, and Venezuela initiated training schools. Some American Protestant groups also began establishing medical missions.[83]

Perhaps typical of the more active missionary denominations is the program of the Seventh-Day Adventist Church. The first training school of this denomination outside the United States was established in Denmark in 1897. After this it rapidly expanded its overseas program. By 1950 the church had nine training schools in Europe; a training school in Ethiopia and Nigeria, several hospitals in Africa, where minimal training for native nurses was given, and training schools in Korea, Japan, the Philippines, Thailand, Iraq, Jamaica, Australia, and Latin America. The denomination, as churches go, is fairly small, but multiply its example by several other churches active in the field, and it is apparent how many missionary activities led to the spread of nursing.[84]

Christian groups were not alone in establishing "missionary" hospitals or training schools. Jewish groups founded training schools in countries where there were Jewish residents. In America the Jewish hospitals were in the forefront of the nursing reform movement. In Israel the Henrietta Szold School of Nursing was set up by Hadassah, a Jewish women's organization, in 1918. This was the first nursing school in which the instruction was in Hebrew. By the end of World War II, seven schools were operating in Israel under Jewish auspices, financed for the most part by contributions from the United States. After Israel won its independence, the number of schools increased.[85]

International Organization

As the nursing movement spread, it became obvious that an international association should be organized. The leader in this was Ethel Gordon Fenwick (Mrs. Bedford Fenwick, 1857–1947), former matron at St. Bartholomew's in England, and one of the leaders in the organization of British nurses. At a Matrons' Council conference in 1899, she proposed to organize an international association of nurses. The Matrons' Council proceeded to call a meeting of nurses in London which founded the International Council of Nurses on July 1, 1899. A provisional committee, composed of members from Great Britain and Ireland, the United States, Canada, New Zealand, Australia, Denmark, Holland, and Cape Colony in South Africa, drew up a constitution which was adopted with some amendments in July 1900. At this meeting Fenwick was elected president, Lavinia Dock of the United States secretary, and a Canadian nurse, Mary Agnes Snively, treasurer. The council sought to encourage the self-government of nurses through their national associations, to raise nursing educational standards, to establish professional ethics, and to increase the public usefulness of its members.

The original plan was to have ultimately one national association from each country represented on the council. At the time of organization, however, the national nursing associations were not sufficiently organized to make this possible. The International Council of Nurses at first then included only individual members. These *councilors*, as they were called, acted as represenative nurses from each country. By 1904 three countries had national organizations eligible for affiliation—the United States, England, and Germany—so these became charter members. Other associations were accepted as they met the standards; an indication of nursing progress in any one country is the date they were admitted into the council. By World War II there were 32 members plus eight countries without national associations that were therefore classified as associate members. After the war the association continued to expand. Headquarters were first in London, then from 1925 to 1937 at Geneva, then back to London until the Outbreak of World War II, when they were transferred to the United States. In 1947 the association again transferred its headquarters to London.[86]

The formation of the International Council of Nurses (ICN) gave nurses a voice in the development of nursing programs throughout the world. It helped set minimal standards in nursing education, although the ICN recognized that each country's nursing programs must develop in accordance with the traditions of that country. With the foundation of the ICN nursing came of age on the international scene.

Six

The Problems of a
Developing Profession

Once it was recognized that a nursing school improved the care of the sick, there was a rapid proliferation of hospital training schools. Unfortunately, much of this mushrooming growth was not particularly beneficial to nursing. There were both a shortage of trained teachers to staff the new nursing schools and a lack of financial support for them. Many of the hospital training school founders considered the trained hospital nurse as simply a substitute for the competent mother or neighbor who cared for the sick at home. Since the average housewife scrubbed her own floors and did the family washing, it was assumed that these and similar chores were part of the work of a nurse. Students were paid little or nothing and had to work long and hard hours for their board, room, and what little instruction they received. Such practices allowed a hospital to be staffed very cheaply and to provide better nursing care than ever before. Because of this type of training, schools were soon started by almost every hospital in the country, regardless of size; this exploited the nursing students, but few people bothered to ask if such procedures might be harmful in the long run—it was enough to establish a nursing school.

This had implications for the whole nature and practice of medicine which have been too often overlooked in the standard histories. Modern medicine is quite obviously hospital medicine, and the key to modern hospitals is nursing. Medical practice before the growth of hospitals generally involved physician visits to the home of the patient where the necessary tasks were performed, including even what was called kitchen surgery, done on the kitchen table. In some of the larger cities, physicians had patients come to them and had special surgeries attached to their office. Hospitals were for the poor and the dying. The discovery of anesthetics and of the importance of aseptic procedures changed hospitals from institutions where people went to die to institutions where they went to get well. Hospitals were no longer only for the poor, but for the middle and upper classes as well. The emergence of nursing coincided with this development and made it possible. For example, when the Nightingale Training Schools were being established in the United States in 1873, there were only 149 hospitals and related institutions in the whole country, and fully one-third of these were for the mentally ill. Fifty years later there were 6,762 hospitals, and hospital beds had increased from 35,453 to 770,375.[1]

Arthur Hertzler, a Kansas physician who wrote his memoirs in the

1930's, recalled the transition from visiting his patients to having them visit him in his office, and finally to establishing his own hospital. In analyzing his reasons for building a hospital, he wrote:

> I had a surgical education but I had to face the fact that a surgeon is not a surgeon if he has no patients. . . . I had done some operating in private houses . . . [but] it seemed to me that if I had a hospital I could augment my surgical practice. . . . I had no intention of building a considerable institution. . . . It was to be a meal ticket . . . until I could build up a city practice. . . . At any rate, almost simultaneously the idea of building a hospital . . . occurred to a number of doctors. . . . As a result . . . many small hospitals sprang up in small towns even when the distance from an established hospital was not great. Actual need, therefore, was not a very compelling factor. I know of one small town which had five hospitals, the number, curiously enough, being exactly equal to the number of doctors located there. . . . At one time Kansas had more "hospitals" per capita than any other state in the Union. . . . After the hospital became a sort of epidemic, many churches established hospitals; either by building a new one in opposition to the private hospital, or by taking over a private one and with this as a nucleus building a sizable institution.[2]

Hertzler utilized one "trained" nurse in his hospital, and she received $40 a month plus room and board. Two "girls," each receiving $2 a week, did the cooking and the laundry. They also received room and board. His assistant received $50 a month and boarded himself, while a janitor, who had charge of general supplies as well, received $25.[3]

Hertzler's personalized account emphasizes the second reason for rapid expansion of nursing: the opportunity for women to earn a living. Room and board plus $40 a month was a lot better than the $2 a week received by the serving "girls" in Hertzler's hospital, and for women who had the choice of being either domestics or nurses there was no comparison. During the late nineteenth century several emerging women's professions appeared, all closely correlated to tasks that women had done in the home or as volunteer activity: nursing, social work, elementary school teaching, librarianship, and secretarial work. All faced similar difficulties in establishing an identity, although nursing had different kinds of problems than the others because of the dominance of the physician in the medical field. Although all five occupations, which appeared when women were entering the world at large, became women's professions, nursing was more so than the others because the hospital training school came to be regarded as a home away from home, and the home for nursing students as established by most hospitals excluded males.

Nurses not only had to overcome the disabilities facing women in general, they also had to demarcate a new area of expertise for themselves, always being careful not to antagonize the physician. Despite the nurse's willingness to be subordinate, the appearance of trained nurses inevitably involved conflicts with physicians and agency administrators, even when members of these groups had encouraged the establishment of nurse training schools. Nurses, nonetheless, assumed much of the responsibility once left solely to physicians, and thereby became a major factor in changing the nature of medicine. The struggle was not easy, since many physicians feared that nurses would undermine their authority, and since nurses themselves, in dealing with the male-dominated profession of medicine, usually tended to avoid a head-on collision by pretending to adopt—or often really adopting—a clearly subordinate role. This was more common in the United States than in Great Britain, where the nurses had established effective independent authority. In the United States, because of the vast proliferation of hospital training schools, it was more difficult to attain independent control in the hospitals, since most hospital nursing, except in the hospitals with less than 50 beds, was done by nurses in training.

Because American nursing had an overwhelming majority of women, it becomes almost a classic case study of a woman's profession trying to achieve recognition and independence in a society dominated by men. For example, it would seem obvious that nursing needed some kind of organization to set guidelines and minimum standards. This, however, was much easier to recognize than to accomplish. Part of the difficulty was that women were not yet recognized as independent individuals. Under English and American common law, a woman was legally under the domination of a male—father, husband, brother, or guardian. Although after the Civil War various American states began to give women statutory relief through a series of laws generally known as the Married Women's Acts, there were still many obstacles to overcome before a women's organization could be established. This partly explains why the U.S. Sanitary Commission, even though its original impetus had come from women's groups, was presided over by men. There were in fact no national women's organizations of any type before the Civil War.

The first were the two suffrage associations organized in 1869; these were followed in 1874 by the Women's Christian Temperance Union. Their membership was never very large. More women belonged to local church associations or groups, but each of these was more or less independent until 1877, when the International Conference of Women's Christian Associations was organized, the forerunner to the modern YWCA. In 1881 a small group of collegiate alumnae met in Boston to form the organization now known as the American Association of University Women, while the National Pan-Hellenic Association of College Sororities was organized in 1891, 24 years after the founding of the first sorority. There were also a few secret and benefit lodges for women which had been established as auxiliaries to the men's societies, primarily because it was thought necessary "to reconcile women to the lifelong pledge of secrecy made by their husbands." None of these groups could be called professional, and in fact the nursing associations were the first professional groups to be organized and controlled by women in the United States.[4]

Nursing Organization

The initiative for organization came from Isabel Hampton (1860–1910), then superintendent and principal of the Johns Hopkins Hospital Nursing School. Miss Hampton (or Mrs. Robb, as she was known after her marriage to Dr. Hunter Robb in 1894) was a former teacher who, believing that nursing offered many opportunities, had entered the Bellevue school in 1881. In 1888 she was made head of the Illinois Training School for Nurses in Chicago, and after serving there for only a short time, she moved on to Johns Hopkins. The dedication that many of the early leaders of American nursing felt toward their profession is indicated by their reaction to Hampton's announcement of her marriage. Many of them regarded this as a betrayal by one of their leaders who was abandoning the battle for nursing and for women's rights to become a simple housewife. Robb did none of these things; although she no longer worked as a nurse, she devoted the rest of her life to nursing and nursing organizations.

The first opportunity for American nurses to associate was afforded by the International Congress of Charities, Correction, and Philanthropy held at Chicago in 1893 as part of the Columbian Exposition. This world's fair, commemorating the four-hundredth anniversary of the landing of Columbus in the New World, was a major event that attracted exhibits and conferences from all over the world. Ethel Gordon Fenwick had come to Chicago in 1892 to prepare for a nursing exhibit at the fair. During her stay in the United States, she and Isabel Hampton planned to include a subsection on nursing as part of the congress on charities. They succeeded, and Hampton managed to have herself appointed chairman of the nurses' committee for arrangements.[5] Thus, it was not by accident that papers by Edith Draper and Isabel McIsaac, both from the Illinois Training School, were devoted to the need for an American nursing organization.[6] The twenty or so nursing superintendents who attended, prompted by Isabel Hampton, then met and called for a convention of nursing superintendents to meet in New York City in 1894 to organize a superintendents' society.

At the 1894 meeting an organization was formally launched with the imposing title of the Society of Superintendents of Training Schools for Nurses of the United States and Canada. Canadian nurses were included at first because Isabel Hampton, as well as several other nursing leaders, including those at Toronto General Hospital, were Canadian. The Canadians later set up their own organization. The first membership rules specifically excluded superintendents of schools affiliated with small hospitals. This "bed rule" was later dropped as membership was also extended to instructors. Lavinia Dock (1858–1956), the nurse historian who attended these early meetings, later recalled that they were held with great solemnity. As befitted women conscious of planning for the future, yet poineering new fields, the nurses argued in great detail over a code of ethics, educational standards, and the future of nursing.

Almost from the first the superintendents felt that a nursing organization with a somewhat broader membership was also needed; a discussion of the formation of a federation of alumnae associations had already been part of the Chicago meeting, and the superintendents now laid plans to bring this about. Lavinia Dock assumed the responsibility for making a study of the bylaws of various professional organizations; since there were no women's professional organizations, except the superintendents' group, she paid particular attention to the men's groups, especially the American Medical Association. This second nursing organization, sponsored by the superintendents' society, started as a confederation of nursing school alumnae associations. Bellevue graduates had formed an association in 1889, those of Illinois Training School in 1891, and those of Johns Hopkins in 1892; other schools had started such organizations or were planning to establish them. Ten representatives of the existing alumnae associations met in 1896 to set up the Nurses' Associated Alumnae of United States and Canada, the organization which became the American Nurses Association in 1912.[7]

Nursing Registration

The major efforts of the Associated Alumnae were concentrated on obtaining state registration of nurses. The idea had been discussed in England, but there had been considerable division of opinion, primarily because of the opposition of Florence Nightingale. Nurses in other parts of the world, however, had already begun to work for some sort of registration. The first registration act was passed in New Zealand in 1901, although a section of the Medical and Pharmacy Act passed in 1891 by the Cape Colony (now part of the Union of South Africa) also included nurses.[8] In the United States, Sophia Palmer, one of the first graduates of the Massachusetts General Hospital School, was an early leader in the struggle for registration. Since she was also the first editor-in-chief of the *American Journal of Nursing* (founded in 1900), she could effectively advance her beliefs. Her first step in this direction was to read a paper before the New York State Federation of Women's Clubs in 1899. She argued that nursing's greatest need was for a law that would control the schools. She asked that the schools be placed under the supervision of the Regents of the University of the State of New York, the pattern for other types of professional licensure in the state. The Regents would then be responsible for approving nursing schools and for appointing a board to examine and register nurses.[9] Lavinia Dock also advocated licensure in an article in the first issue of the *American Journal of Nursing*, although she pointed out that it could not solve all of the problems of the profession.[10] Isabel Hampton Robb, in her presidential address before the third annual meeting of the Nurses' Associated Alumnae, outlined the two priorities of nursing as the support of the growth of the professional organizations and the campaign for registration for nurses in each of the states.[11]

Physicians were already registered in all of the states then in the union. To obtain licensure the American Medical Association and its constituent state organizations had already fought a major court battle resulting in a decision by the United States Supreme Court that occupational licensure was a legitimate function of the police powers of states.[12] This decision also meant that licensure in the United States could not be national as it was in most countries, since the court ruled that the right to regulate occupational groups was a function of the states. This meant that nurses had to mount separate drives for registration in each state.

To facilitate this effort, the Nurses' Associated Alumnae moved to set up constituent state organizations, so that local membership could do the necessary lobbying for the registration acts.[13] This forced the separate alumnae associations to band together, while in those states without alumnae associations, individual nurses were recruited to work for registration. This de-emphasized the individual schools, so that by 1911 the organization changed its name to the American Nurses' Association.

The North Carolina nurses were the first to succeed,[14] and a nurse registration act was passed there in March 1903; other registration acts were passed later that same year in New Jersey, New York, and Virginia. The North Carolina act allowed for licensure by waiver for the rest of that year. Anyone from a "reputable training school," or anyone who could produce a certificate signed by three registered physicians stating that she or he had been working for at least two years as a nurse, was entitled to be listed by the county clerk as a registered nurse. Starting in 1904, however, only those persons who were certified by the Board of Examiners could be listed as registered nurses. The law required the board to make sure that the applicants were of good character, knowledgable in anatomy, physiology, invalid cookery, household hygiene, and medical, surgical, obstetrical, and practical nursing. Certification by the board allowed the applicant to use the initials "R.N." and to have her name entered on the registry kept by the County Clerk.[15]

The campaign in New Jersey met with so much opposition that the statute which passed was weaker. The term "trained nurse" was used rather than registered nurse. Two years of practical and theoretical training were required before applying, but no examination was mandated, and no board of examiners was set up. New Jersey also admitted nurses from "foreign states," if their training were camparable to that offered by New Jersey schools. The New York law created a Board of Examiners appointed by the Regents of the State University of New York from a list of names supplied by the State Nurses' Association.[16] The provisions of the law were those proposed by the members of the nursing organization. Nurses were particularly pleased with the all-nurse board which was considered preferable to the nurse-physician board of North Carolina.

One by one the other states followed suit, so that by 1910 27 states had passed nurse registration acts, and by 1923 all of the states then in the Union, as well as the District of Columbia and Hawaii, had licensure for nurses on their books. The Alaskan and Puerto Rican acts came later.[17] Although state governments had the constitutional right to pass these acts, this does not mean that legislation was ordinarily planned or initiated by members of the legislatures themselves. Rather, the first steps were usually taken by nurses who contacted friendly representatives for their assistance. During the registration drive, programs of local, state, and national nurses' associations often featured "how to" seminars to help nurses with the lobbying process.[18]

The early opposition to nursing licensure tended to come from hospital administrators, from people who ran correspondence courses to prepare nurses, and occasionally from charitable organizations that sponsored home nursing programs. Doctors who administered hospitals or nursing homes were more opposed than active practitioners.[19] Such opposition, nevertheless, was often strong enough to force nurses to retreat from their original goal of protecting the term "nurse" to that of "registered nurse," although it was never enough to stop the movement in any of the states. Often nurses could marshall enough lobbying power to pass a nurse registration act in a single session of the legislature, but if not, they would try repeatedly until the bill passed. Sometimes they accepted a weak bill and planned for revision. One of the most common compromises that had to be made was to accept a board of examiners which included physicians. As the original registration acts were revised, other goals emerged. Increasingly, for example, nurses sought legislative sanction to close schools connected with small or highly specialized hospitals, including mental hospitals, and to make high school graduation a prerequisite for nursing education.

Since none of the original registration acts defined the scope of professional nursing practice, they could be more accurately called nurse registration acts rather than nurse practice acts. A "registered nurse" was defined as someone who had attended an acceptable nursing program and passed a board examination, rather than as one who engaged in a specific type of practice. This emphasized the educational process, and early reform efforts tended to focus on improving the training.[20]

Raising Educational Standards

In the struggle for educational reform, a small leadership cadre of nurses emerged. Its nucleus was the training school superintendents who first assembled at the Chicago Worlds Fair in 1893, although most of them also had some association with either Johns Hopkins or Teachers College, Columbia University. Leadership was assumed by Isabel Hampton, Lavinia Dock, Adelaide Nutting, and Sophie Palmer, their friends, and eventually their students. In 1912 the Superintendents Society became the National League of Nursing Education, and in 1952 it was amalgamated with other organizations to become the National League for Nursing. Despite name changes, its goal of reforming hospital nursing education remained the same for more than a half century.

The superintendents' first effort resulted in a Pyrrhic victory. In her paper read at the Worlds Fair in 1893, Isabel Hampton, then Superintendent of the Johns Hopkins Hospital School, argued that the nursing program should be lengthened to three years in order to improve and standardize the training.[21] The idea caught on quickly; three-year courses were started at the University Hospital in Philadelphia in 1893 and at Johns Hopkins in 1895.[22] Within a decade most nursing schools had followed suit. A few of them coupled the longer training period with a shift to an eight-hour day, which had been started at the Farrand School in Detroit in 1891,[23] but most simply used the extra year as an added economic advantage to the school.

A significant change in the American educational system occurred in 1895, when the Waltham Training School established a six-month preparatory course.[24] The idea had originated in 1893 at the Glasgow, Scotland, infirmary; it was picked up by Waltham and spread from there. Preparatory courses, for example, were established at Johns Hopkins in 1901[25] and at the Lakeside Hospital School in Cleveland in 1903.[26] Most schools did not adopt the preparatory course, which soon became the mark of the stronger schools. Nevertheless, it was a revolutionary change in nursing, since the objective of the six-month course was education rather than service; it allowed students to get some scientific background and to learn nursing procedures before they were sent to the wards.

Collectively, the superintendents also moved on another front. They decided that one of the major defeats in the system was the lack of postgraduate training to prepare potential teachers and administrators. In 1898 a five-member delegation approached James Russell, Dean of Teachers College, Columbia University, about the possibility of starting a course for nurses. Dean Russell was amenable if the nurses could guarantee an enrollment of twelve persons or pay $1000 a year. They accepted, and a course in hospital economics was offered in the Department of Domestic Science in 1899.[27] Members of the Society screened and admitted students, contributed $1000 a year, and taught the course. Teachers College also allowed the students to enroll in psychology, science, household economics, and biology.[28]

The first step to strengthen the program was taken when Anna Alline, one of the two graduates from the first class, took over the administration of the course. Then in 1905 the program was lengthened to two years; in 1907 Nutting left Johns Hopkins to become director of the course. Finally, the program became firmly established in 1910 when it was endowed by Helen Hartley Jenkins.[29] For many years, the Teachers College program was the only source of advanced education available to nurses, and a significant proportion of the nurses who gave leadership to the nursing education and the public health movement in that period went through it. In assessing the contribution of this early Teachers' College course to the development of collegiate education, it is important to realize that its purpose was to prepare a leadership group; it was not designed as an alternate to the hospital training system.

Nursing Texts

Since nursing was a developing field, nurses had to prepare their own texts, gather and collate their own information. The difficulties in establishing nursing as an intellectually respectable discipline are evident from a survey of these early texts. During the first decade of the hospital training school in the United States, some fifteen nursing texts have been identified. All purported to give a "compleat system of nursing" in about 100 four-by-six-inch pages. While the schools also used some of the English handbooks, such as Florence Nightingale's *Notes on Nursing*, the main impression is still primarily of apprenticeship training. The handbook of the Connecticut Training School, which was first published in 1878, continued to sell fairly well until 1913, revealing that nursing itself was not changing as rapidly as the increasing length of the training program would indicate. The outstanding book before 1890 was by Clara S. Weeks (Shaw), *A Textbook of Nursing*, first published in 1885. More than a mere handbook, it was in fact the first comprehensive textbook in nursing. It was intended as a guide to the student nurse, while the earlier handbooks were addressed primarily to the already trained nurse.

In 1887, Lippincott published a four-volume nursing series entitled *Practical Lessons in Nursing*, which included *Fever Nursing, Nursing and Care of the Nervous and Insane, Maternity, Infancy and Childhood*, and *Dietetics*. These were primarily of the handbook variety, which upset some of the early nursing leaders, especially Clara Weeks, because the books, especially the psychiatric volume written by Charles Mills, tended to give only minimal information about disease—lest nurses "make the mistake, not infrequent among them of supposing they are the doctor." The boundaries of nursing care were much debated among early nurses and produced a wide variety of books on nursing ethics, most of which dealt not with ethics, but with the subordination of the nurse to the physician. Some of the nurses believed their own propaganda: when Lavinia Dock's *Materia Medica* for nurses first appeared in 1890, it was not well received by many of her colleagues because they could not see why so much information was necessary.

Gradually, however, the handbook compendium was replaced by more specialized books, modeled after Dock's text. Diana Kimber's *Textbook of Anatomy and Physiology for Nurses* was an important example, and like those of Dock, Weeks, and others, the book was often revised and reprinted. The development of nursing can be measured by the appearance of various textbooks, and it is perhaps significant that the first bacteriology book, that by Mary Reid, was printed in 1904, and the first chemistry book, Lotta Jean Bogert's, in 1924. Mary Sewell Gardner's *Public Health Nursing* was first published in 1916 and was often revised as the study of public health developed. Nursing was slowly but surely extending its intellectual horizons.[30]

Nursing Journals

To maintain contact with the scattered members of nursing organizations, an official journal was planned. Three nursing journals, two in the United States and one in England, had started publication in 1888, but none of them had any particular organizational ties. The English periodical, established by Ethel Gordon Fenwick, eventually became the *British Journal of Nursing*. In America Sarah Post, a Bellevue graduate, who had later studied medicine, started the short-lived monthly *The Nightingale*, which encountered great opposition from organized medicine, both because it was written for nurses and because it was edited by a woman. Somewhat more successful was the journal started by Margaret Francis, Superintendent of the Buffalo General Hospital and head of its training school. She began to publish *The Trained Nurse*, which under this title and that of *The Nursing World* appeared for more than 50 years.[31] As soon as the Nurses' Associated Alumnae was formed, they discussed the need for a journal, but little happened until 1899 when Mary E. P. Davis was made chairman of the periodicals committee. When Davis reported to the Associated Alumnae in 1900, her committee not only had decided to publish a journal, but had established a joint stock company to finance it and had sold shares to nurses and to alumnae associations. Admitting that she had somewhat exceeded her authority, Davis then asked for power to continue. This was given to her; Sophia Palmer was chosen editor, and the first issue of the *American Journal of Nursing* appeared in October 1900. By 1912 the outstanding stock had been purchased by the ANA. When Sophia Palmer died in 1920, Mary Roberts succeeded her, establishing a continuing tradition of nurse editors.[32]

The early *Journal* was organized into departments edited by various nursing faithfuls: Isabel Robb for education; Linda Richards for hospitals and training schools; Davis for sanitation; and Isabel McIsaac for private duty nursing. There were also departments on other nursing interests such as the nursing care of children, food preparation, and prophylactics— disease prevention and bacteriology.

The most colorful of the early contributors was Lavinia Dock, who reported foreign news; she also brought her own personal biases into articles on other aspects of nursing. Since she was an ardent feminist, a socialist, and a pacifist, and had great enthusiasm, her columns are among the most interesting in the early *Journal*. Dock did not approve of World War I; in keeping with her disapproval, she would permit no mention of war in her department of the journal, although war news dominated most of the rest of the magazine. It was only through her mention of the nursing activities in neutral countries such as Denmark that a reader could realize that she knew a war was going on.

Lavinia Dock, perhaps more than any other early nursing leader, recognized the importance of the women's rights movement for nursing, and she was willing to work, march, and be jailed for her beliefs.[33] During the state campaigns for nurse registration, she realized that the lack of suffrage for women was a significant deterrent to their achieving any kind of needed legislation. The solution in her mind was to give both women and nurses more political power. She made a major speech on the subject of the vote at the 1907 convention of the Associated Alumnae,[34] and in 1908 a resolution to support the vote for women was brought before the house of delegates. It was defeated by what was described as a large majority. Disappointed, but not silenced, Dock sought support from the editor of the *American Journal of Nursing*, Sophia Palmer, who answered in an editorial that since suffrage was not a nursing matter, the "*Journal's* editorial policy must be neutral."[35]

Dock was not alone in the fight for suffrage. Lillian Wald, who was also politically sophisticated, gave her strong support, as to a lesser extent did Isabel Stewart, Annie Goodrich, and Adelaide Nutting. Eventually these women were able to convince other nurses of the importance of the vote. Finally, in 1915 the American Nurses Association (successor to the Associated Alumnae) voted to support the Susan B. Anthony amendment which passed in 1920. Nurses were reluctant to do more, however. When the National Women's Party, to which Dock belonged, started campaigning for the equal rights amendment in 1923, organized nursing again refused to support the effort. Most nurses remained apathetic, perhaps fearful of losing what they had already won. In 1950, for example, an ANA committee opposed the equal rights amendment because they did not want to lose the special protection which they believed women had under the law. Such a stance for a nursing organization was contradictory, since most states had exempted nurses (and domestic workers) from protective legislation limiting hours, late shifts, and other "special advantages" accruing to women. The nurses' opposition, however, indicated their ambivalence toward their role as women and professionals in society, and it was not until after Dock had died that the ANA finally supported the equal rights amendment.[36]

Early History of Public Health Nursing

Although the hospital nursing school movement emphasized the care of the sick, a small but growing number of nurses were finding employment in preventive health care. Mary Gardner, the early textbook author in public health nursing, estimated that the 200 public health nurses of 1900 had grown to approximately 3,000 by 1912.[37] This development was important: it brought health care and health teaching to the public, gave nurses an opportunity for more independent work, and helped to improve nursing education.

The district nursing started by Rathbone in Liverpool had been followed by similar efforts in other large British cities. Manchester, as early as 1864, had a Nurse Training Institution to train district nurses. Selected candidates first went to London for hospital training and then returned to Manchester for orientation in district nursing at the Institution. This effort was privately financed; its prime purpose was to care for the "sick poor" in their homes. The nurses dispensed food and medicine and were closely supervised by various middle- and upper-class women who collected the necessary supplies.

In London the earlier idea of visiting the sick as a religious duty dominated the district nursing movement. Although various Anglican and Catholic nursing orders were still active, particularly during epidemics, the largest organization in London specializing in home nursing was the Bible and Domestic Mission. This organization had been established in the middle of the nineteenth century but had concentrated at first on

sending women into the slums of London to read the Bible to the poor or
to lead them in prayers. In 1868 nursing services were added to the Bible
reading. Would-be workers studied the Bible for three months and then
were given four months of practical nursing experience by serving as
attendants in a hospital. The Mission assumed that any woman able to
read the Bible could learn an adequate amount of nursing knowledge by
working in the hospital.[38]

In 1887 as a part of the fiftieth anniversary celebration of Queen
Victoria's reign, a fund was raised by the women of England to provide
training and pay for district nurses. The Queen Victoria Jubilee Institute
for Nurses, organized in 1889, brought together the various existing
groups active in district nursing and gave some organization to the
developing public health movement. The *Queen's Nurses,* as they were
called, were active in both rural and urban areas, and did bedside nursing
as well as teaching elementary health and hygiene.[39]

In the United States the pattern was the same: the sponsorship of
district nursing was first religious, then private philanthropic, and finally
supported by public funds. All three kinds of financing continue to exist,
but the general trend has been toward the government assuming more
responsibility for the health of the people. The older areas of the United
States, especially in the East and parts of the Midwest, still have many old
private charitable institutions, but in the newer areas, particularly in the
West, education, health, and social services were dominated by state and
local governments until the federal programs of the twentieth century.

An example of religious sponsorship is the development of the first
visiting nursing groups in New York City. In 1877 the Woman's Board of
the New York Mission hired Frances Root, a graduate of Bellevue
Hospital's first nursing class, to visit among the sick poor. Her prime duty
was nursing, but she was also cautioned not to "forget the soul's interest"
and to use every opportunity to give godly advice and Christian comfort.
Somewhat less religious was the program begun a year later by the
Society for Ethical Culture, a secular religious group pledged to promot-
ing the highest ethical conduct in all phases of life. Since its nurses worked
out of dispensaries, they had the advantage of medical advice from the
dispensary physicians. The ladies of the Society also made certain that the
nurses had supplies of linen, food, and clothes for patients who might
need them. Since district nursing was emerging simultaneously with the
social worker, originally called friendly visitor, early visiting nurses often
combined both functions.

Two district nursing associations were formed under private philanthropic auspices in 1886. A Boston program was organized by the
Women's Educational Association, which emphasized the teaching of
hygiene and cleanliness, giving impetus to what was called instructive

district nursing. Philadelphia's Visiting Nurse Society was founded in the same year. That almost all the original visiting nurses were graduates of the hospital training schools helped establish the principle that visiting nurses should be trained nurses; this gave the American district nurse a decided advantage over her European counterpart, who was frequently not so well trained.[40]

In 1893 a slightly different kind of nursing developed in New York City under the direction of Lillian D. Wald (1867-1940), a graduate of the New York Hospital Training School. After her graduation Wald supplemented her nursing training by studying in a medical college. She also began teaching home nursing classes on New York's lower East Side, a neighborhood of recent immigrants. One day a small child asked Wald to visit her sick mother. Wald followed the child and found the mother confined to the family's only bed, which was badly soiled by the hemorrhage of two days. To Wald all "of the maladjustments of our social and economic relations seemed epitomized in this brief journey."

Determined to do something about the lack of adequate medical care in the neighborhood and filled with enthusiasm to serve humanity, she convinced two well-to-do friends, Mrs. Solomon Loeb and Jacob Schiff, to finance an effort to help such people. Joining forces with another nurse, Mary Brewster, the two women moved into a top-floor walk-up apartment and offered their services to the neighborhood. To eliminate the stigma of charity, they requested that their patients pay for their services whenever possible. At the end of two years they moved to more permanent quarters—the famed house on Henry Street, paid for by Schiff. Other nurses and social workers joined them, so that the Henry Street Settlement became second only to Jane Addams' Hull House in Chicago as a focus for welfare activities, and Lillian Wald became one of the best-known women in the country.

In 1902 Wald offered the services of one of her settlement nurses for a month to New York City to demonstrate how a nurse could cut down the high absentee rate from illness. The demonstration was convincing; in October of that same year the first nurse was placed on the city payroll. From this tentative beginning arose both the New York City Bureau of Child Hygiene and our whole system of school nursing. Nursing services were further extended by Wald in 1909 when she suggested to one of the officials of the Metropolitan Life Insurance Company that a nurse on its staff could actually save money by reducing mortality rates. The company followed her suggestion by setting up a visiting nurse service for their policyholders, a service that was continued for some 44 years, until the company decided that other nursing facilities had developed to render their service unnecessary. It was Wald, also, who first used the phrase *public health nursing,* a term that soon replaced the various other names by which such nursing had been designated. She was also instrumental in the formation of the Children's Bureau, set up in 1912 as part of the U.S. Department of Labor.

Despite her many achievements, however, she was a controversial figure. She was in favor of the Russian Revolution, and although she did not approve of the Bolsheviks' methods, she remained friendly to their efforts to modernize their country. Her opinions cost her some influential support in the United States, but she never hesitated to speak her mind. Interestingly, Wald was also a strong advocate of prohibition, even after bootlegging had become a national pastime; she argued that the bootleggers harmed only the "idle rich," and she considered herself, in her own words, a member of the 4,000,000 and not the 400.[41]

Once established, visiting nursing expanded rapidly. Most of the large urban areas soon had visiting nurse services of some kind, and following the example of Los Angeles, which had put a nurse on the city payroll in 1897, more nurses found themselves hired by various government agencies in a public health capacity. Encouraging the spread of visiting nursing was the demonstration by Robert Koch that tuberculosis was communicable. In 1903, Reba Thelin was hired by Johns Hopkins Hospital to work in the homes of tuberculosis patients. Her job was to make certain that the patients received the fresh air, rest, and regular meals that were then part of the regime for the disease; she was also to see that the danger of infection was kept to a minimum.[42] Tuberculosis nursing soon became an integral part of public health nursing.

By 1912 public health nursing had become so important that a separate organization became necessary to set standards and to guide its further expansion. The result was the formation of the National Organization for Public Health Nursing (NOPHN), the first nursing organization to admit nonnurses, since it included both public health nurses and interested lay persons and agencies. Lillian Wald's term *public health nursing* was chosen rather than any of the alternative designations because it reflected a hope that the visiting nurse and the newly emerging field of public health and preventive medicine could be linked together. The Cleveland Visiting Nurse Association contributed its quarterly journal to the organization which, as *Public Health Nursing,* was published until 1952, after which a nursing reorganization amalgamated it with *Nursing Outlook.*[43]

The most obvious field in which the public health nurse demonstrated her usefulness and effectiveness to the public was in infant and child care. High infant mortality rates had always been accepted as more or less inevitable, but by 1900 there was an increasing belief that they could be diminished. In 1899 New York City established milk stations to supply fresh cow's milk for sick infants and indigent mothers. Milk distribution programs remained the only operative infant welfare programs until 1906 when the Cleveland Visiting Nurse Association and the Cleveland Milk Fund Association jointly opened a Babies' Dispensary, which offered medical and nursing supervision of both the well and ill child. This service was copied in other cities, and with the formation of the Division of Child Hygiene in the New York City Department of Health in 1908, municipal government became a major factor in the public health nursing field.[44]

Part of the approach in reducing infant mortality rates was to raise the educational standards of midwives, a group for which there were no particular legal standards. Often they were neighborhood women who had had children or who had observed several births, then started delivering babies themselves. A New York City survey published in 1913 indicated that more than 40 per cent of the deliveries were under the direction of untrained attendants, some 3,000 of whom were practicing in the city. Many reformers felt that training and supervision of midwives were absolutely essential before maternal and neonatal death rates could be cut. Any such suggestions were, however, opposed by organized medicine, which felt that midwives should be abolished and the whole field of obstetrics turned over to physicians.

Not all nurses agreed with this, and one of the more notorious of the American nurse midwives was Emma Goldman (1869–1940), whose public career as an anarchist soon took precedence over her role both in nursing and in midwifery. Goldman had become interested in nursing while serving in prison where she had been sentenced for inciting a riot in 1893. The prison physician asked her to help him, and she found she liked nursing. After her release she continued her studies in Vienna where she received diplomas both in nursing and midwifery. When she returned to the U.S. she set up practice as a nurse midwife but soon left to campaign for birth control and more effective social change, although she never entirely lost her interest in nursing.

In general nurses remained ambiguous about midwifery. Shortly after the NOPHN was founded, the training of nurse-midwives was discussed, but no positive action was taken, even though in Europe nurse-midwives were becoming increasingly common. With the establishment of the Children's Bureau in 1912, systematic study of the conditions— mortality and morbidity rates for infants and mothers—was begun. These studies, plus the publicity they received, emphasized the need for better obstetrical care, particularly for the low-income mother. Nurses, unwilling to antagonize organized medicine, still refused to begin programs to train nurse-midwives. A compromise was reached with the passage of the Sheppard-Towner Act of 1921, which provided, among other things, that public health nurses should be employed to instruct local midwives. Various states also began regulating the education, licensing, and practice of midwives; more importantly the states also enacted legislation to utilize the funds appropriated by the Sheppard-Towner Act for public health nursing care of infants and mothers.

Most of the early American development of public health nursing had occurred in the larger cities. Although Great Britain, Canada, and Germany had begun to organize rural district nursing around 1900, very little had been done in the United States. Recognizing this deficiency, Lillian Wald had proposed as early as 1908 that the Red Cross organize country nursing. Wald felt that the Red Cross could do for rural nursing what the visiting nurse associations were doing for the cities, yet at the same time broaden its own activities beyond disaster relief. The Red Cross ignored her suggestion at first, but when Jacob H. Schiff, the New York philanthropist, offered $100,000 for rural nursing, the Red Cross became interested. Approval was given in December 1911, and by 1912 the Rural Nursing Service was under way. Fannie F. Clement, a nurse and trained social worker, was appointed director of the project, which soon began to be called the Town and Country Nursing Service.

Despite the interest in rural nursing, progress was slow, mainly because the Red Cross saw itself not as an employer of nurses, but rather as an agency to secure qualified nurses, to train them, to advise interested communities, and to influence the expansion of rural nursing. Getting local communities to pay salaries, however, was difficult. Mrs. Whitelaw Reid originally contributed some financial support for this, but it was soon withdrawn under circumstances that revealed the exclusive social attitude that has periodically plagued many Red Cross projects. Reid simply refused to contribute more money because she felt that the nurses selected for rural nursing were not ladies, although she added in her letter withdrawing support that "to get on with the village people their not being ladies does not really matter—I suppose the ladies would not like the work." It was largely the decision of the Metropolitan Life Insurance Company to use the existing rural nurses for the service of their policy-holders that enabled rural nursing to continue. By 1916 31 associations were cooperating with both the Metropolitan Life Insurance Company and the Red Cross, but most of the nursing salaries came through the insurance company's payment of 50 cents per call on its policyholders.

After World War I, the rapid expansion of rural health programs only emphasized the difficulties between the nurses and the local Red Cross chapters. Few local chapters really understood the programs, and some of those that did were openly opposed. There was also conflict with community officials over how much control the Red Cross should have. Despite this, between January 1919 and June 1930, nearly 3,000 services were started, although not more than one-third this number existed at any one time. With the entry of federal and state governments into the field in the 1930's, the Red Cross began to withdraw, until by 1947 the whole rural health nursing program was finally discontinued.[45]

A further extension of public health nursing took place in the development of industrial nursing. Probably the first industrial nurse was Philippa Flowerday (later Mrs. William Reid), who was employed by J. and J. Colman in Norwich, England, in 1878. The employees of the company had organized a Self-Help Medical Club to which they contributed a small monthly amount for which they received medical attention. It was part of Flowerday's duties to assist the physician hired by the club, after which she visited the sick employees or their families in their homes. In the United States, the honor of being the first company to employ a nurse is usually given to the Vermont Marble Company, which started a nursing program in 1895, although the John Wanamaker Employees' Benefit Association in New York City and the Frederick Loeser store in Brooklyn started programs soon after. The growth of the program, however, was slow; by 1910 there were still only 66 American firms employing graduate nurses. The big impetus came with World War I when various governmental agencies encouraged the hiring of nurses in order to cut down absenteeism. Most large companies realized the importance of first aid on the job, and although there was some cutback in industrial nursing after the war, the industrial nurse was well established in many of the larger plants.[46]

Private Duty Nursing

Since hospital staff nursing was, except in the smallest hospitals, in the hands of students, the vast majority of American nurses worked as private duty nurses after their graduation. It was toward this group that the ANA concentrated most of its early activities, primarily through the development of nursing registries. Registries of their graduates had been established by Bellevue, Illinois Training School, and other early hospital schools, as well as by some alumnae groups, medical societies, and even strictly commercial employment agencies before the ANA entered the picture. These early registries had several disadvantages. Those run by the hospital schools limited the better jobs to their own graduates, which kept the graduate nurse dependent upon her training school rather than helped her to develop as an independent practitioner. Alumnae groups were likewise restricted, although somewhat independent of hospital control. A few like the Philomena Society (of graduate nurses) in New York City drew from several hospitals, but this soon had little to distinguish it from other commercial registries.[47] Private registries that were open to all nurses not only charged nurses a fee for their service, but failed to distinguish between the trained nurse and the vast number of untrained and semitrained women who were accustomed to refer to themselves as nurses. For the ANA to succeed as an organization, it had to offer services to its members, and the establishment of registries soon became a priority.

The first major breakthrough came when the local county nurses' association gained control of the registry in Minneapolis in 1904.[48] Other associations followed this example either by taking over existing registries or by establishing new ones, although not surprisingly well-established training schools often refused to participate in the central registries, at least at first. Most such opposition had been overcome by the beginning of World War I, but difficulties remained.

Private duty nursing was nursing on a one-to-one basis—i.e., one nurse, one patient. It was also competitive nursing. Janet M. Geister, a Pennsylvania nurse, put it rather succinctly:

> Every nurse is in business for herself. She has to have her own telephone. She has to bear her own losses. Every day there is not a sick patient she is not earning a nickel. Every day that a sick patient fails to get in touch with her she has no income. She has no central organization to which she can go and start work Monday morning and quit work Saturday night. She is running her own little business. If you have ten nurses, you have ten little businesses, you have ten little policies, you have ten methods of work and ten standards of work. Wherever you have individualism you have every different standard of work you can imagine—good, bad, and indifferent. There is no organization to spread all this splendid nursing service over the greatest amount of territory to accomplish the greatest amount of good.[49]

Though prices and hours were usually negotiable, there were limits, and at the turn of the century the nurse worked 24 hours a day, seven days a week, usually in the home of her patient. Standard pay for this in the Eastern industrial states was fifteen dollars a week, although toward World War I it began to rise to 25 dollars. Sleeping and recreation time were at the convenience of the family, not of the nurse. In his lectures given to nurses at Philadelphia Hospital, Theophilus Parvin indicated that in

> some families the nurse will hardly know whether she is fish, flesh or fowl, and the families themselves will labor under the same distressing igno-rance. Some regard her as a friend in need, and treat her with utmost kindness and courtesy; others think her as sort of higher domestic, subject to their orders, instead of having an empire of her own, obeying only the directions of the physician. Some will expect her temporarily to take charge of the house, look after domestic matters, possibly even spend odd minutes in the refreshing labors of a seamstress. Some will have her eat with the family, or at the family table, and others consign her to the kitchen. . . .[50]

Most nurses who stayed in private duty either developed a list of clients or allied themselves with a physician and attended his patients' families at illnesses, pregnancies, child birth, and death. It could be satisfying work, but even at its most satisfying there were long periods when there was no work to be had. When epidemics struck, however, everyone wanted a nurse, and there were not enough to go around.

Undoubtedly, nursing leaders had envisioned nursing registries as run by the ANA as community centers which would improve nursing and strengthen the role of the RN's in the community. Such ambitious plans, however, soon foundered on reality. Not every patient wanted or could afford trained nurses, and registries that emphasized that all their nurses were graduate or registered nurses had to compete with commercial registries that supplied nurses, or at least women who called themselves nurses, at much cheaper rates. The term "nurse" was not legally protected, and many women who called themselves nurses had received their training by correspondence or had done some home nursing and adopted the title. The ANA registries soon found that unless they offered various types of nursing services, the competition among women for nursing jobs made it difficult to impose salary schedules or to limit hours. When the registries competed by offering their listing to all women who wanted to nurse, it proved difficult if not impossible to maintain standards because most women on the registry often were not trained nurses. There was also a wide variation among trained nurses themselves, since many of the nursing schools operated less to train nursing than to staff their hospitals. This meant that hospitals had to have large enough classes to keep their hospitals functioning, and many had little concern about the nurses who graduated from their program. Once a nurse was graduated, unless she taught or became a supervisor, or received further education and became a public health nurse, she *ipso facto* became a private duty nurse. Inevitably the quality of the services varied tremendously, and even the more effective state nurses associations, such as the one in Pennsylvania, found the problems of assisting its members almost insoluble.[51] Although the associations ran registries, they could not protect their members from long periods of unemployment, or when the work was plentiful, as during the 1918 influenza epidemic, nothing could be done to protect nurses who worked in homes from infection, and many nurses were themselves stricken.

The necessary concentration of the ANA and its affiliates on the establishment and management of registries during the early twentieth century also tended to make private duty nurses particularly influential in the organization, which restricted the attention of the state and local groups to the problems of private duty nurses rather than to other problems of the profession. Later, when there were more nursing positions on hospital staffs, this focus made it difficult to mount campaigns to improve the salaries and working conditions in institutions.

Despite these difficulties, the 1925 *American Journal of Nursing* carried an article by a private duty nurse who attacked modern nurses for working only twelve hours a day instead of the 24 hours a day which had been the expected standard in an earlier era.[52] This nurse agreed with those who considered nursing a vocation to serve humanity; since sickness knew no hours, nurses had no right to be concerned with them. Those who did limit their hours or ask for more pay were merely depriving the poor of their services. This humanitarian argument was sometimes buttressed by an economic fear that any complaints might lengthen the wait between cases, and since most families fed the nurse, work under any conditions was sometimes welcome.

A 1926 survey in New York state not only confirmed that the work day had dropped to twelve hours, but also that the economic situation was unfavorable. It was reported that eighty percent of the private duty nurses worked a twelve-hour day, eighteen percent worked a 24-hour day, and two percent worked a different schedule. During the last week of February of that year, at the height of the busy season for nurses, the average New York private duty nurse earned $31.26 which was calculated as equaling 49 cents an hour, slightly less than the 50 cents an hour which charwomen earned at the time.[53]

It seems obvious that the heavy reliance on the private duty approach to the delivery of graduate nursing services had created an unworkable system. Nurses worked long hours, without job security or the peer contact available in an organized institution. Most patients could not afford and did not need skilled nursing services for 24 hours a day. Suggestions were made for more use of visiting nurses or for the development of "group nursing" in the hospitals. However, nurses were themselves too ambivalent and powerless to effect these changes on a large scale. Later events, including the reform of the educational system and the depression, did change the system.

Nurse as Heroine

Despite the difficulties, nursing retained an image for young women that few other occupations open to them had. It was a nurse, Edith Cavell, who became a Belgian heroine during World War I. Lillian Wald, a nurse, was one of the most famous women in America. Clara Louise Maas, another nurse, who had subjected herself to a bite from a mosquito carrying yellow fever, had died a martyr to the cause of disease control. Nurses were where the action was, whether on the local, national, or international scene. When the Ohio city of Dayton was flooded, Mary Elizabeth Gladwin led a group of nurses with their long skirts kilted high, not only to attend to the sick, but to supervise everything from feeding babies to digging trenches. Julia Lide, an Alabama nurse, served in both the Spanish-American War and World War I, in which she was awarded the French *Croix de guerre* for bravery under fire. Nurses traveled to exotic places such as Turkey, Iran, India, China, Africa, to establish nursing schools and do what ordinary women could not.[54] Nurses such as Emma Goldman even became "notorious" anarchists. For women who were still rigidly restricted by concepts of what the proper woman could or could not do, nursing was one way to break the barriers. It attracted large numbers of women who wanted to do something, to be something on their own, and also to serve. It was, moreover, a good background for becoming a wife and mother, and many nurses married physicians, who were themselves in another glamour profession. Stories of nurses and physicians were often romantic, and some of the stories even led to major advances in medicine and nursing.

This happened with the development of rubber gloves, one of the major breakthroughs in aseptic technique. Caroline Hampton, an 1878 graduate of New York Hospital, became a scrub nurse to the famous Johns Hopkins surgeon, William Stewart Halsted, and later married him. Hampton was an excellent scrub nurse, but with the new techniques developed from Lister's experiments, nurses and physicians had to scrub for a long time with harsh soap and then dip their hands in mercuric chloride. Many proved to be hypersensitive to the procedure, including Hampton; she soon developed a dermatitis on her arms and hands. Rather than lose his scrub nurse and fiancée, Halsted contacted Goodyear Rubber Company which had been experimenting with new rubber products. The result was a specially made pair of thin rubber gloves which eliminated the necessity for Hampton to dip her hands in the mercuric chloride. She soon became so adept with her gloves that others, following her example, began using them. Infection dropped from twenty percent to almost nothing, and by 1894 all operating surgeons at Johns Hopkins were ordered by Dr. Hunter Robb, the husband of nurse Isabel Hampton Robb, to wear rubber gloves. Rubber gloves soon bcame standard equipment for medical and nursing personnel and, of course, as a suitable climax for the story, Hampton and Halsted were married.[55]

Seven

Changing Standards in Nursing
Education and Working Conditions

Since one of the major difficulties facing nursing was its apprentice-type training, there were constant attempts to upgrade nursing education throughout the twentieth century. As early as 1895, the Society of Superintendents of Training Schools had urged the establishment of a three-year curriculum and an eight-hour day for student nurses.[1] These programs were combined, less for educational reasons, than because hospitals that adopted the eight-hour day could only have an adequate supply of workers by lengthening the training period. Farrand Training School at Harper Hospital in Detroit was the first to establish an eight-hour day, and soon after established a three-year curriculum.[2] Johns Hopkins also established a three-year program with an eight-hour day (ten-hour night).[3] However, most schools adopted the three-year curriculum without accepting the eight-hour day. The change to a longer training period, meant that student nurses worked long hours, seven days a week, for three years instead of two. Instruction was adjusted to hospitals' needs rather than adjusting floor work to instructional needs. Even in the best schools, when recitations, demonstrations, and lectures, plus the normal unscheduled overtime were included, the work week was usually about 70 hours, which did not include study periods or special emergencies. Johns Hopkins, for example, kept such a regime until after World War I, and it is not difficult to understand why educational standards were often difficult to maintain.[4]

Standards for students inevitably were not very high, since, even if a hospital training school superintendent might have wanted to fail a nursing student, training schools were so subordinate to hospital needs that it was nearly impossible to drop a student who did not want to leave. Many, perhaps most, students dropped out on their own.[5] Student nurses filled almost all positions in the hospital, so that it was not uncommon for schools to graduate students whom the hospital itself would refuse to employ or even to recommend to any employment agency. Most hospitals had very small teaching staffs, who all had other hospital duties. Moreover, teaching was secondary to the needs of the hospital, and it was often a tired teacher who instructed a weary student. One of the earliest nurses to secure released time for teaching was Annabella McCrae, an assistant and part-time instructor in the Massachusetts General Hospital School of Nursing, who in 1912, almost 40 years after the Nightingale schools were established in the United States, was relieved of administrative responsibilities to devote all her time to the organization and teaching of basic nursing procedures.[6]

Problems of Nursing Education

Part of the difficulty with nursing education was simply that nursing was struggling to be accepted as a profession, but its primary difficulties arose because it was a profession dominated by women. Nurses not only had to fight to gain professional status for themselves, but also had literally to force their way into educational and other institutions previously prohibited to women. The other developing professions which also attracted a great number of women—teaching, librarianship, social work—never had to face the same problems that nursing did. Each of the other groups had some close allies in the academic world: social work was more or less applied social science; librarians were important to all the academic disciplines and worked closely with them; and teaching included a tremendous variety of activities ranging from the college and university to the elementary level. Secretaries were another women's occupational group, but their role was better defined than nursing. Nursing lacked allies, both because it sought to create a new field, and because its most natural allies, the physicians, were determined to prevent nursing from becoming an independent profession. None of the other groups was ever dominated by women to quite the same degree that nursing was and is. Teaching always had many men, and while elementary teaching was largely taken over by women, secondary and collegiate teaching and school administration were always dominated by men. Even though the elementary teacher might suffer from many of the same handicaps as the nurse initially did, she had strong allies in other teaching fields, and as soon as they realized that their own professional position was endangered by the lack of status of elementary teachers, they included her in their organizations. Though both library and social work were, like nursing, new and developing professions, neither of them proliferated as rapidly as nursing, and no outside institution managed to dominate them as the hospital dominated nursing. Even though the first few library schools were separate from the university or college, once the universities established their own, they were able to set professional standards much more rapidly than nursing schools were. Moreover, library work, unlike nursing, had always included male executives, and the proportion of men in the field tended to increase, not decrease, as it did in nursing. Social work was established from the beginning in the university; it could set minimum standards much more easily. Secretaries faced many of the same difficulties as nurses but, at least on the higher levels, could establish an effective personal relationship with the boss that could overcome many of their problems.

Post-Nightingale nursing was dominated by women, and the number of men entering the field steadily decreased until very recently. Hospital schools by their very nature, unless they were specifically organized to train male nurses, worked against the recruitment of men. Nursing was also handicapped in its recruitment of men because it was not clearly recognized as a profession. Traditionally, recognition as a profession in the United States has implied some sort of training beyond the baccalaureate degree. Nursing has never quite achieved this and, in fact, has only recently begun to award a significant number of bachelor's degrees. In effect, the comparative slowness of nursing to become part of the university curriculum was one of the factors retarding the very professional recognition that many of the early nursing leaders desired. Several factors made it difficult to get university recognition: (1) its close relationship to medicine; (2) the domination of the profession by women; and (3) the dominance of nursing education by the hospital training schools.[7]

When trained nursing was introduced in America, many of its most vocal opponents were from the medical profession. While almost all physicians recognized the need for better nursing care, and a minority fought for training schools, many feared that the trained nurse would supplant them. A common complaint of physicians in the late nineteenth and early twentieth centuries was that nurses, once trained, were not content with being nurses but instead wanted to become doctors. Dr. Charles Mayo, one of the famed Mayo family from Rochester, Minnesota, as late as 1921, accused nursing of having the most "autocratic closed shop in the country," and of losing sight of the primary impulse of the profession, the alleviation of the world's pain. He wanted to recruit some 100,000 "country girls" to do nursing because city-trained nurses were too difficult to handle, too expensive, and spent too much time getting educated. Mayo later, in an *American Journal of Nursing* article, pointed out that it took almost as long to train nurses as to train physicians, and much longer than it took to train the average chiropractor or dentist. The only result of all this training, he thought, was that the nurse was undertrained as a physician and overtrained as a nurse.[8]

Though Mayo's attack was factually inaccurate and more polemical than persuasive, many of his complaints about nursing education were justified, although they also reflect the insecurities that physicians had about their own education. Though physicians' charges that nurses were not content merely to be nurses would seem to have little basis in actual fact, women who wanted to become physicians were increasingly being shunted into nursing as medicine again erected more and more barriers against them. Moreover, up to about 1920, many nurses were as well educated as the physicians themselves. In the 1870's, few of the medical schools demanded even a high school diploma for admission, and none required a bachelor's degree. Many of the medical programs lasted only two years, while the training period for nurses was being lengthened to a three-year course. It was, therefore, comparatively easy and much more remunerative for nurses to become physicians, although only a few of them actually did. It was not until 1893, when the Johns Hopkins Medical School was founded, that medicine was established on a graduate level, and as late as 1905 only five of the 160 medical schools required college work for admission.[9] Medicine was also divided into sects: homeopaths, eclectics, osteopaths, alleopaths.[10] In 1903 there were 160 medical schools: many were little more than diploma mills, without entrance requirements, hospital connections, or even teaching laboratories.[11]

Nursing was caught in a bind. As medicine sought to improve its own standards, which could only have happened with the development of nursing, nursing either had to trail far behind in its own efforts to improve itself, or face opposition from organized medicine. Inevitably, any attempt to establish minimum requirements, such as a high school diploma, for entrance into a nursing school was bitterly fought both by most of the medical profession and by the hospitals themselves. To allay the doctors' fears, nurses went out of their way to be subservient, including the old custom of standing when a doctor entered a room and of always opening a door for a physician—practices which are finally beginning to disappear.

National reform of medical education did not come until the famous study by Abraham Flexner in 1910, a study that went far toward bringing medicine into the college and university as a true graduate discipline.[12] Increasingly, the medical schools began to conform to the Johns Hopkins pattern, and the weaker and poorer schools were rapidly eliminated. In 1910 only 680, or 15.3 per cent, of the 4,440 medical graduates had a bachelor's degree when they received their doctorate.[13] By 1920 the percentage had risen to 43.5 per cent, and it has been rising rather steadily since that time. On a practical level, then, nursing training in the nineteenth century was often superior to the training of physicians. Isabel McIsaac, of the Illinois Training School, had, for example, instituted clinical demonstrations of nursing procedures as early as 1892, and this was widely copied in nursing circles, but few medical students had actual hospital training until this century.

To put it simply, while physicians and surgeons might hold the "doctorate," their education was not significantly superior to that of the better-trained nurse. The word "doctorate" is put in quotations because many, if not most, of the so-called medical schools had no university or college connections but were what Flexner labeled the "proprietary type," that is, they were private businesses run for profit, lacking university "standards, ideals, and facilities." Before nursing could enter the university or college curriculum, without threatening the security of the physicians, medicine itself had to be assured of a place, which did not happen until well into the twentieth century.

A second obstacle the nurses had to overcome was that so many of them were women, and education for women was only gradually increasing in the nineteenth century. Though female and coeducational academies existed by about 1800, it was not until 1841 that Oberlin, the first coeducational college, gave bachelor's degrees to three women. Several other newly founded colleges and universities followed Oberlin's lead, and some old established schools became coeducational, but not without considerable opposition. Though women's colleges were also developing during the late nineteenth century, few were more than glorified finishing schools. Most girls in the nineteenth century were unable to attend high school until the free public high schools became widespread. A small but increasing number of girls entered the new normal schools, which trained students who had finished elementary school to be teachers. These, however, were not considered colleges and were not very numerous even after 1880. Thus, when the "trained" nurse appeared, there were comparatively few schools that could have offered nurses' training for women on the college level. The universities which did have close ties with medical schools and which might have welcomed nursing students were mostly all-male schools like Harvard, Yale, Dartmouth, and Johns Hopkins. The chief exceptions were the new coeducational state universities, particularly those in the Midwest and West. Teachers College, Columbia, was also receptive, but it was laboring under many of the same difficulties as nursing in its attempt to establish education as an academic discipline. Most of the women's colleges would have little to do with nursing, both because they were seeking to establish their own reputations as academic centers and nursing was too new to be academically respectable, and because many of the women's schools emphasized the training of young ladies and nursing was still often regarded as not quite lady-like.

Against this background it is easy to see why the hospitals quickly seized control of nursing education, and why nursing leaders, including those who wanted professional recognition, felt a need to work from within the structure of the hospital school. Hospital schools were not in themselves bad, as was demonstrated by the many outstanding training schools, but too often hospital needs, even in the best of schools, were emphasized at the expense of the real educational needs of nursing. As the hospital's hold on nursing tightened, it was felt that the only real opportunity to change the pattern of nursing education was through a collegiate school of nursing, especially one in a coeducational school that had both a medical college and a hospital.

The Beginnings of Basic Collegiate Nursing Education

A recent, unpublished dissertation indicates that the first basic collegiate program in nursing was actually established in 1893 at Howard University in Washington, D.C. The program was set up within the Medical Department. Seventy-five students were admitted, and seven were graduated before it was taken over by Freedmen's Hospital Nursing School in 1895. Three factors contributed to the failure of the collegiate program: political in-fighting among administrators, economic conditions, and the then-current consensus that higher education for women was neither necessary nor practical.[14]

The first lasting, basic nursing program affiliated with a university was begun at the University of Minnesota in 1909 by Dr. Richard Olding Beard, a dedicated champion of collegiate education for nurses, who was better able to weather doubts about the feasibility of educating nurses. He fought many verbal battles with physician colleagues, including Charles Mayo, mentioned earlier.[15] Yet, despite Beard's dedication to the nurses' cause, the program was in many ways more similar to the better hospital training schools than it was to the university programs offered in other departments. Although students starting in 1909 were required to meet university admission standards, they worked a 56-hour week on the hospital wards and were awarded a diploma after three years instead of a degree. The curriculum was patterned after the one offered at Johns Hopkins. Students took preparatory work the first semester composed of basic sciences and nursing arts. The second semester included anatomy, physiology, chemistry, materia medica, hospital economics, and ward duty. The second and third years included some basic science, specialty care of patients, and heavy schedules of ward work.[16]

This modest liaison with academia was copied by a few other medical schools, including Cincinnati, Indiana, Virginia, and Washington, when these institutions took over existing hospital schools or started new ones to secure student help to run their university hospitals.[17] In 1916 Cincinnati went further, establishing a degree option and strengthening its university tie.[18] In 1917 a five-year program was also started at Presbyterian Hospital in New York based on an affiliation with Teachers College, Columbia University,[19] and in that same year a similar program began at the University of California.[20] These five-year degree programs included two years of basic sciences at the university, two years of nursing at the hospital, and a fifth year of special training in public health or education. At Presbyterian Hospital candidates who were already college graduates could complete the program in 27 months.[21] By 1923 there were seventeen schools with degree options, including, in addition to those already mentioned: Stanford, Baylor, Iowa, Nebraska, Northwestern, Indiana,

Michigan, Ohio, Washington, Simmons, Mills, Milwaukee, and Downer. Colorado had also started a course, but it soon closed for reorganization.[22] Most of these schools or the hospitals they were affiliated with had retained their diploma options, and enrollment in the degree programs was limited. Nursing, nevertheless, had begun to achieve collegiate status, and the collegiate educators met as a group several times in this period.

Efforts to Improve the Hospital Training Programs

While these pioneer collegiate programs are important, they were not the only significant developments at this time in the eventual reform of nursing education. Equally important were the efforts of nurses to raise the overall standards of education in diploma programs.[23] A significant step in this direction took place in 1917 when the National League of Nursing Education issued its *Standard Curriculum for Schools of Nursing*. This report outlined a three-year sequence including course work in basic sciences and nursing, with experience in caring for patients with medical, surgical, obstetrical, pediatric, and if possible, special disease conditions. The committee recommended that student nurses work no more than eight hours a day and advocated that high school graduation be required for admission.[24] The curriculum was revised and updated in 1927[25] and 1937.[26] Since the standards outlined in these guides were not followed in most training schools, they might better be regarded as calls for change rather than as a description of standards as they were. They were also considered somewhat controversial since there were many nurses who considered it more important to preserve the old emphasis on devotion to duty, which they felt was the cornerstone of the Nightingale model. They feared that to abandon the twelve-hour day for students and hospital nurses or the twenty-hour day for private duty nurses was to abandon the ideals of the profession. Educational reformers thus had to struggle not only against the powerful hospital establishment and the conservative physicians, but also against some members of their own profession.[27]

The Goldmark Report

Consequently, nurses who wanted to improve educational standards sought outside validation of their ideas through a series of major reports done by non-nurse researchers supported by committees of distinguished persons. These reports are fascinating, not only as examples of how the problems were confronted, but also as historical documents. They tend to reflect the thinking of the nursing leadership group at the time they were published, although these ideas inevitably are often attributed to the professional researcher who was hired to spearhead the report. In this respect, as in others, nursing copied medicine. Medicine had first used the report as a reform strategy with the Flexner Report of 1910. Nursing's first major use of the approach was in 1923 when the Goldmark Report was issued. The committee which sponsored it had been established in 1918 with funds from the Rockefeller Foundation. It was chaired by C.E.A. Winslow, professor of public health at Yale, and it included physicians, agency administrators, and nurses.

The committee's first charge was to investigate the educational opportunities open to nurses who wanted to work in the community. There had been postgraduate courses for public health nurses since 1906 when the Visiting Nurses Association of Boston had started the first program. In 1910 Lillian Wald had helped set up a cooperative course involving her Henry Street Settlement and Teachers College.[28] By 1920 there were sixteen five-year collegiate programs.[29] The committee quickly decided that more courses were needed, and that the hospital training programs should also be improved in order to provide a better basis for postgraduate public health courses.

As they discussed the problem further, the committee decided that the inadequacies in basic hospital nursing education were a much more significant problem than any defects in the specialty training for public health. Once this was decided, they enlarged the scope of their investigation to include a study of nursing education. Josephine Goldmark, who had done field research in Cleveland, was hired as secretary and researcher for the committee. She did an empirical study of 49 community agencies and of 23 of the better nursing schools. While the data from this survey were important, they were used primarily as a springboard and as documentation for committee conclusions which were not always based on Goldmark's survey, since other literature and the strongly held opinions of the group members were also considered.

With regard to strengthening hospital nursing schools, the committee agreed with Adelaide Nutting, who had long argued that the basic problem was a lack of adequate financing for nursing education.[30] They also recommended that nursing schools should have separate governing boards, that students should work no more than 48 hours a week, that high school graduation should be required for admission, and that the objective of the training system should be educational not service. If this were done, the committee felt, the training period could be shortened to 28 months and still furnish a better education than three years of service. The committee also recommended training auxiliary nursing personnel.[31]

It is important to note that the committee did not recommend a complete switch-over to university education:

> It should be made quite clear that the Committee does not recommend that
> nursing schools in general should work towards the establishment of
> courses of a character that a university would accept for a degree. We
> realize that the numerical proportion of the nursing profession to be
> contributed by the university school will perhaps always be a relatively
> small one. . . . The value we see at present in the university schools is that
> they will furnish a body of leaders who have the fundamental training
> essential in administrators, teachers and the like. . . .[32]

The Endowed Schools

Although nurses themselves were much interested in the report, and
it was widely discussed in nursing circles, there is little evidence that
hospital boards or administrators were much impressed by it. It did
strengthen the hands of those nurses who were attempting to raise
educational standards, and it did give impetus to the collegiate nursing
program, although the recommendation about auxiliary nursing personnel was more or less ignored by the nurses. Perhaps one of the most
important effects of the study was to establish two schools which were
endowed by the Rockefeller Foundation: at Yale in 1924 and at Vanderbilt in 1930. Winslow, who had chaired the committee, helped arrange
with the foundation for a five-year grant to establish the Yale program as
an experiment.[33] Annie Goodrich, a member both of the committee and
of the informal friendship group of educational reformers which had
developed from the old Superintendents Society, was selected to head the
school. Students entered the program with two years of college work and
took the 28-month nursing course as outlined in the Goldmark Report.
At first, since Yale was an all-male school, the planned bachelors degree
became a point of contention between Goodrich and James Rowland
Angell, the president of Yale. He was willing to accept the school and to
administer the funds for the Rockefeller Foundation, but he baulked at
giving nurses degrees, since they were women and Yale gave degrees only
to men.[34] Finally he capitulated and the first class graduated in 1926 with
degrees, the only women at the time to hold Yale baccalaureates.

To give the Yale students a hospital affiliation, Connecticut Training
School at New Haven Hospital closed its program. Later, however, the
hospital expressed dissatisfaction with the arrangement because Yale sent
its students to the wards only to obtain the necessary clinical experience,
and their object was education rather than service to the hospital. This
forced the hospital to hire graduate nurses to do most of the ward work
and proved more costly than the old system—an effective demonstration
of the reasons why most hospitals were reluctant to support the expansion

of collegiate nursing. Such support, in fact, was not forthcoming until educational standards were sufficiently raised to make training schools a liability rather than an asset. Despite this conflict, Yale, by 1929, had demonstrated the academic worth of its program and $1,000,000 were endowed for it.[35] Vanderbilt was endowed soon after to set up a similar program under the direction of Shirley C. Titus.

Although less directly related to the report, the Western Reserve Department of Nursing Education was also endowed in 1923 by Frances Payne Bolton. The Lakeside Hospital School of Nursing, which was the precursor to the collegiate program, had a tradition of relatively high standards; it had been the third school to adopt the six-month preclinical education plan, and it had participated with Vassar in 1918 in a summer program aimed at bringing college graduates into nursing. Impetus for the school started when some graduate nurses of Cleveland raised money to start the college affiliation. In 1921 the trustees of Western Reserve authorized a department within the university. A five-year option was established to supplement the diploma program, and Carolyn E. Gray became the first dean. The Bolton Endowment put the program on a firm footing and allowed it to engage in educational experiments.[36] In 1934 both Western Reserve and Yale established masters degree programs in nursing, a solution which allowed Yale to become an all-male undergraduate school again for several more decades.

Other Collegiate Schools

In Chicago the board of directors of the pioneering Illinois Training School had concluded that their resources could be better utilized by affiliating with a university. Their undergraduate nursing school was discontinued, its students transferred to the new Cook County School of Nursing, and their assets, valued at $500,000, were transferred to the University of Chicago in 1926. The university developed a graduate program in nursing under the direction of Nellie X. Hawkinson. The Catholic University of America began graduate courses in nursing in 1932. The long-established program at Teachers College, directed by Isabel Stewart, was also undergoing considerable revision in order to prepare nurse educators more effectively. By 1932 there were enough important collegiate schools to begin planning their own organization; and the Association of Collegiate Schools of Nursing (ACSN) was formally launched in 1935.[37]

Unfortunately, simply because a school of nursing was established or associated with a college or university did not in itself make it a collegiate school. In 1935 Lucile Petry of Teachers College indicated in an unpublished report that even though combined programs of basic nursing education and general collegiate education leading to a bachelor's degree had been established in at least 66 schools of nursing since 1916, and new schools were being considered in several other colleges, only 24 of the collegiate schools were an integral part of the college or university. The majority were in effect hospital schools loosely affiliated with colleges. Nursing, even on the college level, was still plagued by the frequent sacrifice of educational objectives to hospital staffing needs. In an attempt to satisfy both the hospital needs and the educational requirements of the university, most of the collegiate schools compromised by offering both three- and five-year programs, and most students were registered in three-year programs.

The Burgess Report

The second major effort to use the report strategy as a reform mechanism occurred in 1926 when the Committee on the Grading of Nursing Schools was established to determine what made a good nursing school. The need and desirability for some standards had long been discussed at meetings of the NLNE; finally in 1926 the NLNE, NOPHN, and ANA cooperated to set up the Committee on the Grading of Nursing Schools, consisting of 21 persons from various positions in the educational and health fields. Funds were raised from the nursing organizations, from contributions by individual nurses and friends of nurses, the most notable being Frances Payne Bolton, and by grants from the Rockefeller Foundation and from the Commonwealth Fund. A five-year study of nursing schools was planned, but this actually took eight years to complete. The purpose of the committee, as defined at the beginning of the project, was to study the "ways and means for insuring an ample supply of nursing service, of whatever type and quality is needed for adequate care of the patient at a price within his reach."

Before the actual grading, the committee decided that a thorough study of the economic conditions of nursing was also needed. This preliminary study of supply and demand in nursing was as important to the development of nursing as the actual rating of the schools. Periodically there had been complaints about the shortage of nurses in the press, by physicians, and even by nurses themselves. When the committee started its investigation, many of its members believed there was a shortage and were concerned about ways to remedy it. Again the services of an outside researcher were secured; May Ayres Burgess, a statistician, directed the project which used large-scale questionnaires to gather data. The first questionnaire sent to nurses, physicians, patients, nurses' registries, agencies, and hospitals revealed a surplus, not a shortage of nurses, particularly in private duty, and although the investigation demonstrated that there were many patients who were not receiving adequate nursing care, there were more than enough unemployed private duty nurses to care for them. In fact, there was not enough work available for the nurses being graduated each year. Based on the statistical evaluation of the samples, the committee concluded that nursing unemployment would get worse rather than better and emphasized that most nurses were not really earning an adequate income or working desirable hours.[38] In view of these findings, the committee rather bluntly asked if "hospitals [have] any social justification for running any but very high type schools in the fact of an apparent over-production of nurses, not all of whom are reasonably acceptable to society?"

Two sets of questionnaires were then sent to all nursing schools accredited by the states in which they were located. In order to get the cooperation of the various schools, information and ratings were kept confidential. As a result in the first report, made in 1929, some 70 per cent of the queried schools replied,[39] and on the second made in 1932, about 80 per cent replied.[40] The data were used to substantiate recommendations and to rate schools. The committee urged that unaccredited and small (less than 50 beds) hospitals close their schools. They argued that no school should continue to operate in a hospital which did not employ a minimum of four registered nurses, including one instructor who was at least a high school graduate. They further recommended that the school should close if it worked its students more than eight hours a day or 56 hours a week, or expected them to carry head nurse and supervisory positions, or kept no records, or sent students to do private duty nursing for the profit of the hospital.[41]

The moral persuasion of the committee was buttressed in this period by an even worse unemployment situation than had been documented in the 1928 report. Some graduate nurses were so desperate that they were willing to work for board and room, and many were sent to work in hospitals with their wages paid by federal make-work projects.[42] Under these circumstances "altruism" triumphed, and many small hospitals closed their schools and "hired" graduate nurses. The number of schools fell from a high of 1,885 in 1929 to 1,781 in 1932[43] and to 1,311 in 1940.[44]

Unemployment

The predictions of increasing unemployment for nurses made by the Grading Committee turned out to be all too accurate. The depression that followed the stock market crash of 1929 created widespread unemployment throughout society, and nurses were no exception. People did not stop being sick, but few could afford private duty nurses. Public health and visiting nurses carried a heavier case load than ever before, but not many agencies could afford to hire more nurses. Though the ANA had earlier set up a relief fund to aid nurses in financial difficulty, it had been severely taxed by payments to the many nurses who had contracted tuberculosis and were unable to work; the depression caused such widespread demands on the almost negligible fund that the profession was simply unable to give any relief to unemployed nurses.[45]

Various solutions to the problem were discussed, and many were tried. One of the plans receiving the most publicity was the effort in Chicago to set up hourly programs of home nursing. Concern that persons with moderate means who needed a nurse would be unable to pay for a whole shift led to a proposal that nurses visit a patient for an hour or more rather than for a whole shift. The plan was backed by the Rosenwald Fund, but the service was abandoned after an eighteen-month trial period. The effort failed because those patients of moderate means who could be satisfied with a part-time visit of a nurse were already using the visiting nurses, and those who needed more nursing care needed it for longer periods of time, even though they could not afford it.[46]

As most of the privately financed plans failed to meet the demands on their services, the federal government, particularly under the administration of Franklin D. Roosevelt, intervened. One of the first New Deal attempts to combat the depression was the National Recovery Administration, popularly called the NRA. Part of the program of this agency was to encourage employers to hire more workers to do the existing work by reducing the work week. Since the twelve-hour day was still common for private duty and hospital nurses, the ANA, following the lead of the NRA, advocated a "share the work" plan whereby employed nurses would voluntarily cut their working day to eight hours, which would allow three nurses to work instead of only two.[47] Unfortunately, nursing income was already marginal and the plan in effect meant that any nurse who shared her job would take a cut in pay which she could not easily afford. Probably this would not have been too difficult to work out if nurses had been employed in hospitals, but most nurses were engaged in private duty, and the nurse who did share her job still had to wait a long period on the registry before being assigned to a case. As a result, most nurses were reluctant to share what little work they had. Although the plan did not work very well, the publicity given to shorter hours and the demonstration that a nurse could do better work in eight hours than in the longer twelve-hour day did help nurses to consider curtailing the normal working day.

Under regulations of the Federal Emergency Relief Act, which was passed in 1933, bedside care for indigent patients was considered a legitimate use of public funds. Although only a few private duty and public health nurses were hired under these provisions, the ruling set a precedent for further governmental support of nursing services.[48]

Much more effective in aiding nurses than the NRA, which was soon declared unconstitutional, was the WPA (Works Progress Administration), created in 1935 to give work to unemployed workers. Nurses as a result were employed in existing public health organizations, hospitals, and sanitoriums on a wider scale than ever before; new programs for crippled children were set up; and widespread immunization programs were started. By 1936 over 2,000 professional nurses were employed by the WPA in various public health programs, and another 1,800 nurses were doing bedside nursing and servicing WPA projects.[49] Additional benefits to nurses and to the nation's health in general came with the passage of the Social Security Act in 1935. This initially provided pensions to the needy aged, old-age insurance, unemployment insurance, benefit payments to the blind, dependent mothers and children, and crippled children, and for expanded health programs. These health programs were administered through the United States Public Health Service (USPHS) and the Children's Bureau, both of which increased the employment opportunities for nurses in public health. The depression-born government programs radically changed the public health field, emphasizing the shift from voluntary philanthropic agencies to public ones, so that today most such services are provided by official agencies.[50]

One of the leaders in these new programs was Pearl McIver. Hired in 1933 by the government as a public health nursing analyst, she assisted local health agencies to use unemployed nurses. When the Social Security Act was passed, McIver became the public health nursing consultant for the USPHS. The new service drew heavily on the NOPHN for ideas and standards in public health nursing, and Dorothy Deming, who had been editor of *Public Health Nursing*, also became a consultant. Over the years amendments to the Social Security Act have further increased the public health programs administered by the federal government.

It was during the depression that most nurses ceased to be private practitioners and became employees. As the small hospitals closed their nursing schools, they started hiring graduate nurses. In 1927, it was reported that 73 per cent of the hospitals connected with a nursing school had no graduate nurse employees; by 1937 that number had decreased to 10 per cent.[51] The effects of this change can also be shown by the increase in general duty nurses from 4,000 in 1929 to 28,000 in 1937. By 1941, when the National Census of Nursing Resources was taken, more than 47 per cent of the 173,000 active nurses in the United States were engaged in some kind of institutional work (including teaching), while only 27 per cent remained in private duty.[52]

This sudden transformation of hospitals from training schools for students to major employers of nurses caught the nursing profession somewhat unprepared. Even though an increasing number of nurses found employment in the hospitals, the majority of them considered it the least welcome type of nursing. This unpopularity resulted less because hospitals demanded long hours of work (so did private duty), than because they demanded a control over their employees that would have been unheard of in any other profession, including in many cases the requirement that nurses live in the nursing homes on hospital grounds. Even when working hours began to be reduced, and nurses were allowed to live away from the hospitals, nurses were still required to work the "split shift," so that while they technically worked eight hours a day, they had to stay at the hospital for twlve hours. It was not until 1936, when the NLNE in cooperation with the American Hospital Association issued the *Manual of the Essentials of Good Hospital Nursing Service*, that there were some recognized minimum standards for nursing practices in hospitals without schools of nursing.[53] Nursing, however, still lagged behind all the other professional groups and most of the nonprofessional ones in establishing an eight-hour day.

Changes in Medicine

Nursing was also involved in the explosion of new medical discoveries and techniques which by themselves outmoded the older concept of the private duty nurse in the home. In the process, medicine became more intimately connected with the hospital than it had ever been before. Childbirth, for example, which had previously occurred in the home, now required hospitalization. Developments in anesthesia, in obstetrical surgery (for caesarean sections), in special equipment, in better aseptic techniques, together with the changing nature of the American family, all contributed to this move. So did the invention of the incubator and other devices for infant care that could only be found in the hospitals.

Hundreds of new surgical techniques and operations were developed which allowed the surgeon to operate on the chest, brain, heart, and other parts of the body that before would not have been operable. Aiding the surgical breakthrough were not only improvements in asepsis and anesthesia, but in the development of transfusion, which became a routine procedure after the discovery of the blood groups by Karl Landsteiner of Vienna in 1901. New inventions and recording devices also changed the nature of surgery. With the development of the rapid frozen-section method, first introduced in 1905, surgery also became a diagnostic tool.

Medicine was also changed by breakthroughs in the pure sciences such as chemistry. Chemotherapy has been used throughout human history, but in the past most of the drugs had been symptomatic rather than specific. Quinine was one of the first specifics to be discovered, and this led to the search for others. The man who did most to revolutionize chemotherapy was Paul Ehrlich (1854-1915), who believed there was a special chemical affinity between certain drugs and certain cells. To prove this he began the hunt for a chemical compound that would destroy the syphilis spirochete without killing the patient. After testing 605 chemical combinations, he discovered "606," or Salvarsan (arsphenamine), in 1910. Seeking an even less toxic combination, he researched several hundred more until he found Neosalvarsan (neoarsphenamine). It was not until 1935 that the next major breakthrough in chemotherapy came with the discovery of sulfonamides by Gerhart Domagk. This was followed by the perfection of penicillin and other antibiotics. The discovery of penicillin dates from a chance observation by Sir Alexander Fleming in 1929, but the practical development of the drug did not come until 1939. Since that time numerous other antibiotics, including the cephalosporins, the erythromycins, the tetracyclines, and others have been developed which made it possible to deal successfully with infections caused by most gram positive and some gram negative bacteria as well as with the spirochete of syphilis. Pneumonia is an example of the effect on nursing of such discoveries, since its victims had required days of close observation by the private duty nurses. It is now no longer such a serious nursing problem.

Almost as important as developments in biochemistry and chemotherapy were discoveries in biophysics. X-rays, first observed by Wilhelm Konrad Roentgen in 1895, completely transformed both diagnostic techniques and the treatment of certain diseases. The electrocardiograph was invented by Willem Einthoven of Leyden in 1903, and the electroencephalograph by Hans Berger of Jena, Germany, in 1929. First x-ray, then radium, tracer elements, and then radioactive isotopes began to be used for treatment and diagnosis.

Preventive medicine was materially aided by discoveries in nutrition. The first major development in this field was the realization of the need for accessory foodstuffs, which soon came to be called *vitamins*. Large-scale elimination of rickets resulted from this discovery, and diseases such as pellagra, beriberi, and pernicious anemia were finally brought under control. These successes, when combined with the extension of immunization programs to include diphtheria, whooping cough, tetanus, and polio, and with successful campaigns against yellow fever, malaria, hookworm, and typhus (through the discovery of DDT and other insecticides), changed hospitals from places for long-term patients into centers of diagnosis, cure, and relief.

Health Insurance

Coinciding with the changes in medicine was the growth of health insurance. Since health insurance usually paid only for claims incurred during hospitalization, many diagnostic and minor surgical procedures that could have been done in the doctor's office were transferred to the hospital. In part the new emphasis on hospitalization recognized the changes in American life. The decline in the size of families, the change from a rural to an urban society, the increase in mobility, all forced Americans to be dependent upon institutions for services previously given by relatives or neighbors. Though certain lumberjacks and miners had some form of health insurance as early as 1900, the movement for large-scale insurance plans arose with the depression.

Before then various fraternal orders had organized health insurance plans, and some states had required payment of disability benefits or compensation for loss of earning from vocational or industrial accidents, but the large-scale group insurance plans date from the one established at Baylor University Hospital in Dallas in 1929. For $6 per year per person, the hospital agreed to provide 21 days of hospitalization to each of 1500 local schoolteachers. The plan proved so successful that it was soon extended to include several thousand other residents of Dallas; similar plans soon appeared in California, New Jersey, Minnesota, North Carolina, Louisiana, Ohio, and the District of Columbia. Organized about the same time as the Baylor University Hospital Plan were the Farmers' Union Cooperative Hospital Association, Elk City, Oklahoma, the first consumers' cooperative formed specifically to provide medical care through group prepayment, and the Ross-Loos Clinic, a physician-owned group practice prepayment clinic in Los Angeles.

By 1934, hospital insurance groups had been organized in some 40 cities, more than 100 hospitals were participating, and there were about 100,000 subscribers. By 1936 the number of subscribers had increased to 450,000. At that time the American Hospital Association received a grant from the Julius Rosenwald Fund to establish the Hospital Service Plan Commission. It advised hospitals or communities considering establishing voluntary, nonprofit hospital care insurance plans and was a clearing-house of information for executives of existing hospital service associations. The commission adopted the blue cross as its symbol, and hospital insurance plans approved by the commission were known as Blue Cross Plans. The first published list of the 41 nonprofit organizations conforming to the established standards revealed an enrollment of 1,500,000 in April 1938.

For a plan to get the Blue Cross seal, benefits had to be guaranteed to the subscribers through contractual arrangements with a group of member hospitals. Usually the plans utilized already tested techniques such as payroll deduction, waiting periods for benefits, maximum benefits stipulated in advance, and selection or exclusion of certain conditions for coverage. The health insurance plan business skyrocketed during World War II, since many defense plants and other industries, unable to raise wages above certain maximum levels decreed by the government, instead offered so-called "fringe benefits," particularly health insurance and paid vacations. As a result, by September 1946 there were 22,882,211 Americans paying their hospital bills at 3,483 member hospitals through 81 voluntary, nonprofit, prepayment plans in 44 states and the District of Columbia. Private companies, which had previously ignored the field, also offered health insurance plans and health plans became a key issue in the various industrial contracts negotiated by the large unions after World War II. The first large group of private physicians to offer a medical plan was the California Physicians Service in February 1939, although county medical societies in Washington and Oregon had set up their own plans somewhat earlier. Michigan, Pennsylvania, and various other states followed the example of the California physicians; this led the American Medical Association to set certain standards for approval, and those plans found acceptable were allowed to display the shield of approval, hence Blue Shield policies. These policies soon became an integral part of most Blue Cross group practices.[54]

While the growth of the hospital insurance industry helped finance improved institutional care, including nursing care, the heavy emphasis of the American insurance carriers on hospitalization was in the long run to have some negative consequences. Office diagnostic procedures such as x-rays and laboratory procedures and even some minor treatments were transferred to the hospital, so that they would be covered by insurance. This increased hospital usage and made the hospital an even more crucial center for medical practice. Unfortunately, however, since hospitalizing patients meant putting them to bed and caring for them as if they were sick, this practice eventually helped to escalate health care costs.

There were a few pioneer group health plans which were able to avoid this trap by offering comprehensive care including ambulatory care, so that they did not need to put well people to bed to carry out diagnostic and treatment procedures. Pioneers in this field were the HIP (Health Insurance Plan) in New York which covered public employees, the Kaiser Permanente plan on the West Coast which started as a medical plan offered to Kaiser workers during the building of the Hoover Dam, Ross-Loos which was also on the West Coast, and the Group Health Insurance in the Washington, D. C. area. These plans were also able to save significant costs because of their cautious approach to surgery and their emphasis on preventive health care.[55]

Eight

Government and Nursing

Increasingly in the twentieth century, the dominant force affecting American nursing, or for that matter American medicine, science, and higher education, has been the U. S. government. When the Nightingale movement was beginning in the United States, nurses sought the support of various state governments to achieve registration, but little attention was paid to the federal government. Today, however, the federal government, through its training programs, its capitation, construction, and research grants, its hospitals and other institutions, and its financial support of medicare and the various categorical programs, determines how nursing will function. This governmental role is true not only in the United States, but in most of the rest of the world and symbolizes the changing nature of modern society in which everyone is so interdependent on everyone else that one of the major tasks of government is to hold us all together.

In the past, when the federal government's association with nursing was restricted, governmental interest was most acute in wartime. American wars thus serve as a good starting point for discussing the growing governmental intervention in nursing, although as early as 1891 matrons (nurses) in the Indian service had been classified as civil service employees. The turning point in the relationship between nursing and the U.S. government occured during the Spanish-American War (1898). When war with Spain appeared imminent, the Associated Alumnae offered its services to the government. Instead, the Surgeon-General turned the nursing service over to the Daughters of the American Revolution, although he appointed a woman physician, Dr. Anita Newcomb McGee, as director. Although the government obviously recognized nursing as something that women could do, it did not yet realize the real distinction between a trained nurse and a supposedly natural female talent for taking care of the sick. McGee's appointment is also symbolic, since the government believed that a physician, even a woman physician, should be in charge of nursing. Despite the devoted service of McGee, who was named acting Assistant Surgeon General of the Army, both nursing and medical services were poorly organized, and the trained nurses who responded to the call for nurses were badly handicapped. Individual nurses such as Anna Carolina Maxwell, who was in charge of Sternberg Hospital at Camp Thomas, Chickamauga Park, Georgia, did outstanding service, but this was despite the system rather than because of it. Many of the nurses were greatly distressed over their inability to perform adequate nursing or to impose even minimum hygienic standards; many more soliders succumbed to these last two deficiencies than died from actual battle wounds. All told, some 1,563 nurses served in the war.[1]

It was shortly after the Spanish-American War that American nursing gained its first authentic martyr-heroine, Clara Louise Maas, mentioned earlier. Maas volunteered to be infected with yellow fever as part of a research project. After contracting a mild case the first time, she again volunteered in order to secure full immunity. But the second infection was fatal, and she died August 24, 1901, ten days after her second exposure. Her training school, originally the Newark German Hospital Training School, was later renamed for her.

Investigations conducted after the war tended to prove that the difficulties were not caused by a lack of trained nurses, but rather by a lack of effective organization. As a result there was a campaign to improve nursing organization in the armed forces. As the first result of such efforts, Congress established a permanent Regular Army Nursing Corps in 1901 and a Navy Nurse Corps in 1908. The first Army superintendent was Dita Hopkins Kinney, an 1892 graduate of Massachusetts General, who had served as a contract nurse in the Spanish-American War. The nurses' lobbying for a Regular Army Nursing Corps had estranged them from the Red Cross, in part because the Red Cross felt that army nursing should be under its control. When Jane Delano (1862-1919), a Bellevue graduate, became the second superintendent of the Army Nursing Corps in 1909, the army and the Red Cross agreed on a plan of cooperation which lasted until the end of World War II. Delano was head both of the Red Cross Nursing Service and of the Army nurses, although the Red Cross position was at first unpaid. When she resigned from the Army in 1912, she devoted her full time to the Red Cross, but through her contacts, the Red Cross managed to obtain a quasi-governmental status within the Army nursing groups.[2]

Shortly after the United States entered World War I (April 6, 1917), representatives of the ANA, NLNE, and NOPHN met in Philadelphia to plan what role nurses should take in the war. Little was accomplished at this initial meeting except to assure President Woodrow Wilson of the support of American nurses. Shortly after the meeting had adjourned, however, Adelaide Nutting convened an informal group of nurses which designated itself a National Emergency Committee on Nursing; this soon became the official Committee on Nursing of the General Medical Board of the Council of National Defense. Its first task was to organize a census of nurses in the United States. This census, not finally completed until March, 1918, reported that there were 66,017 registered nurses and 17,758 nurses who were not registered, a combined total of 83,775. It was also expected that approximately 23,000 nurses would be graduated in 1918.[3]

Since the census took so long to complete, the committee went ahead without it, trying to bring nurses into the war effort, and making plans and offering advice on how best to meet the expected nursing shortage. The United States government was no better prepared for war than the nurses, and much improvisation was needed to meet the sudden demands. To make matters worse, nursing itself was in turmoil because of what had been regarded before the war as a tremendous surplus of nurses. In retrospect there was less a surplus of nurses than an inefficient use of them, since all of the problems of nursing unemployment were in private duty. In times of crisis, as in epidemics and wars, however, there were never enough nurses to go around. Even while there was a "surplus" of private duty nurses, there was a shortage of nurses qualified to fill the administrative, teaching, and public health nursing positions. The services themselves were still on a peacetime basis when war was declared. There were around 400 nurses on active duty in the Army Nursing Corps and about 150 more in the navy. Listed on the Red Cross rolls were an additional 8,000 nurses who, under the arrangements made by Delano with the Red Cross, were regarded as reserve nurses for the armed forces.

As the armed forces increased their mobilization, whatever preparations nurses might have made quickly proved inadequate. The Army raised its estimate of nursing needs from 10,000 in the middle of 1917, to 22,000 at the end of the year, and to an estimated 50,000 by the middle of 1919. Almost immediately there was a demand for nurses to staff the army hospitals cropping up at temporary bases erected across the country. Ultimately a total of 21,480 nurses served in the Army Nurse Corps (10,000 of them overseas) and another 1,500 in the Navy Nurse Corps. Several thousand other nurses served directly under the Red Cross.[4]

One way of meeting the rising demand was to lower standards: age requirements were reduced from 25 to 21, membership in the ANA was no longer required, and graduates of state-approved schools with less than a daily average of 50 patients were also admitted into the corps. As the nurses went off to war, civilians also began to experience a nursing shortage To increase the supply of nurses, several committees recommended that college-trained women be given a speeded-up nursing program. Vassar College was the first school to initiate such a program; as a result of an effective recruitment campaign by Vassar officials and alumnae, some 400 graduates of 115 colleges took the summer preliminary course in nursing offered at the college in 1918. The students who completed this course were then required to undergo two years of additional training in nursing theory and practice in selected hospital schools. Most of the women who completed the Vassar course reported to the assigned hospitals, but only a minority remained to complete the course once the war ended. Stimulated by the Vassar example, about 50 other institutions were planning similar programs when peace ended most such efforts.[5]

Considerable friction developed between the armed forces and the Red Cross, both of which recruited nurses. Part of the rivalry occurred because the army wanted to control its own nurses and not have them act separately as the Red Cross groups often did. Despite the efforts of the various nursing organizations, the Red Cross, and the federal government, however, the supply of nurses was still inadequate. This led to rather drastic measures. On February 9, 1918, the Surgeon-General requested that the Red Cross begin training a large number of aides to become paid workers in the military hospitals in the United States.[6] This would eliminate the Red Cross, at least in part, from its competition with the army by having it concentrate on another nursing program, and yet enable the Red Cross to maintain and expand a project it had proposed as early as 1915. At that time the National Committee on Red Cross Nursing Service had begun a series of special courses in elementary hygiene, home care of the sick, and other simple nursing procedures, for the average housewife. Organized nursing, while opposing the program, had reluctantly consented to participate after it appeared that the Red Cross would proceed without them. When the Surgeon-General indicated that such aides would be used in base hospitals, the nursing associations mounted a campaign of open opposition. At least part of their opposition came from experience with nurses' aides in Europe. When America entered the war, wealthy American expatriates in England and France had become the leader of volunteer nursing groups; when trained nurses arrived, the volunteer women were arrogant and domineering toward them. This struggle continued until the volunteers were simply outnumbered and forced to cede control to the registered nurses. Another part of the nurses' opposition undoubtedly resulted from their fear of the peacetime economic competition of these aides, many of whom undoubtedly would have competed with the trained nurse for jobs. Most of the opposition, however, arose from the concepts that the nursing leaders had of nursing itself. If nursing was a profession, as it claimed to be, and something more than just woman's work, as too many people still regarded it, then nursing required intensive training. In essence, the struggle over nurses' aides was part of the struggle of nurses to establish themselves as a professional group.

The question of nurses' aides was discussed at the convention of national nursing organizations in Cleveland in May, 1918; rather than reject the plan outright, some nurses under the leadership of Annie Goodrich (1866-1954) countered by proposing an Army School of Nursing. This meant that most of the nursing care in military hospitals would be done by student nurses just as it was in civilian hospitals. The Army School was opposed by Delano, by Dora E. Thompson, Superintendent of the Army Nurse Corps, and by the American Hospital

Association. There was much debate over the merits of the two conflicting plans, but the nurses finally voted in favor of an Army School of Nursing. Goodrich had already presented the plan to the War Department, but shortly after the convention adjourned, the whole scheme was disapproved by the Secretary of War, Newton D. Baker. The nurses immediately established a special committee, including Frances Payne Bolton, to meet with the Secretary, who like Bolton was from Cleveland. Baker reversed himself and approved the Army School program with the proviso that the Student Nurse Reserve was also to provide students for civilian schools of nursing. Goodrich was appointed dean in May, 1918, and applications were accepted immediately. Because of her active recruitment, there were 1,578 students on duty in 32 military hospitals by the end of the year. Although many students resigned, married, or returned to other occupations at the end of the war, 512 nurses were graduated in 1921 from the Walter Reed General Hospital, Washington, D.C. and from the Letterman General Hospital, San Francisco. By 1923 only the Walter Reed unit was still operating, and this was soon transferred to the school that the United States Public Health Service had established at Fort McHenry in 1922; this in turn was closed in 1931.[7]

Even though the Army School of Nursing was not a permanent institution, and different methods of recruiting nurses were utilized in World War II, nursing in effect had been recognized as a profession by the government. It still had many handicaps to overcome, but its position was considerably more secure in the 1920's than it had been in 1900. This was most evident in the growth of the federal government as a large-scale employer of nurses. Nursing services were established in the Hospital Division of the U.S. Public Health Service in 1919, the Veterans Bureau in 1922, and the Indian Bureau in 1924. In all of these the registered nurse was the key, and while nurses under the civil service classification act of 1923 were classed as a subprofessional group, new fields of employment were rapidly developing. Some 20 years later the ANA managed to have nursing recognized as a profession in the civil service.[8]

World War II

Between World War I and World War II, nursing had weathered the depression and the problem of an oversupply of nurses. This had resulted in improved nursing education and in the closing of many weaker schools. As war approached in Europe and the Far East, however, the depression problem of an oversupply of nurses began to change into a potential wartime critical shortage. At the 1938 biennial convention of the three nursing organizations, future demands were indicated by the announcement of the Army Nurse Corps that it was increasing its strength from 600 to 675 nurses. Although the United States had passed the Neutrality Act in 1938,[9] Presidential pressure had been exerted on Congress to approve a peacetime draft in order to increase the number of men under arms. Nurses were active in this preparatory phase of the war.

In the summer of 1940, Julia C. Stimson, then president of the ANA and a former head of the Army Nurse Corps, called together a group of nurses representing all the national nursing organizations, the American Red Cross Nursing Service, and various federal agencies.* The result of this meeting was the Nursing Council of National Defense (later changed to the National Nursing Council for War Service). This was the first time in American nursing history that all the national nursing organizations agreed to coordinate their efforts in the same direction.[10]

The Council set to work on a nationwide survey of all registered nurses in the United States, a first step toward planning how best to use nurses, patterned after the World War I effort. Theoretically such information had been available previously from the state boards of nursing examiners, but in fact existing information was unreliable. Many nurses were registered in more than one state, giving a misleading picture about the total number of nurses; but existing information was further complicated because in many states nursing registration was done only once: after a nurse had registered, it was difficult to learn whether she were active or still capable of or interested in nursing. At times the records even continued to carry the names of dead nurses.

The U.S. Census of 1940 had included nurses among the professional groups surveyed, but while reliable, this information also was misleading, since students had been counted with graduate nurses. Realizing the importance of such a survey for the country's defense needs, the U.S. Public Health Service agreed to pay for the project. All registered nurses were sent questionnaires, and over 75 per cent of the 460,000 questionnaires sent out were returned by July 1, 1941. Although some of the returns were unusable, the census disclosed that there were 289,286 registered nurses in the United States, of whom 173,055 could be considered actively engaged in nursing. Of these, some 100,000 were theoretically eligible for military duty—that is, they were unmarried and under 40. Before actual eligibility could be determined, however, their professional qualifications had to be examined, and they had to pass a physical examination. Most of the inactive nurses were married or had

*Included in the Nursing Council were the American Nurses Association, National League for Nursing Education, National Organization for Public Health Nursing, Association of Collegiate Schools of Nursing, National Association of Colored Graduate Nurses, plus the Nursing Service of the American Red Cross. Government agencies included the Children's Bureau, United States Army Nurse Corps, United States Navy Nurse Corps, United States Public Health Service, Nursing Service of the United States Veterans Administration, and the Nursing Service of the Department of Indian Affairs.

family responsibilities, but some 25,000 of them said they were available for full-time nursing duty if needed. Despite these numbers, it was obvious to the planners that in war there would be a critical shortage of nurses.[11]

With the advent of the peacetime conscription, the army began activating more nurses; the first reserve nurse to go on active duty was sworn in on October 8, 1940. By April, 1941 a peacetime recruiting peak had been reached when 589 nurses entered the Army in a single month. Enlistments fell off in July, 1941 and did not pick up again until after the Japanese attack on Pearl Harbor, December 7, 1941, which marked the official entrance of the United States into war. All enlistments into the Army Nurse Corps were handled throughout the war by the Red Cross Nursing Service. The navy, at first dependent upon the Red Cross, soon launched its own program. Even through 104,500 nurses were processed for military service, and about 70,500 assigned to duty by 1945, the increasing need for nurses led President Roosevelt in January 1945 to request a draft of nurses, and a bill to that effect was in Congress when the war ended. It seems clear that nurses would have been drafted if the war had lasted much longer.[12]

The war also demonstrated the weakness of a recruitment system based on the Red Cross as a semi-official body. There had been considerable antagonism between the military and the Red Cross throughout the war. The Red Cross Reserve before the war had not really included nurses eligible for military duty; instead it had been a sort of national registering body of nurses when there were no national minimum standards. As a result the so-called first reserve of enrolled nurses (nurses eligible for military service) was composed mainly of people essential to the maintenance of nursing school and nursing services, only a few of whom would have been eligible for military duty. Even after the Red Cross had reorganized its reserve, there were still difficulties because nurses were the only women on active duty in the armed forces, and the military had never quite decided how to handle them. However, the shortage of manpower forced the military to set up some special women's units including the WAAC's (Women's Army Auxiliary Corps), later simply WACS; the WAVES (Women Accepted for Volunteer Emergency Service); the SPAR's, whose name was derived from the Coast Guard motto, *Semper Paratus*; and a women's unit in the Marines. While the members of these units were concentrated in non-combat areas, they facilitated the integration of nurses into the armed forces by demonstrating that the structure could include women. By the end of the war, the Red Cross and other special recruitment groups were dropped, and the armed forces undertook their own recruitment.

The changing status of women in the military also raised the question of rank for nurses. In 1920 army nurses and in 1942 navy nurses were given "relative rank"—they carried officers titles, but were accorded less power and pay than their male counterparts. In 1942 relative rank was altered to give the same pay and allowances as officers of comparable rank in other branches of the service, although its status was still considered lower. At the same time Julia O. Flikke, Superintendent of the Army Nurse Corps, was promoted to full colonel, the first woman to hold this rank. In 1944 relative rank was replaced by regular commissioned rank for the duration of the war; finally in 1947 permanent commissioned rank was given to nurses.[13]

On the surface this struggle for rank may seem to have had only symbolic significance, but it was essentially a struggle to gain the power that was needed to plan and deliver good nursing care. During World War I the Superintendent of Nurses, while nominally in charge, had to have all orders signed by an officer in the personnel division of the medical department. This ambiguous status in the highly structured military system caused inefficiency and indirection. When regular rank was finally achieved, nurses won the right to manage nursing care, including both the care they themselves delivered and the nursing functions of enlisted corpsmen. In gaining this managerial power, military nurses set the direction for all members of the profession toward more autonomy and more responsible managerial positions.[14]

During the war nurses were stationed in 50 different nations and were awarded 1,900 honors ranging from the Purple Heart to the Distinguished Service Medal.[15] While some of the nurses who were stationed in the Philippines were evacuated when the islands fell, 66 remained behind. Members of this group were in a hospital attacked by the Japanese; 37 months later they again came under fire from the Americans when the area was recaptured.[16] Nurses landed at Anzio under fire and dug their own foxholes; they appeared on the Normandy beachhead shortly after D-Day. Wherever American troops were stationed around the world, nurses in fatigues became a common sight. The fatigues, in place of the nurses' regular uniforms, facilitated their work in tents or other makeshift facilities.[17]

As the military absorbed more and more nurses, civilian needs also grew. Hospitalization had changed from a luxury to a necessity, so that nursing had to expand to meet not only the tremendous military demands but also previously nonexistent civilian ones. Government programs, such as the Emergency Maternity and Infant Care Act, passed in 1943 to give maternity care for the wives of enlisted servicemen in the lower grades, also tended to increase the demands on nursing resources. To meet them nurses as well as government officials proposed a series of programs. The first to pass Congress was a nurse refresher course designed to prepare inactive nurses for active practice. This initial program, in effect from July 1, 1941 to June 30, 1943, also gave special grants to teachers and to nurses who were preparing for supervisory positions. The great importance of the program, however, was that it marked the first direct federal support of nonmilitary nursing education, thus setting the precedent for other programs.

The next government entrance into nursing education was a massive one, the sponsorship of the United States Cadet Nurse Corps. The Nurse Training Act—commonly known as the Bolton Act, after Frances Payne Bolton, then a congresswoman from Ohio—passed Congress in 1943. The act offered prospective nursing students a free education, uniforms, and a small monthly stipend for a maximum of 30 months. Participating institutions had their students maintained at government expense for the first nine months, tuition fees paid throughout the program, and further government assistance in expanding residential and educational facilities. Under the direction of Lucile Petry, director of the Division of Nurse Education, Office of the Surgeon-General, more than a hundred nursing schools were approved for participation within the first year of the program, and hundreds more were added to the approved list before the program ended. Between July 1943 and October 15, 1945, the final date for admission to the corps, almost 170,000 cadets entered 1,125 participating nursing schools; two thirds of the entering class graduated. As a result of this massive program, the U.S. Cadet Nurse Corps became the largest uniformed women's service in the United States. Though not technically on active duty, each student nurse had to promise to enter the armed forces upon graduation or to do critical civilian nursing.[18]

Although the Cadet Nurse Corps can be considered regressive because it solved the nursing shortage in the traditional way—with student services—it also stimulated educational change. Since the Bolton Act required that actual education be accelerated to 30 months instead of the then common 36-month training period (although cadets often served an extra six months in army camps or in their own school to meet state board registration requirements), nurse educators were forced to reexamine their objectives, curricula, and teaching methods to achieve the shortened course. For some of them this conscious planning of an education also was a new experience. The infusion of federal funds also allowed schools to improve facilities and to hire new and improve old faculty since additional monies were allocated to finance faculty education. Participating schools were also required to cut the students' work week to 48 hours (including both class and clinical time) and were forbidden to discriminate on the basis of race or marital status. All of these precedents were important for the improvement of nursing education.[19]

Aids for Nurses

Despite the increasing amount of government funds given to nursing education and the widespread use of student nurses to staff hospitals, the shortage of nurses was still critical. To help solve this problem, hospital administrators, the armed forces, the Red Cross, and reluctantly nurses themselves turned to the training of auxiliary nursing personnel. Such personnel had been recommended to the nurses by the Goldmark Report, had been advocated even earlier by various Red Cross societies, and in fact had often been employed by hospitals for some time, but the war brought this movement to the fore.

In 1919 Mabel Boardman, a director of the Red Cross, had proposed an organization of volunteer aids using the title *Ladies of Saint Filomena*, to allow the Red Cross to benefit from the good will and satisfaction of a group of women known as Red Cross "ladies." When some of her fellow directors objected to the title, *Ladies of Service* was used instead. A pilot program was begun under the direction of the nursing service in the District of Columbia in 1919; in April 1920 the program was enlarged, but the name was changed to *health aids*. Nurses were reluctant to see the program extended, however, as were some other groups within the Red Cross. The growing unemployment problems of nurses weakened the program further, so that it limped along with very little success. In 1938 when Mary Beard became director of nursing service for the Red Cross, the training program was changed, however, and so was the name to *nurses' aids*. The revised program called for a ten-week course in the hospitals. Graduates of the first class were awarded Red Cross pins on April 23, 1940. Nurses were the chief instructors for the course, with additional lectures being given by other medical and health authorities, after which each aid served briefly in the hospital. The program was introduced into other areas by the Red Cross, but the big impetus for expansion came in 1941 when the Office of Civilian Defense asked the Red Cross to train 100,000 nurses' aids a year. Prospective aids took a training course of 80 hours, including both theoretical and practical instruction which had to be completed within seven weeks. After certification, they were obliged to give a minimum of 150 hours of service on a prearranged schedule subject to hospital discipline.

By the close of 1945, the 212,000 women who had been certified as aids had contributed over 42,000,000 hours of service in nearly 3,000 hospitals. The importance of the aid program is difficult to estimate, but it helped to change nursing. To use their "aids" effectively, nurses had to make a real distinction between skilled and nonskilled nursing care, which most nurses had not previously been called upon to do. As a result, the aids began to perform many of the errands, light cleaning, and tray-carrying that nurses had previously done themselves, and even performed some of the less technical nursing procedures. Many of the aids proved so adept at their tasks that hospitals wanted to keep them; and in order to do so, they offered to pay them. The pay issue was hotly debated within the Red Cross; in mid-1942 a directive permitted aids to become paid hospital workers, but those who did had to resign from the Volunteer Nurses' Aide

Corps and return their Red Cross insignia. This directive caused such a strong reaction that the Red Cross was forced to change its policy in 1943, so that the aids, both paid and unpaid, continued to wear the Red Cross and Office of Civilian Defense insignia, as well as the blue pinafores, white blouses, and blue-and-white caps of the corps. Many of the women who became paid aids eventually became practical nurses when licensing for practical nurses was instituted in their state. In sum, the wartime use of nurses aids was the important first step in the stratification of the nursing role into registered and practical levels.[20]

Male Nurses and Nursing Heroines

Despite the critical demands for nurses during the war, male nurses were often overlooked by both the government and the public. The laws organizing the Army and Navy Nursing Corps had designated the nurses as females. As a result, during World War II when nurses at first held relative and finally regular rank, male nurses were kept in enlisted grades. Many were not even assigned to jobs that used their nursing knowledge, although the navy had a much better record in this respect than did the army.[21] Not until 1955 when Edward L. T. Lyon, a graduate of Kings Park New York State Hospital School of Nursing, was commissioned a second lieutenant in the Army Nurse Corps, did military policy change.[22] Such action was probably symbolic of the changing status of male nurses in general.[23]

Nurses continued to serve in the armed forces after World War II, but since neither the Korean War nor the Vietnam War involved total mobilization, they were not as influential for nursing as World Wars I and II. Moreover, since the pattern was now set, and nurses were an integrated part of the armed forces, fewer precedents for nursing were created. Vietnam did produce another nurse heroine, however, the French nurse Geneviève de Galard-Terraube, who served at Dienbienphu during the siege of 1954. Galard-Terraube had been trapped at Dienbienphu on March 27, 1954, when her Red Cross helicopter, the last to reach the fortress, had been crippled on takeoff. She spent 51 days at the fortress caring for wounded French soldiers. She was ultimately released by the Viet Minh forces, and the French gave her the Cross of the Legion of Honor.[24] For Americans the major influence of the Vietnam war was the realization of how effective medical corpsmen were in reducing the number of fatalities from wounds. This was a significant factor in the physician assistant programs which encouraged nurses in growing numbers to be nurse practitioners, a development discussed later in this book.

In the meantime, the federal government had increasingly begun to enter the medical field. Some government intervention only indirectly effected nursing, such as the enactment of the Hospital Survey and Construction Act of 1946 (better known as the Hill-Burton Act), which led to a major renovation and extension of health care facilities throughout the United States. Improving hospitals largely depends upon skilled nursing, but it was not until the Nurse Training Act of 1964 (Title VIII of the Public Health Service Act) that the government directly aided students and schools of nursing, programs which have since continued in one form or another. The significance of government intervention in this area can be illustrated by the more than $334 million from fiscal year 1965 to the end of fiscal year 1971 which was awarded for scholarships, loans, trainees, construction, basic support for nursing schools, and projects to improve nursing education and recruitment. Schools of nursing first became eligible for Project Grants for Improvement under the Nurse Training Act of 1964, and this series of grants was continued after 1968 under the Title II of the Health Manpower Act.[25]

The government also encouraged research in nursing and in improving nursing education. The Division of Nursing Resources within the U.S. Public Health Service started an extramural program of nursing research and research training for nurses in 1954. One of the first results was a Research Grant and Fellowship Branch, later called the Nursing Research Branch. Under the leadership of the Research Branch, a series of special conferences reported on and criticized current nursing research. In 1958 the Division of Nursing offered fellowships to nursing faculty members and future faculty members to pursue advanced degrees. Special grants were also given between 1958 and 1966 to nursing schools with graduate programs, and when this program was phased out, it was replaced by one general support for nursing research.[26] The Nurse Training Act of 1971 and subsequent acts emphasized aid for special programs. These grants encouraged experimentation in nursing education and the delivery of health care to underserved populations. They helped develop nurse practitioner programs and instituted programs to bring more minority group members into nursing. The impact of the federal programs has improved nursing education, facilitated the development of a research tradition, and encouraged nurses to expand their work role.

A basic assumption behind the federal support has been that better nursing education could improve the health care delivery system. Conversely, every change or planned change in the health care delivery system has a momentous impact on nursing. The movement towards some form of socialized medicine or national health insurance (the current term) has been a long time incubating. Proponents of national health insurance started campaigning as early as 1915 when several of the more advanced industrialized nations already had some type of national plan for health care delivery. In 1935 President Roosevelt deleted the health insurance provisions from the original Social Security Act because his advisors felt that medical opposition would threaten the legislation. During the next 25 years, several health insurance bills were introduced and defeated. Finally, in 1960 the Kerr-Mills bill provided payments to the states to help defray the cost of health care for welfare patients. In 1965 the Medicare-Medicaid legislation provided hospitalization for persons over age 65 who were covered by social security. The legislation allowed the eligible patients to purchase physician services for a nominal monthly fee and extended the Kerr-Mills coverage to the blind, to the disabled, and to dependent children.[27]

Although organized nursing supported national health insurance, organized medicine fought long and hard against government intervention in health care. Inevitably the Medicare bill was a compromise between advocates and opponents. One of the more costly legislative compromises added a layer of administration between the government and the provider, namely the insurance companies. Another compromise which also proved extremely costly allowed physicians and other providers to charge their "customary" fees. These two compromises helped to gain the support of the insurance industry and of physicians, but the price of such concessions has been a rapid escalation in cost.[28] A reform package passed in 1972 amended the social security act to mandate Professional Standards Review Organizations to monitor provider fees and patient care practices. Unfortunately, nurses did not lobby effectively for their opinions, and since most congressmen apparently believed that physicians were the only important health workers, the PSRO's were strictly physician bodies until 1976. In that year a few nurses were allowed to join screening bodies and began to help set standards for health services.[29]

The 1972 social security revisions and subsequent legislation provided financial incentives for the development of Health Maintenance Organizations as alternatives to total dependence on the fee-for-service system. These amendments also expanded patients' services, since family planning and health screening services were mandated for Medicaid recipients and better benefits were provided for disabled persons. These expansions, however, are piecemeal, and comprehensive planning is needed. Tentative steps have, however, been taken. The Health Services Agency law of 1975 replaced three previous programs—the Hill-Burton Hospital Construction Act, the Regional Medical Program, and the Comprehensive Health Planning Act of 1966—with new, stronger planning and development systems from the local to the national level. Local boards carry significant power to monitor federal funds spent for health care. This appears to be the precursor for national health insurance, since it provides the mechanism for implementing such a law without the massive inflation in health care costs created by the 1965 Medicare-

Medicaid legislation. An interesting departure from previous programs of this type requires that 51 per cent of the members of the local planning boards be consumers, while the other 49 per cent must represent providers.[30] Though hospital councils have tended to decide the membership of the boards, nurses have usually managed to have at least one representative on the local board who can help plan future improvements in the health care delivery system. As government increasingly enters this system and exercises a growing influence over nursing education and practice, it is particularly important that nurses find effective ways of sharing in the decisions on the directions to be taken.

Nine

Specialization and Stratification

World War II was a watershed for American nursing: it marked the massive government entry into the nursing field, as reported in the last chapter; it coincided with the shift from private duty nursing to hospital nursing; and it encouraged a change in the status of nurses. Nurses had not only achieved officer rank, but because they were often the only women on or near the battlefield, they became heroines for women everywhere. It was almost pro forma for any movie, play, novel, or short story about men at war to include nurses. Even though the military imposed rather rigid discipline, to many nurses it was far freer that the life they had known as a civilian nurse, and few wanted to return to the old nursing of long hours, low pay, and a regimented life.

Organized nursing was not unaware of possible changes in the nurse's role, and at the height of the war, planning had already begun for peacetime nursing. The initial result of these plans was the publication in 1945 in the *American Journal of Nursing* of "A Comprehensive Program for Nationwide Action in the Field of Nursing."[1] Following the now established tradition, a series of proposed studies was outlined; these studies were a springboard for much of postwar nursing development.

Undoubtedly the most influential of the various studies was Esther Lucile Brown's *Nursing for the Future*. Brown, a social anthropologist who had already studied nursing as an emerging profession, was chosen by the National Nursing Council to analyze the changing needs of the profession. When she started the project, she was director of the Department of Studies in the Professions of the Russell Sage Foundation, and her research was supported by both the Sage Foundation and the Carnegie Foundation for the Advancement of Teaching. To obtain data, Brown visited nursing schools around the country, attended workshops, and consulted with a nursing advisory committee, a lay advisory committee, and individual physicians and hospital administrators.[2]

Brown's ideas were not unique. Documents of the period and the report itself suggest that certain nurses on the professional advisory committee were particularly influential, among them Luicile Petry of the United States Public Health Service, Blanche Pfefferkorn, director of the Department of Studies of the National League of Nursing Education, and Sister M. Olivia Gowan, dean of the nursing school at Catholic University of America. These same documents also suggest that the leadership in nursing education was much more diffuse that it had been a few decades earlier when it was dominated by a small group of Eastern superintendents.[3] While this diffusion of power left the profession without an easily identifiable elite, it undoubtedly provided better leadership for educational improvement.

Although the recommendations of the Brown Report reiterated most of the suggestions made in previous reports, there were significant differences. The Goldmark Report, for example, had suggested—but not stressed—that nursing be more stratified; the Brown Report urged that nurses be divided into professional and practical levels. Practical nurses, according to the report, could be trained in vocational programs, while the professionals should be educated in colleges or universities or, at the very least, in hospital schools that maintained some affiliation with institutions of higher education. This particular recommendation was the first major public call for the preparation of all registered nurses within the mainstream of higher education rather than in peripheral institutions like hospital training schools.[4] Earlier recommendations on collegiate education for nurses had reserved such training for a relatively small elite rather than for nurses in general.

Based upon the use of nurses in the armed forces and within the Veterans Administration, Brown postulated that the nurses of the future would be required to assume more supervisory and administrative duties, act as physicians' assistants, and assume more responsibility for preventive medicine. If nurses were to fulfill this expanded role, she felt that they should not waste their time and energy on activities that other, less-skilled workers could do. Her report therefore recommended that auxiliary personnel, particularly practical nurses, be trained to work within the nursing team and that the professional nurse be used for the specialized nursing of the acutely ill, for supervision, for administering institutional nursing services, and to assist the physician; professional nurses should do the planning, administration, and supervision within the community health services, teach health, and undertake the administration, teaching, and research within the schools of nursing. For nurses to fill these functions required changes in education. The prewar hospital training programs were inadequate because they left too many nurses ignorant of the broader issues and events in both health and society.

Parallelling the Brown Report was a study by the Committee on the Function of Nursing, a group strongly influenced by Eli Ginzberg, a professor of economics at Columbia University. In *A Program for the Nursing Profession,* Ginzberg pointed out that it was an elementary principle of economics "never to use high-priced personnel for low-priced work." He argued that since nursing had developed when employment possibilities for women had been extremely limited, nurses originally had been a very inexpensive source of labor. Inevitably the student nurse had been treated more or less as a slave, while the graduate nurse compared to a freedwoman without means. Conditions, however, had changed since the nineteenth century, and nursing had to change with them. In the process organized nursing had to face up to serious problems, more serious than any other professional group, but unfortunately for nursing, most nurses, he felt, lacked the education needed to meet the crisis. While Ginzberg, like other researchers, foresaw a shortage of nurses in the immediate future, he bluntly stated that a major reason for the expected shortage was the "traditional tendency to minimize economic incentives in rewarding nurses." He recommended in part that nurses use auxiliary nursing personnel for duties that could be performed by the less-skilled; he also urged nurses to begin serious research about nursing.[5]

Practical Nurses and Nursing Reorganization

Predictably these reports accelerated the development of the licensed practical nurse (LPN) or, as in Texas and California, licensed vocational nurse (LVN). Practical nurses, as is evident from the previous chapters in this book, are at least as old as civilization itself. In fact "nurse" had been so widely utilized as a term for female attendants on the sick that all efforts in the post-Nightingale period to restrict its use to registered nurse have proved unsuccessful. Though organized nursing had opposed the use of nurses aids* in World War I, they had not been particularly successful in stopping their use in other fields. Moreover, in their attempts to gain licensure for RN's, organized nursing inadvertently encouraged the advent of the practical nurse, at least in some states. Virginia, for example, had passed a law in 1918 licensing attendants, and a few other states had followed suit, although technically most such laws concerned attendants in mental hospitals rather than practical nurses in general hospitals.[6]

A radical change occurred in 1938 when New York revised ieaeerarce ais, The New York statute differed from earlier nursing laws in three important ways: it stratified the nursing role into the practical and registered (or professional) level; it defined the scope of practice for each of these levels; and it prohibited other persons from being employed as nurses.[7] Where earlier practice acts had defined nurses in terms of their qualifications, New York now defined them in terms of their functions. Since in 1940 there were an estimated 190,000 so-called practical nurses in the country, the New York revisions were imitated as a model by many health care professionals.

---

*The spelling of aid varies according to the period. In the earlier literature the spelling was always aide. By the postwar period there was considerable variation and we have chosen to use aid.

Concurrent with the passage of the New York law, nurse directors of some of the training schools which offered instruction for household or practical nurses met and drew up plans for their organization. From this and subsequent meetings came the National Association for Practical Nurse Education (NAPNE) formally organized in 1941, just in time to help deal with the escalating nurse shortage of World War II. During the war, the NAPNE joined the National Nursing Council, marking the beginning of organized cooperation between the practical and professional nurses. The wartime experience also demonstrated the usefulness of nurses' aids both to nurses and to the medical profession as a whole, while hospital managers endorsed them as an effective way to cut costs. After the war all the interested groups were willing to work with the Vocational Education Division of the U.S. Office of Education to analyze the role of the practical nurse. This analysis, published in 1947, was followed in 1950 by the "Practical Nursing Curriculum," an accreditation program and an organized push for recognized legal status.[8] By 1950 29 states had licensed practical nurses, and by 1960 all the states and territories had statutes dealing with this new group of nurses.[9]

Simultaneously, practical nurse associations began to appear. The first had started in New York in 1940, and by 1949 enough states had associations to form the National Federation of Licensed Practical Nurses (NFLPN). Many of the original practical nurses were licensed by waiver, that is, they received their license because they had worked as practical nurses for a specified number of years before the act was adopted and thus were included under so-called "grandfather" clauses. All nurses licensed after the passage of the laws, however, had to be graduates of approved schools, and inevitably both the number of schools and the number of practical nurses increased rapidly—by 1954 there were 125,000 LPNs. Many of the practical nurses licensed by waiver had worked as nurses' aids during the war. With the development of practical nurses, the aid was increasingly relegated to nonnursing duties.[10]

Restructuring the Nursing Organizations

Another result of the postwar studies of nursing was to restructure the nursing organizations. The number of such organizations had proliferated as various new nursing needs appeared, usually with no cooperative planning between the existing groups. Early in 1944 the joint boards of the three older nursing organizations (ANA, NLNE, and NOPHN) voted to undertake a joint survey of their organizational structures. They were soon joined by the National Association of Colored Graduate Nurses (NACGN), the Association of Collegiate Schools of Nursing (ACSN), and the American Association of Industrial Nurses (AAIN), which had been organized in 1942. Following standard nursing practice for initiating any innovation, the joint group hired an outside consulting firm to help plan the restructuring. The resulting report, however, was unsatisfactory, and although it contained a two-part option, it met with significant opposition at the 1946 biennial meeting. One plan called for a single body of professional nurses but with autonomous subgroups for the various nursing specialities; an alternative plan established two organizations, the ANA and a second group tentatively called the National Organization for Nursing Service to include those outside the profession. Rather than split organized nursing, the report was returned to committee and to various state organizations for further study and recommendation. Finally, at the 1952 biennial, nursing was included in two restructured organizations, the American Nurses Association and the National League for Nursing (no longer the National League for Nursing Education). When the final plans were effected, the National Association of Colored Graduate Nurses had already been absorbed into the ANA, while the NOPHN and the ACSN had agreed to join the reorganized NLN. The AAIN, however, decided to withdraw from the proposed union and go its own way, although a separate section of industrial nurses was also included within the ANA.[11]

Racial Integration

Like most other occupations, nursing had often drawn a color line. Most of the early hospital training schools had refused to admit Black students, and separate schools for them had been organized at Provident Hospital in Chicago in 1891 and at Howard University and Freedman's Hospital in 1893. By 1920 there were 37 segregated Black hospital schools. Segregated nurses' training labored under the same handicaps as other segregated education including being underfinanced. While 24 of the 37 schools were eventually accredited, about the same proportion as existed nationally in schools of all types, there were still problems. A 1925 study found educational facilities for Black nurses to be inadequate and offered little hope for improving them. Most of the Black hospitals simply lacked the facilities of their white counterparts, and even with dedicated personnel the handicap to equality was nearly impossible to overcome. A 1928 study conducted by the American Medical Association, for example, found that Negro hospitals were inadequate, while conditions under which Negro nurses trained were described as deplorable.

Martha Franklin, a graduate of the Woman's Hospital of Philadelphia, an integrated nursing school, had organized the National Association of Colored Graduate Nurses in 1908, but in 1920 it had only 375 members. It was not until the Rosenwald Fund entered the field that the status of Black nurses began to improve. The fund offered fellowships for graduate study, gave financial aid to the NACGN itself, strengthened training schools, and encouraged agencies to employ Black nurses, an important action when discrimination in the job market was rampant. Unlike almost every other national organization, the ANA had never drawn a color line, and even though the number of Black nurses on its rolls was never very large, this at least was one barrier that did not have to be broken. Yet, while the ANA itself had no official discriminatory policy, many of its state affiliates did, and since membership in the ANA was through state nursing associations, large numbers of Black nurses were unable to join, particularly in the South where most Blacks lived and worked.

In the 1930's the initial work of the Rosenwald Foundation was supplemented by the U.S. Government, particularly through the dedicated efforts of Mary McLeod Bethune, director of the Division of Negro Education in the National Youth Administration (NYA). Under her direction the government began offering support to Black nurses, and the organized NACGN nurses began to have a greater share in organized nursing. During World War II, the NACGN was included as a constituent member of the National Nursing Council, and through its lobbying the Council itself pressured the U.S. Government to use Black nurses more effectively. Such pressure was extremely important since the U.S. Government, despite the efforts of individuals such as Bethune or Eleanor Roosevelt, was one of the bulwarks of discrimination: throughout the war the armed forces themselves were segregated. Hardly any Black nurses had been allowed to enlist in World War I, and almost no Black nurse had been encouraged to join the Red Cross reserve. Under pressure, however, government policies began to change, albeit slowly, until in 1943 a campaign was organized to put more Black nurses into the Army Nurse Corps. By the end of the war, some 600 were on duty. The navy, traditionally more restrictive in its policy toward Blacks than the army (which included the Air Force in World War II), had just begun to induct Black nurses when the war ended. Not until the Truman administration were the armed forces fully integrated, and nurses, whether Black or white, could only then enter on more or less equal terms.

Despite its own tolerance of segregation in the armed forces, the U.S. Government increasingly sought greater integration. Probably the most effective program in breaking racial barriers in nursing schools was the Bolton Act establishing the Cadet Corps, which barred institutions from discriminating on the basis of "race, creed, or color." Some 2,000 Black students enrolled in the Corps, and, although many schools only eliminated their more overt discrimination, the number of nursing schools actually admitting Black students increased to 76 in 1946. Barriers had been formally dropped in more than 300 schools by 1951. The removal of discrimination forced the existing segregated Black schools either to improve or close their doors. One that did close was the school of nursing associated with Meharry College in Nashville, Tennessee, whose director felt that there was no longer a need for segregated nursing education.

Organized nursing also began to deal more effectively with its own discrimination. At the 1946 biennial, the delegates recommended that all state and district associations eliminate racial bars to membership at the earliest possible date. The Tennessee State Nurses' Association was the first to comply, and by the end of 1948 six other states had followed suit. To put further pressure on recalcitrant states, the ANA provided individual membership for professionally qualified nurses who were excluded from local associations because of race, color, or creed. Encouraged by the success of these efforts, the ANA suggested in 1949 that the functions and responsibilities of the NACGN be absorbed by the ANA. The NACGN voted to accept this suggestion unanimously at its convention and in 1951 celebrated its dissolution with a banquet in New York City. This move suggests that nursing was ahead of other professions that were still divided by race, although in the mid-1960's some Black nurses questioned the wisdom of dissolving the NACGN, and the Council of Black Nurses was established to articulate minority concerns again.[12] In 1951, when the NACGN was disbanded, approximately three per cent of the nursing students were Black; by 1975 eight per cent of the registered and fifteen per cent of the practical nursing students were Black. The baccalaureate and associate degree programs were the most open to Blacks; most colleges participated in minority recruitment, so that nine per cent of their students were Black while only five per cent of the Diploma students were Black.[13] In the last few years there have also been schools that have actively recruited students with Spanish surnames. Visible minorities still have fewer members than their percentage of the general population warrants, but the situation is improving.

Rising Standards and Changing Directions

Restructured and newly integrated, organized nursing had greater strength. An immediate sign of this was the strengthening of the National Nursing Accrediting Service, a body first established in 1948. Through this the profession finally was able to bring some national minimum standards into nursing education. One of the first efforts of the NNAS had been a project to classify schools, and the first result was the *Interim Classification of Schools of Nursing Offering Basic Program* which appeared in 1949 and was followed in 1950 by *Nursing Schools of Mid Century.* This project used the strategy developed by the Grading Committee in the 1930's; nursing schools were promised anonymity if they would furnish data about themselves. A surprising 97 per cent of all schools (1156) participated in the questionnaire, and each participant was given an individual report indicating how it compared to the other schools. Schools were divided into two major groupings, although there were many unclassified schools whose standards, finances, or other aspects were regarded as too inadequate to be classified. Group I, the better schools, included approximately 25 per cent of all schools, while Group II, schools meeting minimal standards, included about 50 per cent. Most of the unclassified schools had few students, since 85 per cent of all students were enrolled in schools in the first two categories.[14]

A further impetus to establishing uniform standards was the State Board Test Pool. Though originally begun in 1938, standardized tests were not developed until 1945, when 25 boards of nurse examiners were participating in the State Board Test Pool. By 1950 all boards were members. Uniform testing had the merit of establishing minimum standards for nursing, and further encouraged borderline institutions to improve their educational standards or face notoriety. The test board pool has also facilitated movement of nurses between states. Geographic mobility is easier for nurses than for other professional groups which have retained individual state tests with individual standards.

Higher standards in nursing education, which required schools to expand their physical facilities, hire more teachers, improve their libraries, give their students more instruction and less work time, led to increased cost. Rather than spend the additional monies, many hospital schools closed or sought college affiliation. Since hospitals could no longer use their students for many of the menial tasks necessary to operate a hospital, they had to use auxiliaries. Many hospitals switched to training practical nurses or gave short courses to prepare aids and attendants. The number of hospital nursing schools began—and has continued—to decline rapidly. Less than 30 per cent of the programs preparing registered nurses are now hospital based.

Further Stratification of the Nursing Role and Nurse Education

Nursing also became increasingly stratified. Besides the aids and LPN's, RN's themselves began to split into at least two functional levels: a basic and an advanced or specialty level. These two levels can be identified as (1) associate degree or diploma level RN's, and (2) baccalaureate level. While there had been some cleavage between diploma and baccalaureate nurses in the past, this had not really divided the nursing role. Both types of nurses did essentially the same job, although those with college degrees tended to do most of the teaching and administration. The growing stratification of today seems a result of the major effort to prepare registered nurses in the community colleges.

In 1951 Mildred Montag proposed to train nursing technicians in the junior colleges where she felt that the curriculum would emphasize education rather than the service goals accepted by most of the hospital training schools. When she wrote, the two-year community colleges were beginning to expand rapidly, and in an attempt to extend their own role, some of them had already become affiliated with the hospital training programs.[15] Following Montag's study, a private donor funded a five-year experimental program involving eight participating schools. The first two project schools, the Orange County Community College in Middletown, New York, and Farleigh Dickinson College in Rutherford, New Jersey, opened in 1952. Other programs were started in Michigan, Utah, California, and Virginia in the next three years. The last school to join the original project was the Monmouth Memorial Hospital school in Long Branch, New Jersey, which in 1955 reorganized its existing training program to fit the community college model.[16] Graduates of the pilot programs demonstrated clinical competence and did well on state board examinations,[17] although some state regulations and laws had to be changed for them to be licensed.

The growth of community college nursing education was further encouraged when the W. K. Kellogg Foundation funded projects in 1959 in California, New York, Texas, and Florida. Included in the grants were monies to prepare potential faculty members for community college programs and funds for continuing educational classes for faculty members already teaching and for needed consultation. By the time the project terminated in 1964, more than 100 schools had been assisted.[18] From this point community college nursing zoomed. By 1973 there were 574 programs in operation,[19] and by 1975 they were preparing most registered nurses. In 1962 students from associate degree programs constituted 3.7 per cent of the graduating registered nurses; a decade later they were 37 per cent of the graduating class.[20]

While the growth of baccalaureate education has been considerably less dramatic, it has also been significant in the past few decades. By 1940 76 schools offered at least a degree option, although most graduates of such schools probably contented themselves with the diploma. As late as 1949, when West and Hawkins surveyed nursing education, the five-year pattern was still dominant, although with many variations. Some schools had finally begun to shorten their program to conform to the college norm of four years. West and Hawkins found 111 programs administered by four-year colleges and universities: 61 of these offered only a degree; 45 offered both degree and diploma options; and eight of the collegiate schools, despite their college affiliation, gave only a diploma. There were also 95 schools run by hospitals that had arrangements with colleges to offer their students degrees. Altogether there were 201 baccalaureate programs.[21] Another study found a significant contingent of RN's, possibly as many as 10,000, who had enrolled either as full-time or part-time students in baccalaureate programs not attached to their original nursing schools.[22] Obviously, both individual nurses and various training schools sought the advantages of the degree whenever possible.

Nursing, however, even as part of a degree program, was usually regarded as an educational stepchild. Margaret Bridgman spoke for most nursing educators in 1953 in her book, *Collegiate Education for Nurses*, when she suggested that degree programs should not consist of separate hospital and college segment but should be coordinated. The major in nursing, she argued, should be an upper division major like other academic subjects. She found the double option plan educationally untenable because a single class could not be simultaneously pitched to both upper division and lower division, nor to the wide varieties of students in such programs who ranged from those with collegiate prospects to those academically ineligible for college.[23]

Increasingly, baccalaureate education moved in the direction called for by Bridgman, who in part was echoing the earlier recommendations of Esther Lucile Brown. Since nursing educators as a group were far more powerful than they had been a half century earlier, colleges were more willing to heed them than the hospitals had been. Educators attempting to improve their programs had also been aided by the formation of the National Accrediting Service in 1949 on an interim basis and by the development of the permanent accreditation program in 1952 as part of the National League for Nursing.[24] Curriculums were strengthened; faculties became more like other university departments in terms of degrees and publications; and many of the double-option schools were closed. As one of the first results of the closing of the double-option schools the number of degree program declined, so that in 1960 there were actually fewer than there had been a decade earlier. But the surviving programs were stronger. The 158 baccalaureate-only programs (out of the 172 degree programs) of 1960, had risen to 258 basic degree programs in 1970, only one of which offered a diploma option.[25]

The Problems of Turf

As the collegiate nursing education became dominant, new problems emerged, largely because of the division of nursing between the associate degree and baccalaureate programs. The kernel of the debate concerned the differences between the two. Montag had argued that the associate degree should be terminal, but in fact many transfers occurred in all disciplines between community and four-year colleges. Nursing could only have been a terminal degree in a community college if it had been abolished in all four-year colleges, which no one in nursing wanted. Though Montag believed that the objectives, content, and teaching methods of the community college programs were so different from those used in baccalaureate programs that "the ladder concept of curriculum development was indefensible,"[26] she simply misunderstood community college education. Unfortunately, her philosophy was supported by many nursing educators who knew little about community colleges. Other educators found the refusal of nursing educators to build baccalaureate nursing on the junior college base to be simply obstinate. Since these same nursing educators had often argued for the community college courses, they soon found themselves at loggerheads with state legislatures or with other academics.

To solve the problem, many tried to distinguish the two programs by identifying separate roles and functions for the two types of nurses. Associate degree nurses were seen as competent technicians working under physician supervision to help the patient recovery, while the baccalaureate-level nurse was supposedly able to take a broader view of patient care with an emphasis on social and psychological problems.[27] This point of view was published in 1965 by the Committee on Education of the American Nurses' Association in which the professional nurse was given responsibility for total patient care, while the technical nurse was supposed to understand the "physics of machines as well as the physiological reactions of patients."[28] The professional nurse's relations to machines or in the biological aspects of patient care were more or less ignored, as was the responsibility of the technical nurse for the patient's social and psychological problems. Since, however, nursing educators in both the four-year and two-year schools were often prepared in the same graduate schools and saw nursing in much the same way, this theory was unrealistic. It did, however, help baccalaureate educators resist the career ladder concept.

If community college graduates had accepted their imputed terminal status, any dichotomy that nursing attempted to impose, regardless of its rationale, probably would have been successful. A significant number of community college graduates, however, refused to accept such definitions and argued that they as registered nurses should be allowed to achieve the baccalaureate degree without starting over.[29] This difference between reality and the stated ideal had appeared early in the Kellogg project,[30] and as the number of associate degree students increased the problem compounded.[31] Not until the Lysaught Report recommended removing the unnecessary impediments between the collegiate programs was organized nursing willing to modify its standards.[32]

A 1973 report of the NLN indicated that 82 per cent of the generic baccalaureate programs were offering some type of advanced placement to registered nurses from diploma and associate of arts programs, although this was often little more than tokenism. There were, however, thirteen career ladder programs for registered nurses in 1973, and several more have opened since then.[33] Some of these programs were quite flexible: students could attend one year to become a practical nurse, two years to be licensed as a registered nurse, or take four years to earn a baccalaureate degree.[34] Such developments are still controversial.

Spliting nursing education in two also caused divisions at work. The nurses with associate of arts degrees did not seem to mind sharing responsibility for basic patient care with diploma nurses. The functions of nurses with baccalaureate degrees, however, remain somewhat more problematic,[35] in part because of the misleading rhetoric of some of the early nurse advocates of such programs. Before the broad-scale development of collegiate nursing education, those nurses who had an academic education were quickly drained off into teaching or administration and were only rarely involved in patient care. As nurses gained more education, the academic and top administrative roles were increasingly monopolized by nurses with masters or doctors degrees, so that it became necessary for the baccalaureate-level nurse to concentrate on patient care. Much of the nursing literature in the 1960's dealt with the special skills of the baccalaureate nurse for meeting the social and psychological needs of the patient, but few hospital administrators were willing to pay more for the liberal education and better scientific background of the baccalaureate nurse. To them an RN was an RN, whether she had two, three, or four years of education. In fact many administrators would have substituted LPNs for RNs, if this had not meant losing their accreditation. Some of the baccalaureate nurses found jobs as public health nurses, but this source of employment begun to dry up as more agencies demanded nurse practitioners for community health positions.

It would seem logical to justify a baccalaureate program by including at least beginning specialty orientation,[36] but this, too, has proven controversial. Still, as of this writing there are several programs preparing nurse practitioners or beginning clinical specialists at the baccalaureate level.[37] Obviously, graduates of baccalaureate programs who have skills in diagnosis and treatment, or who can care for a specialized group of patients, have less difficulty distinguishing their role from that of basic nurses. The career ladder bachelors degree programs are particularly well suited to incorporate such concentration because students have already acquired their basic nursing skills by their senior year. While this diminishes the time available for the broad liberal education so earnestly sought by nursing educational theorists of the recent past, it seems to accord with trends in other baccalaureate professional education and is increasing as of this writing.

Still another problem associated with the changing pattern in basic nursing education is the minimal amount of clinical practice normally received by the college graduate. The great strength of the hospital program was the total immersion of the students in the clinic; college graduates seem rather raw in comparison. New mechanisms such as internships are developing to deal with this problem, but here again nurses face the traditional problem associated with such programs in the past—student exploitation.[38]

Graduate Education

As college education, either at the associate or baccalaureate levels, became the norm for nurses, an increasing number took advanced degrees. Such degrees, in fact, were essential if nursing was to be accepted in the college community. A 1953 survey had indicated a serious shortage of nurses with higher degrees. This was most evident for teachers in college programs where only 36 per cent of the faculty had earned a masters degree, 51 per cent were at the bachelors degree level, and thirteen per cent had no degree at all.[39] For nursing to equal other university departments, a significant number of nurses had to pursue advanced degrees.

Another difficulty for nursing was that many of its advanced degree holders had their degrees in education. This made nursing radically different from almost any other profession where the terminal degree was either in the field itself or was a research Ph.D. Only education itself had more educational degrees than nursing. One of the reasons for this was that Teachers College, Columbia University, had started accepting graduates of the nursing baccalaureates into their masters degree programs as soon as they were eligible for admission.[40] To pursue graduate work in other fields would have required another specialty, so that inevitably education became a favorite degree field. In 1926 the University of Chicago opened a graduate program to prepare administrators and teachers, and in 1932 the Catholic University of America started offering graduate courses in nursing. As indicated earlier, both Yale and Western Reserve had experimented with using the masters degree as the basic professional degree, but had abandoned it.[41] Although Yale again offered a basic masters degree to prepare registered nurses in 1975, the leap from diploma education to a masters degree for the same basic job was too great to be justified by most employers.

Education degrees were also traditionally earned on a part-time basis, since most were designed for teachers or administrators who would attend over several summer sessions. Since other disciplines were less willing to tolerate this long drawn-out process, nurses rarely entered these fields. Edith S. Bryan was one of the first nurses to earn a doctorate, in 1927 in psychology and counseling from Johns Hopkins. Other nurses followed, but before 1950 only an estimated 28 nurses had ever obtained a doctorate in any field. By 1970, however, 535 nurses had obtained doctorates. Degrees in education continued to outnumber those in all other fields.[42]

Graduate education received an important boost from the U.S. government in 1956 when the first Professional Nurse Traineeships were established. This act and later revisions provided federal funds to prepare registered nurses for teaching, administration, supervision, and clinical specialties at the baccalaureate, masters, and doctorate levels.[43] Such government support produced a rapid increase in the number of master of nursing degree programs. In 1972, for example, there were 80 such programs with an annual output of 2,200 graduates.[44] Nursing doctorates also increased until the total number finally exceeded 1,000 in 1973.[45] It is estimated that within the next decade the nursing faculty will have as many doctorates as in any other university department.

An Abstract for Action

Objective support for many of these trends in education was given by a report prepared by the National Commission for the Study of Nursing and Nursing Education in 1970. The report was financed by the W. K. Kellogg Foundation, the Avalon Foundation, and a private donor. An outside researcher, Jerome P. Lysaught, was selected as director of the project. The study was broader than earlier nursing studies including nursing practice as well as education. The first report of the commission, titled *An Abstract for Action*, recommended more research in nursing education and practice and better use of current and future research data. It repeated the recommendation made by Esther Lucile Brown in 1948 that all nursing education become part of the educational system rather than a hospital adjunct. On the other hand, Brown had also recommended that nursing be stratified. That had been accomplished, but had caused new problems. Consequently, the Lysaught Report recommended the development of a career ladder or other mechanisms for facilitating mobility between the many levels of nursing. Joint committees of nurses, physicians, and other health professionals were recommended to remedy the lack of communication between nursing and other health professions. Finally, the report recommended better salaries for nurses, so that more highly qualified persons could be recruited and retained.[46]

Changing Fields in Nursing

As nursing education changed, so did the role of nurses. Among the major determinants of the role of nurses have been the beliefs and attitudes of physicians. There have been periodic boundary disputes between the professors of medicine and of nursing. One of the more interesting controversies has concerned midwifery. Throughout most of our recorded history, midwifery had been something that women as a group were supposed to know about, and most physicians had ignored it much as they had ignored the nursing role of women. The post-Nightingale development of nursing occurred simultaneously with that of obstetrics and gynecology as medical specialties. In England and on the Continent, nurses and physicians collaborated to develop a system in which nurse midwives handled normal deliveries and obstetricians dealt with problem deliveries. This movement was less successful in the United States because the medical profession was more determined to dominate the field.[47] Thus American nurse midwives were ordinarily able to practice only where physicians were unavailable or unwilling to serve. The Sheppard-Towner Act of 1921 emphasized the official exclusion of nurses. While assigning public health nurses the task of teaching and improving the practice of lay midwives, it made no provisions for nurses themselves to practice. Instead, the legislation encouraged replacing lay midwives with physicians.

Because of these attitudes, it was not until 1932 that the first American school of nurse-midwifery was established, as part of the maternity center of New York City.[48] It was at this school that most of the American nurse-midwives received their training, although, since many of them were prevented from practicing by state laws, they had to teach or work in hospital maternity wards. Probably the most notable American experiment with nurse-midwifery in the interwar period took place in Kentucky under the direction of Mrs. Mary Breckridge. A native of Kentucky and a graduate of St. Luke's Hospital in New York, she studied the health needs of the hill people of Kentucky and concluded that there was an urgent need for better antepartum and obstetrical care for mothers. She went to England to take the courses in mid-wifery, and on her return in 1925 helped organize the Committee for Mothers and Babies. Her first center was in Hyden, Kentucky, and others soon followed, each designed to serve about 800 people. The rule of the service was that if a husband could reach the nurse, then the nurse could make it back to the mother, a task that sometimes proved not only exciting but dangerous. Most of the original midwives came from Great Britain, although American schools for nurse midwives were eventually established in New York, Tuskegee, Alabama, Philadelphia, and New Mexico. The Kentucky service, which changed its name to the Frontier Nursing Service, also began training midwives in 1936, a program that was increased when the outbreak of World War II forced the recall of most of the British nurses. In the postwar period, the expansion of roads into the mountains and the spread of hospitals, many of which were organized by the United Mine Workers, led to a temporary decline in the importance of Kentucky midwifery.[49]

Indeed, almost everywhere the growth of hospital obstetrical units effectively undercut most of the midwifery programs in the United States, since hospital privileges everywhere were limited to physicians. Under medical pressure and without much opposition from organized nursing, many states stopped licensing midwives both nurse and lay. Before the nurse midwife was entirely eliminated, however, there was a reaction, and nurses joined with other women to challenge the physician monopoly. The renewed growth of the feminist movement in the sixties contributed to this challenge, but so did the high infant and maternal mortality in the United States, at least as compared to other developed industrialized nations. The natural childbirth movement also encouraged the acceptance of midwives, since comparatively few obstetricians could afford to spend the time involved in giving the support services for natural childbirth. Since most nurse midwives were women, many mothers could not only rely on their expertise but could more easily identify with them. Midwifery, which had almost disappeared, began to revive in the 1960's, and by 1975 there were over 1,500 certified members of the American College of Nurse-Midwives. To be certified by the College, nurses must have taken course work in an approved program preparing them to give total care to the woman throughout the maternity cycle as long as the delivery is a normal one.[50]

Changes in the state nurse practice acts have supported the resurgence of nurse midwifery. While in 1965, nurse midwives were specifically authorized only in New Mexico, the eastern counties of Kentucky, and New York City,[51] by 1976 nineteen states and the District of Columbia had revised their practice acts to authorize nurse midwifery. An additional 26 states allowed nurse midwives to practice without separate, specific recognition. In some of these states, the general provisions written to expand the nursing role could be used, while in others the old lay midwifery statutes were considered sufficient. This meant that in 1976 there were only five states which still restricted the practice of nurse midwives.[52]

Similarly ambiguous has been the status of the nurse anesthetist. A nurse, Edith Graham, had begun giving anesthesia at the Mayo Clinic in 1889;[53] after Graham's marriage to Charles Mayo, another nurse, Alice Magaw, succeeded her as anesthetist. Until Graham had started as anesthetist for the Mayo brothers, interns had usually given anesthetic, but the Mayos found that a trained anesthetist served far better than any intern, and as Magaw herself later put it, "No one can learn to be a surgeon while giving the anesthetic."[54] By 1904 she had given ether or chloroform using an Esmarch in 14,000 cases without a single death.[55] In 1909 a course for nurse anesthetists was established in Portland, Oregon.

Schools quickly proliferated, although unfortunately many of the programs suffered from the same exploitation that occurred in other hospital programs: student anesthetists were an economic boon to most institutions since they gave significant service to the hospital in return for their training.

As medical anesthesiology developed, the legality of the nurse-anesthetist was questioned. In 1917 an appellate judge in Kentucky ruled that nurse anesthetists were not practicing medicine when they worked under the direction of and received remuneration from physicians.[56] The question arose again in 1934 when a group of California physicians sued a nurse anesthetist, Dagmar Nelson, employed by St. Vincent's Hospital in Los Angeles. The physicians claimed that she was practicing medicine in violation of the California Medical Practice Act. Both the court decision and the appeal were in favor of Nelson on the technical grounds that since the operating surgeon was in charge, the nurse anesthetist was not practicing independently.[57] This last decision did much to lessen the pressure from physicians, but it also emphasized the subordinate role of the nurse. Although only four states now mention nurse anesthetists separately in their practice acts, there is a consensus that the expanded definitions of the role of the registered nurse which have been written into state licensing acts in the last decade cover the practice of nurse anesthetists.[58]

The American Association of Nurse Anesthetists, founded in 1931, has worked to raise the standards of the group. In 1933 they established *The Bulletin of the National Association of Nurse Anesthetists,* and in 1952 they started an active accreditation program. By 1972 there were more than 200 schools of anesthesiology and approximately 800 graduates a year.[59] Gradually, too, physician anesthesiologists have become more cooperative; they now seem to realize that there is room in the field for both specialists.

While in most fields the role of the nurse is expanding, there is at least one nursing role, that of the airline stewardess, which has become less important in recent years. United Air Lines started to employ nurses as stewardesses in 1930, and the other lines soon followed suit, as did railways and steamships. During the wartime shortage of nurses, however, the airlines increasingly recruited nonnurses, and as air travel became safer and cabins were pressurized, the need for nurses disappeared altogether.

On the other hand, the role of the psychiatric nurse was expanding. The advances in this field are closely correlated with advances in neurology and psychiatry which had developed as medical specialities in the late nineteenth century. One of the most important neurologic pioneers was Jean Martin Charcot (1825-1893), a physician at the Salpetrière asylum near Paris. Students flocked to France to study Charcot's innovations in treating the diseases of the nervous system. Probably his most famous pupil was an Austrian, Sigmund Freud (1856–1939), who, though originally a neurophysiologist, became much more interested in the psychological causes of disease. Through his investigations in Vienna, Freud developed psychoanalysis and became one of the founders of modern psychiatry. Though never entirely ignoring the organic causes of mental diseases, Freud emphasized the importance of sex repression and childhood experiences in his psychotherapeutic methods. Through his challenging concepts and his ability as a writer, Freud's ideas spread throughout the Western world. Pupils of Freud, such as Carl Gustav Jung (1875–1961) and Alfred Adler (1870–1937), modified his teachings into their own system of depth psychology.

The growth of psychiatry combined with other innovations in the treatment of the mentally ill revolutionized the nature of mental hospitals. Brain surgery, the controversial shock treatment (which developed in the 1930's), the equally controversial insulin therapy, and especially the post-World War II growth of tranquilizers greatly facilitated the treatment of psychotic patients. Control of syphilis eliminated many of the deteriorated syphilitics who had filled the "insane asylums" of an earlier period. Neurotic and even mildly psychotic patients could now be treated in outpatient clinics. Mental hospitals, which even as late as World War II more often resembled prisons than hospitals, became places of treatment instead of simply custodial institutions. Particularly important in this change were nurses, who, influenced by the milieu therapy, suddenly realized that they were crucially placed to serve the social and psychological needs of the patient, needs generally ignored by the physician. Nursing schools seized the opportunity to broaden their curriculum by giving their students sophisticated course work in the social and behavioral sciences, and an increasing number of nurses received master and doctoral degrees in this field.

Not all expansion of the nursing role was in the social and behavioral sciences, however, and one of the most radical changes occurred in the developing coronary care units. These units originated from a shift in interest from the causes of myocardial infarctions to effective treatment. In 1950 more than 25 per cent of those hospitalized with myocardial infarction died in hospital, and another 50 per cent of those afflicted died without ever reaching medical aid. Research revealed that the anticoagulant therapy, the main treatment for many years, was not effective in reducing deaths from myocardial infarction since only a small number of such deaths resulted from embolism. In fact, nearly half the deaths were caused by arrhythmias.[60]

This realization coincided with the discoveries of William Kouwenhoven and his associates that the heart could be massaged through the intact chest[61] and of Bernard Lown that a fibrillating heart could be controlled by the direct application of an electric current across the myocardium.[62] A mobile crash cart was equipped with a defibrillator and external pacemaker and manned by a team of trained personnel, but the survival rate still remained discouragingly low because of the length of time between the discovery of the arrested patient and the application of the new techniques. The solution was the coronary care unit, the first of which opened in 1962 at Bethany Hospital in Kansas City, Kansas.

It was recognized very early that the units were not effective unless their staff could recognize and terminate arrhythmias. Though originally conceived as a physician responsibility, the coronary care units soon became a nursing specialty, since the key to success was soon seen to lie in the nurses who kept the long vigils, provided the routine care, performed the specialized tasks, skillfully identified arrhythmias, and could act promptly and independently.[63] The result was a new role for nursing which demanded that the nurse assume multiple responsibilities in the system of care, some of which overlapped with medical responsibilities. To do this effectively, nurses had to begin to collaborate with physicians instead of remaining merely subordinate to them.

The nurse's role was even further expanded by the development of the nurse-practitioner, the first formal program of which was established by Henry Silver and others in Colorado in 1965.[64] In a sense nurse practitioners are older than 1965, since public health nurses were already working in expanded roles,[65] and since nurses in outpatient settings had been responsible for the long-term management of patients with chronic illnesses at Massachusetts General Hospital since 1962.[66] Nurses themselves, however, were ambiguous about some of these programs, and there was considerable debate about whether the nurse practitioner was really a nurse since she did so many things that nurses traditionally had associated with the doctor's role.

While nurses debated, the job of physician's assistant was created. According to the early publicity associated with the development, after two years training they would provide not only primary care, but would outrank nurses and be paid almost double what nurses with more education were paid. The physician's assistant program developed from an analysis of the use of medical corpsmen in both the Korean and Vietnam wars. Corpsmen had, after some initial training, acquired great expertise in treating the wounded, and yet in civilian life, they had little opportunity to use their skills unless they went to medical school, which lack of education made difficult for most of them. In 1965 Eugene Stead started a two-year program at Duke University with four ex-corpsmen who, after taking courses in the basic sciences and the less complex medical subjects, would become physicians' assistants and give primary care.[67] The second major physician's assistant program was the Medex course for ex-independent duty corpsmen set up in Washington state.

This program was federally financed to provide technical assistance to primary physicians, particularly in rural areas where the shortage of doctors was acute.[68] The number of physician's assistant programs then increased rapidly until in 1972 there were 50 accredited programs, and 37 states had allowed them to practice.[69] With the end of the Vietnam War, however, the number of independent corpsmen radically declined, and schools had either to revise their requirements or find other sources of students.

As the physician's assistant movement became less important, the number of nurse practitioners grew. Physicians suddenly seemed to realize that they were overlooking the most natural source of primary care for their patients—the nurse. The American Academy of Pediatrics was the leader, sponsoring conferences, research, and statements supporting practitioners whom they termed "nurse associates."[70] In 1971, after negotiations, the Academy issued a joint statement with the American Nurses' Association suggesting guidelines for short-term courses for the preparation of nurse practitioners or associates. Although these negotiations were broken off for a year, in 1974 the Academy again supported the idea of nurse practitioners and in 1977 established testing procedures and certification of Pediatric Nurse Practitioners. The American Medical Association followed the lead of the Academy and in 1970 officially supported the expansion of the role of the nurse.[71] Starting in about 1970 various agencies within the Department of Health, Education, and Welfare funded experimental practitioner programs. Most of these projects were operated outside of the nursing schools in extension programs, or they were joint projects of schools of medicine and schools of nursing. Though these programs demonstrated the utility of the practitioner and developed curriculums, their experimental status gave them shallow institutional roots. As soon as the grants terminated, so did most programs. The most recent trend has been to integrate practitioner preparation into the ongoing nursing education program, a more effective long-term approach. Basic physical and psychological diagnostic skills are now considered part of baccalaureate education, while advanced nurse practitioner training is becoming a masters level specialty.

Ten

Economics of the Profession
And Its Changing Image

Nursing, at least in the United States, traditionally was not a well paying profession, primarily because it was dominated by women, and women in America have always earned less than men. This is no less true in the 1970's than it was in 1900. A 1976 study by the Survey Research Center at the University of Michigan, for example, found that the average working man made seven dollars per hour while his female counterpart earned $4.34. Moreover, when work hours were adjusted to account for total break time and time spent for on-the-job training, the wage disparity increased ($8.48 for men and $4.86 for women). Not only did women work for less, they also tended to work harder. The Michigan study found that based on reports of level of energy expended at work, women averaged 112 per cent over men. Of particular importance to nursing historically was that unmarried women received the least amount of break time and scored highest in the work effort scale.[1]

Anti-discriminatory legislation and the growing efforts to achieve equal pay for equal work may lessen the gap between men and women, although women still remain at the lower end of the pay scales. Since nursing was a woman's profession, it was perhaps inevitable that nurses would be underpaid. Nursing, however, as indicated elsewhere in this book, labored under more serious handicaps than most of the other women's professions because nurses lacked the male allies that social workers, librarians, and teachers had. They were also handicapped compared to secretaries who worked for businessmen while most nurses worked in charitable institutions. In fact, it has only been since the 1940's that hospitals as a group changed from charitable to non-profit or even profitable institutions.

Another handicap was the Florence Nightingale image. Nursing was a special calling, and nurses were regarded as specially committed to the needy. As women, nurses were also not supposed to be militant, but submissive, accepting, and passive.

Furthermore, most nurses were ambiguous about their own role and status. Nurses regarded themselves as professionalsn and it was part of the inculcated rhetoric of nursing during much of the twentieth century that professionals did not strike or agitate for better working conditions. In this sense nurses were similar to teachers, librarians, social workers, and other groups who, while striving to be professionals, increasingly were not self-employed. Physicians and dentists were also professionals, but since most of them were self-employed, they could simply raise their fees and their income by group action. Even when most nurses were self-employed, they were put at a financial disadvantage because of their inability to control the designation of nurse. Though many people would pay extra for a "registered nurse," many would not, and trained nurses often found themselves competing with women who also did housework and family care on the side.

Another factor was that nursing education was dominated by the very group that employed nurses, the hospitals, and as long as it was possible to use student nurses in key nursing roles, any potential long-term struggle for higher wages or better working conditions could be sidetracked simply by increasing the number of student nurses. When the University of Chicago hospitals and clinics, for example, in the immediate post-World War II period found it difficult to hire enough nurses, the university seriously contemplated establishing a hospital training school unaffiliated with the university, a model pioneered by Johns Hopkins. By this time, however, educational standards for nurses had been raised sufficiently, so that a new training program proved too costly. In fact, even long established programs found it difficult to meet the rising educational standards, if only because it had become increasingly hard to charge the cost of long-term training programs to patients. Expensive nurse training programs also raised hoepital costs, so that it became more difficult to compete with those hospitals without such programs unless the cost of training programs had been amortized over the years, there were large endowments for training, or as in many Catholic hospitals, a religious community was willing to undertake the training as part of its own program.

Until World War II there was also a surplus of trained nurses for the available jobs. Only in national emergencies such as the influenza epidemic of 1918–1919 was there a shortage. Part of the surplus was on paper since many women who trained as nurses followed the standard conventions of the day by marrying and leaving the job market. Many continued to be available for temporary work, occasionally taking cases from the registry to help finance special family purchases or meet a particular family need. They were not, however, full-time nurses. Their potential availability, nonetheless, tended to depress the wages and working conditions of others, since any basic improvement in these conditions caused many women to reenter the job market.

Inevitably, the result was low pay for long hours. A survey done by the Department of Labor in 1946–1947 indicated that nurses worked longer hours, did more night and shift work, carried more responsibility, received less overtime pay, had fewer fringe benefits, and were paid lower salaries than most workers in industry or in comparable occupations.[2]

Collective Bargaining

Despite these ideological handicaps, nurses gradually came to realize that if they were to make more money, they had to take more decisive action. Collective bargaining seems to have begun in California during World War II spurred by the massive population growth in that state. As the center of the rapidly expanding aircraft industry, California also became a center for wartime shipbuilding, for steel manufacture, and for other heavy industrial products; it was also the major shipping point for the war in the Pacific. Workers were recruited from all over the United States to come to California, and to attract them, wages escalated, limited only by government ceilings on wages and prices. Nurses, who also moved to California, did not seem to benefit, however. As dissatisfaction grew, several groups of nurses saw labor union affiliation as a way of improving their condition,[3] and their efforts to unionize led the California State Nurses Association to seek to become a bargaining agent in its own right from the War Labor Board. The CNA efforts were quickly terminated when it was found that the ANA did not yet allow its constituent state organizations to act as bargaining agents.[4]

Finally, in 1944, the ANA Board of Directors stated that although the national organization had to remain aloof, the state association was free to bargain.[5] The ANA also formed a committee to study the employment conditions of registered nurses. Shirley Titus, then executive director of the California State Nurses' Association, chaired the committee,[6] and as an enthusiastic supporter of collective bargaining, she was able to convince them.

Following the 1946 report of the committee, the House of Delegates of the ANA adopted an economic security program which included collective bargaining for state and district nurses' associations. The specific program committed the association to work for the 40-hour week, for minimum salaries, for increased participation of nurses in planning nursing services, and for eliminating racial barriers in nursing.[7] Speculation has it that the program was also designed to prevent mass entry of nurses into labor unions, an assumption borne out when the ANA also precluded its members from joining any other organization that could act as their bargaining agent. The impact of the economic security program as it was adopted, however, was unlike that of any labor union of the time, since the nurses deliberately voted to weaken their effectiveness by including a clause that "Under no circumstances would a strike or use of any similar coercive device be countenanced."[8]

When the statement became policy, hospitals were under the provisions of the 1935 Wagner Act which obliged them to bargain with their employees. In 1947, the Taft-Hartley Labor Management Relations Act specifically exempted non-profit hospitals from the necessity of recognizing bargaining rights of employees. Although the Taft-Hartley Act technically did not make collective bargaining illegal, when combined with nursing's voluntary pledge not to strike, that was the initial effect, since nursing apparently could not force hospital management to negotiate.[9] It took time for nurses to realize that this no-strike pledge eliminated their trump card, since even at the 1950 ANA Biennial the no-strike pledge was reaffirmed.[10]

Despite these difficulties, there was some collective bargaining and minor improvements in salaries and working conditions. By 1952, five state nurses' associations had been named as bargaining agents for groups of nurses employed in California, Minnesota, Pennsylvania, Washington, and Wisconsin.[11] Moral persuasion and public-relations campaigns were the chief weapons in these negotations, methods which sometimes proved effective simply because the salaries of nurses were so low in comparison to other trained workers that the sympathy of the public could be enlisted against reluctant administrators.[12]

Perhaps it was inevitable that some nurses would find the limited methods of moral persuasion insufficient. In 1952, when negotiations broke down between nurses and the management of the Union Labor Hospital in Eureka, California, all but one of the nurses resigned.[13] In 1961, nurses in Kewanee, Illinois, exasperated with their low salaries and the substandard care received by their patients, petitioned the hospital administration and the board of directors to meet with them or with representatives of the Illinois Nurses' Association. When their request was refused, 24 of the 46 nurses resigned, and the nurses' state association supported them. The decision to walk out took great courage because most public opinion, including hospital and medical opinion, was hostile.[14] That same year, at an institution in Bradenton, Florida, five nurses were summarily fired when the nursing staff informed the administrator that it was unhappy with the institutions' personnel policies. The Florida Nurses' Association took the case to court and forced the administration to discuss grievances.[15] Thus, gradually, dissident nurses forced their organization to develop tools other than public-relations campaigns and moral persuasion.

In 1962, economic security efforts received an important boost when President Kennedy issued an executive order establishing collective bargaining as a right for federal employees.[16] Since, at that time there were approximately 22,000 civilian nurses employed by the federal government,[17] this move allowed collective bargaining for many cases. Although it was possible to choose a union to represent them, most nurses chose state nurses' associations as their bargaining agents.

In 1966, 20 years after the inception of the ANA Economic Security Program, some modest economic gains could be noted. The average salary in 1966 for general duty nurses was approximately $5,200,[18] about two and one half times the 1946 salary of $2,100. Since the cost of living had nearly doubled in this period,[19] the salary gains were not sufficient to make nursing really competitive with other jobs requiring comparable education or even with the same demanding work schedules. It was in 1966, however, that nurses finally seemed to overcome their fear of using direct action.

In New York City, in that year, nurses employed in the nineteen municipal hospitals decided that their situation had become intolerable. Salaries and working conditions were so poor in relation to other New York institutions that the registered nurses had steadily left city employment. To demonstrate their discontent, nearly 1,500 (or about half) of the nurses employed by the Department of Hospitals resigned. Five days before the resignations were to take effect, the nurses' demands were met, starting salaries were increased from $5,150 to $6,400 with differential pay for evening and night shifts, academic preparation, and experience.[20]

In the San Francisco Bay area, after again investigating the possibility of leaving the California Nurses' Association to join the Teamsters Union or the AFL-CIO, nurses decided to stay with the professional association. When they met strong resistance in their negotiations with administrators, the nurses established informational picket lines. After stormy and prolonged negotiations, they decided to submit mass resignations. Under this pressure the California Nurses' Association Board of Directors voted to revoke the no-strike policy. With a new weapon at their disposal, Bay-area nurses were able to negotiate a contract raising their starting salaries from $5,280 to $7,200.[21]

Other nurses also struck. Two of the collective bargaining victories of 1966 were studied by sociologists who offered further insights into some of the problems facing nurses. Ada Jacox interviewed nurses who participated in a Youngstown, Ohio, strike. She found that at first the Youngstown nurses had hesitated to participate in any collective bargaining because they considered it "unprofessional." Jacox, intrigued by the concept of being unprofessional, found that these nurses also classed as unprofessional many other activities such as wearing a uniform on the street, participating in politics, or wearing jewelry on duty. Professionalism for nurses, she concluded, seemed to be associated with "ladylike" behavior, rather than the knowledge, power, and self-direction which sociologists traditionally had associated with the term.[22] With such attitudes it took many disappointments to force nurses to take action, and Jacox found that even after a string of disappointments, it was only the strong support of Youngstown's friendly unionized steelworkers that finally led the nurses to strike.

The collective bargaining of the Cook County Hospital (Chicago, Illinois) nurses was studied by Ingeborg Mauksch. She found that the nurses felt driven to collective bargaining by their inability to control the deteriorating standards of patient care.[23] Both of these studies traced the slow realization by nurses of the importance of their own power, and it was a painful realization for nurses as a whole. During the first half of 1966, the ANA economic security unit reported 143 "situations" involving close to 19,000 nurses who joined forces to negotiate better salaries, improved working conditions, and more power over nursing care.[24] Symbolic of the changes in 1966 was the vote by Pennsylvania nurses to revoke the no-strike pledge.[25]

Although in most of the 1966 negotiations nurses neither resigned nor struck, simply that they seemed willing to consider these alternatives added a new dimension to their relations with hospital administrators. Strikes by nurses, mass resignations, and hospital labor disputes of any sort were meticulously reported in *Hospitals*, the official journal of the American Hospital Association. Since hospital management was kept so well informed of events around the country, enlightened administrators began to improve conditions before their own hospitals were struck.

In 1968 the ANA finally repealed its no-strike pledge,[26] a move strengthened by the repeal in 1969 of the no-strike policy of the National Federation of Licensed Practical Nurses, a policy initially instituted in 1958.[27] These repeal actions were somewhat belated since work stoppages had already occurred. Nonetheless, a strike differs from a mass resignation, if only because striking workers do not necessarily lose their tenure and retirement benefits. Mass resignations ordinarily are more drastic than strikes; they are acts of desperation by workers who find a situation intolerable.

Even with the repeal of the no-strike pledge, nurses labored under great handicaps, since hospitals had no obligation to bargain with employees. This changed in 1974 when the Labor Relations Act was finally extended to include employees of non-profit health care institutions. In effect, hospitals and other health care agencies were required to bargain with employees; to guarantee this, negotiations were monitored by the National Labor Relations Board.[28] While the full impact of these changes has not yet been felt, it seem clear that nurses have finally reached a favorable economic position and have begun in their bargaining goals to include more emphasis on the control of nursing practice,[29] an essential mark of any profession.

Though most practical nurses have chosen unions as their representatives, if only because of the unions greater expertise in bargaining, the majority of registered nurses seem to be selecting state nurse associations. To meet these needs, the state associations have had to expand their budgets and hire professional staffs to handle their burgeoning economic activities. This change has not been welcomed by all nurses, including most supervisors who find themselves in a rather dubious legal position if they continue to belong to an organization which represents their employees. This has led many administrators to resign from the ANA.[30] Inevitably, this has changed the organization, which can be expected to become more responsive to the rank and file in the future.

The new militancy of the American nurses also had an international impact. In 1974, under the sponsorship of the International Labor Organization and the World Health Organization, representatives from nursing, government, management, and labor met in Geneva. They drew up recommendations to guide the United Nations in preparing public policy. The basic premise was that nurses should have "economic and social status which will reflect the importance of their role in health care." This included the right to collective bargaining, a 40-hour work week, reasonable pay, and education within the general educational framework rather than in isolated noneducational institutions.[31]

Nurse Practice Arts

As nurses became somewhat more militant and as the possibilities for expanding their role developed, they also began to demand the revision of nurse practice acts. Traditionally, nurses had dealt with the problems inherent in the feminine role of nursing by engaging in what has come to be called the "nurse-doctor game." The classical description by Leonard Stein revealed how physicians and nurses spent their professional lives "playing a game" in which physicians repeatedly seek and receive advice and help from nurses but in such a way that the physician's omnipotent aura is always preserved.[32] The charade was necessary because of the restrictions of the nurse-practice acts. The original nurse registration acts, which had been written early in the twentieth century, were primarily designed to distinguish the newly established RN's from more traditional nurses. In 1938 a new and second phase in nursing licensure began when New York state mandated the licensure of all who sought to give nursing care. This act defined two levels of nurses, registered and practical, and made it illegal for any others to practice. In order to enforce the law, it was necessary to define what nursing was, and this definition added a new element to the nurse practice acts.

In the New York licensure law, a registered nurse was defined as someone who was compensated for professional services, which included observing patients and carrying out nursing procedures and those medical procedures ordered by physicians. Over the next few years, several states passed similar statutes, until by 1955 about half the states had followed the New York lead.[33]

In an effort to help the nurses in all states obtain mandatory licensure, the American Nurses' Association in 1955 adopted a model definition of nursing:

The practice of professional nursing means the performance for compensation of any act in the observations, care and counsel of the ill, injured, or infirm, or the maintenance of health or prevention of illness of others, or in supervision and teaching of other personnel, or the administration of medications and treatments as prescribed by a licensed physician or dentist; requiring substantial specialized judgement and skill and based on knowledge and application of the principles of biological, physical, and social science. The foregoing shall not be deemed to include acts of diagnosis or prescription of therapeutic or corrective measures.[34]

By 1967, fifteen states had incorporated this language into their laws; six other states had used it with only slight modifications.[35] Although the model definition was in some ways an accurate reflection of the nurse's role in 1955, to disclaim any act of diagnosis or prescription was unnecessary and blocked any expansion of professional responsibility. There is no evidence that individual physicians or the American Medical Association overtly forced nurses to renounce their diagnostic and treatment function in their own practice acts. Instead, it seems that the nurses themselves sought to avert any possible opposition even before it could develop by denying themselves responsibility to make decisions.[36] In effect, nurses were writing into law the old nurse-doctor game.

Since, however, nurses had to make diagnostic and therapeutic decisions, some system was needed to help them get around their own disclaimers. One means was through the joint statement, the first of which was promulgated in 1957 when members of the California nursing, medical, and hospital associations announced that nurses could do venapunctures to start intravenous fluids.[37] Though joint statements had no legal status and could not contravene written statutes, they unofficially legitimized the changing nursing roles. Other state associations followed the California example.[38] Volunteer health organizations also became involved. In 1966, for example, the Michigan Heart Association approved the use of defibrillators by coronary care nurses.[39] In 1970 joint practice commissions were set up in several states at the urging of the National Commission for the Study of Nursing and Nursing Education. These bodies also sanctioned new responsibilities for nurses.[40]

As the pressure for expanding the nurse's role in the acute and ambulatory setting mounted, the common law protection offered by the joint statements seemed legally frail, if not absolutely illegal. Moreover, most nursing schools were reluctant to prepare nurses for roles not legally sanctioned. To allay these fears, a special committee was appointed by the Secretary of Health, Education, and Welfare. In 1971 this committee saw no legal barriers to expanding the role of the registered nurse.[41] Rhetoric is one thing, however, and legal fact another, and the statement merely added to the confusion. The Attorneys General of Arizona[42] and California[43] stated that nurses could not legally diagnose or treat patients in their states since this was clearly forbidden by the nurse practice acts.

Statutory revision was necessary, and the third and current phase in nursing licensure dates from 1971 when Idaho became the first state to revise its practice act. Three states amended their acts in 1972, five in 1973, twelve in 1974, nine in 1975, and two in 1976. Other states continue to follow. Virginia assigned regulatory responsibility for nurses with expanded functions to the Board of Medicine.[44]

The Idaho revision assigned the task of regulating nurses with expanded roles to the boards of nursing and medicine by inserting the following clause after the traditional prohibition against diagnosis and treatment:

> "except as may be authorized by rules and regulations jointly promulgated by the Idaho state board of medicine and the Idaho board of nursing which shall be implemented by the Idaho board of nursing."[45]

Following the passage of the amendment, the combined boards developed regulations. Nurses wishing to perform acts of medical diagnosis or treatment in Idaho are required to show their agency that they have obtained the necessary special education. Then and only then must the committees of nurses and physicians or dentists in each facility draw up standardized policies and procedures to guide the new nursing functions.[46]

The second approach to developing the nursing role was first used in 1972 when New York adopted the following definition of professional nursing:

> The practice of the profession of nursing as a registered professional nurse is defined as diagnosing and treating human responses to actual or potential health problems through such services as case-finding, health teaching, health counseling, and provision of care supportive to or restorative of life and well-being and executing medical regimens prescribed by a licensed or otherwise legally authorized physician or dentist. A nursing regimen shall be consistent with and shall not vary any existing medical regimen.[47]

The New York approach differs from that of Idaho in its assumption that all (or perhaps most) nurses are seeking more responsibility for diagnosing and treating patients, not just those nurses who are defined as practitioners or specialists. This approach became popular when other states revised their laws. Regardless of whether the Idaho or the New York model is followed, most states have revised their practice acts to provide for a significant expansion of the nursing role, and the remaining states have begun to follow. The effect has altered the legal position of American nurses making them more responsible for decision-making, more accountable for their own practice, and perhaps even weakening the traditional nurse-doctor game.

Also helping to challenge this game has been the increase in the number of "men nurses," a term used by nurses in part because of their dislike of the various specific references to female, such as the original designation of the Army Nurse Corps, Female. Professional male nurses have existed in the United States for almost as long as female ones. The School for Male Nurses was established in 1886 in connection with the New York City Training School for Nurses on Blackwell's (Welfare) Island.[48] Other schools specifically for men followed; a small number of schools were co-educational. By 1910 about seven percent of all student and graduate nurses were men. This was the high point. For the next 30 years the percentage declined: it was only two percent in 1940.[49] Undoubtedly, one of the reasons for the decline was the stigma of being part of a woman's profession. A more important reason, however, was simple discrimination. Almost every nurse training school demanded that its students live on the hospital grounds in nursing residences. The few nurses who were employed in the hospital, including often the nursing faculty, also lived in these homes. Most nursing residences adopted rather stringent regulations about what student nurses could do, and most did not allow their students to stay outside of the residence after 9 P.M. unless they were on duty or had special permission. Men were usually not allowed beyond "the parlor" or "sitting room."

Though restrictive requirements were often part of the dormitory living for women on college campuses, it seems in retrospect that nurse training schools were especially severe. With such regulations, no hospital training school would have considered housing male students in the same dormitory with females; thus, every training school had either to establish separate wings for their male students, allow male student nurses to live away from the hospital, or refuse to admit men all together. Most opted for the third choice. A few schools housed male students in the quarters reserved for interns or residents, but this usually proved unsatisfactory because the male student nurses not only suffered from the stigma of being in a woman's profession, but the additional loss of status associated with being a nurse while living with "doctors." Inevitably, most male nurses were graduates of separate nursing schools. These schools included the Mills Training School for Male Nurses established in 1888 and affiliated with Bellevue Hospital, and two schools established by the Alexian Brothers, one in Chicago in 1898, and the second in St. Louis in 1928. Most male nurses were graduates of hospital schools associated with mental institutions.[50]

None of the male nursing schools originally affiliated with the Associated Alumnae, the predecessor of the ANA, and when the ANA was reorganized between 1916 and 1922, no provisions for male nurses were made. Not until 1930 were the membership bylaws revised to include properly qualified male nurses.[51] Men in nursing suffered from some of the same types of discrimination that women traditionally had suffered in other fields: they were regarded as second-class citizens. As mentioned earlier, the laws authorizing the Army and Navy Nursing Corps designated nurses as female. During World War II, despite the critical shortage of nurses, male student nurses were unable to get deferments from their draft boards to finish school, although engineering, medical, and other types of students often received this privilege. No government program encouraged male nursing within the armed forces. As a result the number of men in schools of nursing, never very large, dropped from 725 in 1939 to 169 in 1945.[52]

At the low point of male nursing, the ANA finally took corrective action by organizing the Men Nurses' Section in 1940. After the war the number of male nursing students slowly began to increase, first in the psychiatric hospitals, but then more noticeably in the baccalaureate and associate degree programs where the housing and dormitory situation was not the problem it was in the hospital schools. By 1972, 2,460 men had enrolled in associate degree programs, and there were 3,159 in 1975. Baccalaureate nursing programs had 1,386 enrolled in 1972 and 1,916 in 1975.[53] Gradually, the barriers both imagined and real have been dropped. A major factor in attracting more males was simply the improvement in salaries and working conditions recounted earlier in this chapter, although census data indicates that male nurses generally were and are paid much more than nurses in general.[54] Part of this disparity was caused by the scarcity of male nurses, although simply being male probably accounted for much of the differential since men continue to make more money than women. If this disparity is not eliminated soon, tensions between male and female nurses will escalate. Some of these tensions have already increased, particularly among nursing educators who have reported that male students are not as submissive as their women students. Males also reject those aspects of nursing theory that they associate with the subordination of nursing to medicine.[55]

The United States was not the only country where nursing became predominantly a women's profession, and male nurses in other countries have had even more problems. In Great Britain, for example, men risked being called sister or matron. As late as 1966, the London *Daily Mirror* headlined a man's appointment as head of nursing services in a British hospital, as "Mister Matron." Despite these difficulties, which might challenge even the strongest male ego, Great Britain had more male nurses proportionately than did the United States, although, as in this country, most practiced in mental hospitals. As salaries and wages for nurses improved, however, more British men found nursing a rewarding career.

In short, expanding the nurses' role was rather a circuitous process. To earn more money, nurses were forced to question their traditional role and to assign some of the less skilled tasks to less qualified personnel, the LVN, aid, or orderly. As nursing redefined itself, some of the more restrictive provisions of the earlier nurse practice acts had to be eliminated. Once these were removed, more nurses specialized, and thus earnings were increased, although the two did not always occur at once. In fact, better pay required more effective organization and collective bargaining. As nurses became more self-confident, nursing itself became more attractive to men, who increasingly began to enter the profession. As part of their re-evaluation, nurses became aware of a "nurse-doctor game," and under the growing influence of feminism, began to challenge it, a challenge that has been supported by the growing number of male nurses.

Eleven

The Second Hundred Years

Although nursing and health care projects were introduced throughout the world after the reforms of Florence Nightingale, nurses themselves rarely helped to plan these programs because internationally the profession was too weak. This difficulty plagued nursing until the end of World War II. The International Council of Nurses (ICN), established in 1904 with great expectations, had been rendered inoperative by World War I. This meant that nursing, lacking the necessary international voice, had no direct influence on the health organizations of the League of Nations. Indirectly nurses were allowed to participate through the League of Red Cross Societies (LORCS), founded in 1920,[1] but the most valuable contribution of the LORCS to nursing was the establishment of a course in public health nursing at London University.[2] Later, courses in nursing administration and education were added, and over the years the program brought a limited number of nurses to London each year—some 200 nurses from 41 countries by 1933.[3]

The ICN, which had adopted a plan of international conferences every three years in 1909 at its London meeting, had met in Cologne, Germany in 1912, and planned to meet in San Francisco in 1915, a meeting cancelled by the outbreak of World War I. As an emerging international group, nursing was more disrupted by the war than most other professions, and even the Grand Council, the board of directors plus representatives of member organizations, did not assemble until 1922 in Copenhagen. Finally, in 1925 an International Congress was held at Helsinki, but by that time the international health organizations had solidified. The 1925 Congress voted to establish a journal, the *ICN,* later renamed the *International Nursing Review,* and to move the headquarters of the organization to Geneva for proximity to the League of Nations. Financial difficulties shifted the headquarters back to London in 1935, while the outbreak of World War II only added to the monetary crisis. The journal was suspended, and some of the records were moved to the United States.[4]

The major accomplishment of the ICN in this interwar period was to establish the Florence Nightingale International Foundation as an endowed trust within the ICN. Nurses and nursing organizations contributed about $200,000 to memorialize Nightingale's contribution to nursing. One of its major projects was continued support of the program for nurses at London University, from which the LORC had withdrawn. After World War II, the foundation published a series of studies on nursing education. In 1956 the foundation was dissolved and its remaining funds were used by the ICN to encourage research in nursing and for fellowships for nurses who wished to undertake advanced studies. As the ICN grew internationally, it took on the tasks of improving nursing education, nursing practice and service, and bettering the social and economic welfare of nurses throughout the world.[5] Most importantly it also serves as a nursing presence in WHO, the World Health Organization.

The United Nations

Despite the disorganization of World War II, nurses found themselves in a much better position to assert their right to participate in international health planning at the end of World War II than they had been after World War I. Undoubtedly, this strength was partially the result of a growing awareness of the value of nurses, especially in those countries that had influence and power in setting up the United Nations. The almost moribund ICN also profited from the lessons of World War I, and a small group of officials began planning activities before the war ended. One of the results of this planning was the publishing of the *International Nursing Bulletin,* the first issue of which appeared in October 1945. Plans were also made for an international congress, which met in 1947 in Atlantic City, New Jersey to plan for the future.

Part of the effectiveness of nurses within the newly organized United Nations was also the result of the special interest of Thomas Parran, the American chairman of the committee that planned the World Health Organization (WHO), and Brock Chisholm, the Canadian who served as its first director. The ICN was given both the right to participate in the Assembly and the committees of WHO and the right to submit memoranda to the Director-General. Nurses were made part of the committees, conferences, and medical teams being organized as projects to be sent throughout the world. An Expert Committee on Nursing was also established within WHO to promote nursing in underdeveloped areas and emerging nations. Each of the six regional offices of WHO had a nursing office under the direction of a chief nurse, while nurses were employed in almost every project. Nurses within WHO were soon running demonstration units in many countries, the success of which led to the establishment of training schools and the improvement of nursing practices in many of the newly independent or underdeveloped countries.[6]

Without WHO, nursing would undoubtedly have suffered serious setbacks, since nursing in much of Asia and Africa had been identified either with Christian missionaries or with Western colonialism. When these areas became independent, they often tried to remove all trace of their former colonial status, including nursing schools, while Christian missionaries were expelled. Since, somewhat paradoxically, these same nations were tremendously impressed with the medical and scientific advances of the United States and Western Europe, they nevertheless wanted to improve their own health care practices. WHO was an effective alternative, allowing nurses to work with newly established governments without threatening their integrity or independence.

Egypt (United Arab Republic) and the Middle East

Perhaps Egypt is typical of what happened in many parts of the world. In Egyptian hospitals English nurses up to the end of World War II had held almost all supervisory positions. Under them were Egyptian "nurses" of two classes: the upper-level nurse, who received three years of nurse training after completing the ninth grade of school, and their assistants, or lower-level nurses, with two years training after completing the sixth grade. There were also hospitals run by French and Italian nuns and some American missionary schools, which used American hospital training programs as models but adjusted their standards both to the lower educational level and to the low status of Egyptian women at that time. When the British (and the French) were forced out of Egypt in 1956, nursing immediately dropped in quality because none of the Egyptian nurses had been trained to be leaders. Moreover, a few women in Egypt had become considerably emancipated, going to college and entering professions, so that the old style of nursing, which demanded twelve-hour days and six-day weeks and made the nurses into little more than doctors' servants, was no longer an attractive occupation. The Egyptian government, foreseeing a possible decline in nursing and wanting to raise nursing standards, turned to the WHO to help it improve nursing practices. The result was the establishment of two WHO-sponsored collegiate nursing schools, first at Alexandria University, and later at Cairo University. These new-style nurses not only had to contend with the Egyptian physicians who still tended to look down on the nurses, but were also opposed by the old-style nurses who quite naturally felt threatened by the better-qualified nurses. This tension was not eased by the college-trained nurse being the educational equal of the Egyptian physician, since medicine in Egypt is an undergraduate major. Despite these tensions, however, the new-style nurse survived, and graduates of the collegiate program went abroad to the United States, England, Scotland, Canada, and elsewhere to earn advanced degrees before returning to Egypt to continue the struggle to improve nursing. As the number of Egyptian graduates increased, they were invited by other Arab countries, many of them newly rich from oil, to improve their programs. Egyptian nurses went to Kuwait, Libya, Saudi Arabia, and other countries, establishing new nursing programs wherever they went. Occasionally, the WHO programs were supplemented by American nurses who went abroad under the Fulbright or other such programs as faculty members in the new national schools.[7]

In general, however, the emerging nationalism in the Middle East and elsewhere made it difficult for any outsiders other than a WHO nursing team to be in control, although individual nurses outside these programs could also be effective. The country with the most advanced nursing in the Middle East, Israel, has had almost no influence on its neighbors because of its isolation from the Arab world. Israeli nurses are equal to those of the most advanced nations of the world, and could, if given an opportunity, assist their sister nurses in neighboring countries, but as of this writing there is little contact between the two. Somewhat more influential in effecting nursing change in the Middle East is the nursing school associated with the American University of Beirut in Lebanon. This school, established as part of the American Hospital in Beirut in 1905, later affiliated with the American University where it offered an optional degree program. In 1950 after Lebanon became fully independent from France, the nursing school established a one-year training course for area nursing leaders in an attempt to improve nursing practice. Unfortunately, the effectiveness of the American University's program was limited by the continued domination of American nurses. Moreover, though the University had become increasingly secular, it was still associated with the Christian missionary movement in the minds of many Muslims, although the university had a significant number of Muslim faculty and students. Antagonisms between Muslims and Christians in Lebanon run deep, as was indicated by the civil war of 1976. Though the American University is an integral part of Lebanon, it is now difficult to predict whether it will continue to have much influence on nursing outside of that country.

Nurses in Africa

African nursing shares many of the same problems as nursing in the Middle East, but the problems are compounded because in many of the newly independent countries the old colonial administration did little to advance indigenous nursing. This was true in much of Portuguese Africa and in the Belgian Congo, now Zaire. A school of nursing was established in the new Republic of Congo through the monetary assistance of the Rockefeller Foundation, but its growth was limited by the strife within the country. After it was reorganized as Zaire, however, health services were also reorganized.

In French Africa, the French as a rule gave little support to public health or to education except in those areas where there were large numbers of French settlers, such as Algeria and Morocco. Those few Africans who did receive an education in the French colonies, however, probably received a more sophisticated one than elsewhere in Africa; the schools which existed there were officially recognized as part of the French educational system, equal to any school in France. Unfortunately, few Africans in French Africa became nurses. Many of the health centers were staffed by male nurses, so-called, who received an apprenticeship training, but by American standards the title of nurse was little more than a courtesy. It was not until 1951, for example, that a nursing school was opened in Dakar, French West Africa, and the training followed the state course of nurses in France.

It was in French Africa that the most famous medical missionary of modern times, Dr. Albert Schweitzer, spent most of his adult life. Schweitzer, who was internationally known as a theologian, musician, and writer, rendered important service to the natives, but his African nurses were inadequately trained to meet the demands of modern medicine. It was not until after his death that necessary nursing reforms could be introduced. It was in places like Africa that the WHO performed its most valuable services to nursing.

WHO Also Has Problems

Obviously, for a country to participate in a WHO project it must belong to the United Nations. The most populous country in the world, China, was excluded for a long time, and this international isolation meant that Chinese nurses have also been isolated. Although China has always been an independent country, various outside powers such as England, France, and the United States exercised great influence on the internal affairs of China during the nineteenth and early twentieth centuries. Western missionaries entered China in great numbers to establish nursing and other schools, but when the Chinese Communists took over, both missionaries and nurses were called agents of foreign imperialism. Most of the nursing schools (there were more than 300) were closed when the missionaries were expelled; nursing practice inevitably suffered. Unfortunately, China could not call upon the WHO for help in improving nursing because, until the Nixon administration, the United Nations dealt only with the Chinese government-in-exile in Taiwan.

Estrangement and isolation encouraged the Chinese to return to their own traditions, and Chinese physicians used acupuncture and other traditional remedies and began to blend traditional and Western medicine. It is not yet clear what role Western-style nursing will have in this new medicine, but as the animosities between China and the West lessen, it seems likely that nursing in China will change, again becoming more Western.

In general, the WHO nursing programs have essentially adopted American and Canadian rather than British nursing practices. As a result most of the nursing programs in underdeveloped countries have tended to look to Canada or the United States for leadership once schools were established. This complicates the issue of nursing in China and in many other Communist and neutral countries.

It is important to realize that there are certain basic differences between American and British nursing education. The American model emphasizes an intellectual approach, with great attention to the social and behavioral sciences; the British have emphasized nursing techniques, including midwifery. Since the development of the nurse practitioner and clinical specialist, American nurses have begun to reassess their system and to pay greater attention to the biological sciences and to the techniques of physical assessment, but they have retained their basic emphasis on collegiate education. On the other hand, British nursing has been unwilling and unable to establish itself in colleges and universities to any great extent. Rather, it has retained an apprenticeship model of training.[8] While this model may be functional for some underdeveloped countries, the collegiate plan looks more attractive to those countries that need nurses for a highly responsible role.

Canadian nursing bridges the gap between the American and the British because it has elements of both in its educational system—and it also has a developing collegiate program. Canadians have also been more acceptable to many of the neutralist countries than Americans simply because they are regarded as neutral themselves. (This was particularly true during the American involvement in Vietnam, which resulted in a massive wave of anti-Americanism in many third-world countries.) As a result, many WHO schools and teams have been directed by Canadian nurses. As indicated, however, American nurses did serve in the WHO programs, and these programs were often supplemented by Fulbright lectures, Peace Corps work, or by special American projects when requested by the host country. Despite suspicions of the United States, large numbers of foreign-trained nurses have nevertheless come to the U.S. for further training or for graduate study under programs financed by the WHO, private foundations, the universities themselves, and even by the American government.

Russian Nursing

Although much of the world belongs to what is sometimes called the

Soviet zone of influence, the Russian (or Soviet) pattern of nursing has been largely ignored in the West. In the nineteenth century, developments in Russian nursing seemed to be somewhat influenced by the West. While Florence Nightingale and her nurses were caring for British soldiers in the Crimean War, Russian women were serving on the other side. Probably the best known of the Russian nurses was Ekaterina M. Bakunina, a Moscow society girl who volunteered to serve as a nurse after hearing an appeal from the Grand Duchess Elena Pavlovna in 1854. After a brief period of observation in hospitals, she donned the habit of the Order of the Exaltation of the Cross and went off to the Crimea. The Russian nurses suffered from greater handicaps than the British, and some seventeen of the 160 women who volunteered died, mostly from typhus. The nursing order continued to exist until 1894 when it was absorbed by the Russian Red Cross.[9]

Russian nursing was radically reorganized when the Communists seized power during the 1917 revolution. Men and women were declared equal, and distinctions between professional and manual workers were abolished. Though the effectiveness of such a declaration can be debated, it effectively divorced nursing from two of the struggles which have dominated its history in much of the rest of the world: the battle for equality for women and the attempts of nurses to be recognized as a profession. Russian nurses, however, have had other problems.

As part of their reorganized medical practice, the Soviets established three categories of medical workers: lower, middle, and higher. This set up a vocational ladder in which the unskilled were separated from the skilled, and the skilled and semiprofessional from the professional. The lines between the three groups, however, were and still are not clearly drawn. In fact workers on the lower rung who qualify by additional preparation and experience can advance to the next highest level. People who initially join at the middle level can move to the upper level as their training and experience increase. On the lowest level are the aides and orderlies who have four years of general education and some practical training. Nurses belong to the middle level along with midwives and feldshers (semi-physicians who care for lesser ailments and do minor surgery). The middle-level group have eight to ten years of general schooling plus a three- or four-year course in their specialty. Physicians, the top-level practitioners, have ten years of general schooling and four or five years of training.

Nurses, feldshers, and midwives are all trained in technical institutes associated with regional medical centers. In 1972 there were 635 of these centers, 21 of them in Moscow. All the institutes used the same textbooks and the same audiovisual aids. All of the teaching is done by professors from the university or teachers from pedagogical institutes. Clinical subjects are taught by hospital physicians who are expert in the practical aspects but not necessarily in teaching. Nurses are trained either for general nursing or for nursing children. Midwifery is a specialized course. In the first year, students spend most of the time in the classroom; only 164 hours are spent in the hospital, where the emphasis is on housekeeping. In the second year students take care of patients and are taught how to give injections and handle technical equipment. The third year is devoted to extensive preparation for the state examination. Training for feldshers is similar to nursing but requires an additional year since they have special preparation for relatively independent practice, especially in the villages. The midwife training program is similar to that of the feldsher but with greater concentration on obstetrics. Nurses who become head nurses or anesthesiologists are given further training at special institutes. They can also take special courses in physical therapy, surgery, obstetrics, pediatrics, anesthesiology, psychiatry, and neurology.[10]

The chief difficulty with the Russian system is that it does not provide a professional identity for nurses, since doctors, nurses, feldshers, aides, and other medical workers all belong to the same organization. Instead nursing acts as a halfway house between other goals. The more ambitious nurses do not seek leadership in nursing organizations or attempt to improve nursing practices, but instead move on to the highest category, that of physician. Nurses also lack control over their own training. There is, however, a career ladder. It has been estimated that about one-third of the physicians in the Soviet Union (almost all of whom are women) served first as nurses, midwives, or feldshers.

After World War II Soviet influence was established in many areas of the world, sometimes influencing Western-trained nursing and sometimes establishing the Soviet pattern. In countries such as Poland, which had a strong and independent nursing system before it became part of the Soviet bloc, nurses remain much more Western even though they are regarded as middle-level medical personnel. In general the ICN has not had much influence on the Soviet nurse, and she has been left out of many of the UN agencies which have set their personnel standards along Western lines. This isolation of the Soviet nurse has handicapped a truly international communication and movement of nurses.

Latin America

Modern nursing was slow to develop in Latin America, mainly because of middle-class prohibitions against working women and a resistance of the middle and upper classes to recognize the importance of any sort of manual labor, the category to which they assigned nursing. Early Nightingale schools were established in Brazil and Argentina. The Ana Neri School in Rio de Janeiro was founded in 1923, largely through the efforts of American nursing. Brazilian nursing was long dominated by Americans, and it was not until late in the development of Ana Neri that Brazilians themselves took control. In 1943 the school became part of the University of Brazil. Other collegiate schools were established later, but this only divided Brazilian nursing into three rival groups in which the university-trained nurses found themselves in a decided minority.

The influence of the United States was also evident in Argentine nursing education. In 1918 a hospital school was started at the Parmenio Piñero Hospital in Buenos Aires. In 1937 Standard Oil Company set up a nursing school in Salta, Tartagal. The first university school opened in 1940 in Rosario under the direction of the medical faculty who recruited an American, Jean Martin White, as its first director.[11]

Chilean nursing has also been relatively progressive. The Chilean Association of University Nurses became a member of the International Council of Nurses in 1953. Uruguay has attempted to improve its nursing practices by requiring nine years of preliminary education for admission, but in much of Latin America the nurse is still regarded as a servant for the doctor. Perhaps the Rockefeller Foundation has been most influential in setting standards for nurses in Latin America. It was, for example, under its auspices that the University of Mexico School of Nursing was established in 1935.[12] Cuba, which had a low standard of nursing, established its first collegiate school in 1976; its first class is to graduate in 1980. In Cuba, despite strong Russian influence, the American-Canadian model of nursing is still predominate. This is probably significant for the development of nursing in other underdeveloped and emerging countries associated with the Soviet Union. Also influential has been the growth of nursing in the Commonwealth of Puerto Rico. Nurses here belong to the ANA and to the NLN and are increasingly important in transmitting the ideas and practices of modern nursing to the Hispanic world. In recent years WHO projects have also created a demand for better-trained nurses throughout the area.

Japan

Japanese nursing has changed quite radically in the last few years and has had considerable influence in Asia. Though Christian missionaries had opened nursing schools in the nineteenth century, the real impetus for improving the care of the sick came from the Japanese government as part of a program for military preparedness. In this the Japanese followed the plan of the German Red Cross to staff its military hospitals. A Red Cross hospital and training center were built in Tokyo, and ladies of the imperial family and the high nobility were encouraged to take courses. Some even took the two-year course of training, which qualified them as full-fledged nurses. During World War I the Japanese Red Cross units met British and American nurses, who were then their allies, which further broadened the Japanese nursing program.

Nursing suffered a severe setback during World War II, however, when the needs and demands of the war effort forced the Japanese to ignore most of the legal regulations about nursing. Moreover, many hospitals were destroyed. During the American occupation of Japan, there was a reorganization which included an attempt to relate nursing schools to institutions of higher education. This development coincided with a partial emancipation of the Japanese woman, and nursing became involved in the drive for equality. In 1947 special regulations were adopted for public health nurses, midwives, and nurses, which brought nurses and midwives together under special licensing provisions. Nursing, however, still had difficulties, and a 1953 *Report on Nursing and Midwifery in Japan* indicated many of the same problems that affected American nurses in their relation to physicians. The Japanese system of admitting the family of the patient together with the patient himself makes for a different hospital situation than Americans are accustomed to, but the effect is to allow nurses to become as far removed from actual patient care as many already are in American hospitals. This type of patient care is widely practiced in much of the world, and makes it somewhat easier for the American professional nurse to be grafted onto the existing system, since there is less need to develop all the auxiliary personnel now part of the American scene.[13]

Nursing in the British Commonwealth

Quite obviously Canadian nursing is of high quality, but then so is that of Australia, New Zealand, South Africa, and other English-speaking areas of the British Commonwealth. Perhaps somewhat more surprising, British forms of nursing also remain the ideal in India, Cyprus, and other non-English-speaking countries of the Commonwealth.

Until the British withdrew from India, the majority of trained nurses came from missionary schools and were Christian or Parsee women, who were outside of the caste restrictions that so handicap development in much of modern India. Unfortunately, when India gained its independence (though it still remained in the Commonwealth), it had fewer nurses than physicians, which made it extremely difficult to maintain standards. Though the various five-year plans in India have called for improving nursing practices and extending nurse training, many of the missionary schools were closed as foreign support for them was withdrawn or Indian pressure was exerted against outsiders. There are collegiate schools of nursing at New Delhi and elsewhere, and the few college-trained nurses have positions of great responsibility. There are also several hospital schools, but the mass poverty and social disorganization of much of India make effective nursing extremely difficult except in very limited areas. Indian nurses are among the leaders in trying to bring various methods of family planning to the people, something that nurses around the world are just beginning to realize is of major concern to nursing itself.

Since it is not our purpose to examine each country in detail, Australian nursing can be considered representative of the British Commonwealth. Australia has had two levels of nurse: the registered nurse, with three years' training, and the nursing aid or enrolled nurse, with one year's training and practical experience. Basic nursing education generally was provided in hospital schools of nursing, following the British rather than the American model. Each state in Australia has a Nurses' Registration Board which is responsible for setting the required curriculum and for final examinations leading to registration. Australia, in the 1970's, started to develop baccalaureate programs to move its nursing into Colleges of Advanced Education. Until recently there have been few generalized public health nurses in the American sense; but rather, specialized nurses have provided well-baby care in baby health centers, care in child health centers for children with physical or emotional problems, school health services, and home nursing services. The generalized community health nurse is just developing. As in the United States, nurses are expanding their role, and in 1973 the Karmel Committee, reporting to the Australian Universities Commission on Medical Education, recommended that nurses be encouraged to work in an expanded role in conjunction with physicians in community health centers and as practice nurses in large group practices. There is an Australian precedent for this since so-called bush nurses have long been the main source of medical care in vast stretches of central Australia.[14]

Since Canadian nurses exercise so much influence upon the world scene it is also important to understand contemporary nursing in that country, which is both like and unlike the American system. Canada has two main classes of nurse: the registered nurse and the registered nursing assistant. There are also untrained personnel such as orderlies, nurse's aids, practical nurses, and psychiatric aids. As in the United States there are a variety of educational programs for registered nurses ranging from diploma programs in hospitals and community colleges to baccalaureate programs and advanced degree programs. Unlike the United States, however, the Canadian government itself began to intervene early in nursing, and government reports did what ANA-sponsored reports such as the Brown or Lysaught Reports did in this country. In 1969, for example, a Task Force Report on the Costs of Health Services in Canada underlined the importance of more efficient use of registered nurses, suggesting ways of assigning specific tasks to less costly personnel. The Canadian Nurses' Association then stated officially that manpower needs could be met effectively and economically by expanding the role of the nurse.[15]

In April 1971, a national conference agreed that the registered nurse was the most logical physician's assistant,[16] thus giving Canada a strong start on the nurse practitioner program. In April 1972 the Committee on Nurse Practitioners recommended guidelines to the Department of National Health and Welfare for developing educational programs for nurse practitioners to serve as initial contact for entrance into the system of care, to assess the individual's health status, and to determine the need for medical, nursing, and other intervention.[17] Later the Canadian Nurses' Association and the Canadian Medical Association endorsed expanding roles for nurses.[18]

The first major research project on the results of using nurse practitioners as an alternative to physician care was done in Canada. In 1974 David L. Sackett and his associates reported a study in which 1,598 families were randomly assigned to nurse practitioners or physicians for primary ambulatory care. At the end of a year no significant differences were found in the two patient groups in mortality, morbidity, or on measures of physical, social, and emotional well-being. Nurse practitioners were able to handle about 67 percent of the patient visits without referrals; the remainder were passed to physicians for more definitive treatment.[19] In short, as Canadian nurses have become increasingly influential internationally, they have also pioneered many areas of nursing practice and education.

Each country or cultural area, however, tends to make its own response to the demands for better care of the sick, and even within Western Europe there are significant differences. Though Continental nurses were strongly influenced by the Nightingale model, they were slower to modify their earlier practices than the English, perhaps because few had had as bad a system as England before the Nightingale school emerged. Because their nursing systems were better, attempts to improve on the English model led to strong opposition from physicians and from those women accustomed to acting as nurses. Tentative beginnings toward change were disrupted by both World Wars and by the interwar economic depression. Even France did not pass a law protecting the title of state registered nurse until 1946. In that same year the Italian Nurses Association was reorganized. Italian nursing's earlier efforts toward reform and improvement had been hindered by a three-way struggle between the state diploma nurses (a minority), the nuns, and the various untrained practical nurses who made up the vast majority. Finally, in 1954 a National Registration Board for Nurses was established to bring some order out of the chaos.

Scandinavian nursing was much more advanced than French or

Italian. After World War II Sweden reorganized and improved its whole nursing program by requiring high school education for admission and intensifying both the theoretical and the practical instruction. Danish nurses were even further advanced, since as early as 1938 they had had a postgraduate school of nursing education at the University of Aarhaus. Scandinavian health care also has been particularly effective in preventive medicine and in social and health insurance.

Increasingly, nurses everywhere began to resemble one another, facing many of the same problems. Belgian nurses, for example, in 1971 organized themselves to query physicians about nursing functions. In interviews the nurses asked the physicians whether nurses could properly perform certain specific procedures. Uniformly the physicians replied that nurses could, that they did them every day, and that without nurses to perform these functions hospitals could not operate. None of the tasks about which the nurses questioned the physicians, however, were legally permitted. Belgian law, for example, did not allow nurses to give intravenous injections, although nurses regularly did so. Despite general concurrence by the physicians about the expanded scope of nursing functions, and the nurses' willingness and ability to engage in these functions, official rules were slow to change.[20] In short, Belgian nurses found themselves exactly where American nurses were before they began to demand a revision of nurse practice acts as discussed in the last chapter.

American Nursing

Since this is the case, it is important to understand some of the concerns of both American and Canadian nurses who, in nursing education and practice, are among the world leaders. American nurses have already fought many of the battles that European nurses are just beginning to fight, although the time lag between the two North American groups and their sisters elsewhere is no longer as great as it once was. Nonetheless, the paths set by American and Canadian nurses will probably both be followed elsewhere and help to set the standards for the WHO and other international agencies, thus serving as examples to nurses everywhere.

Assisting these two groups to dominate the world scene has been the influence of American and Canadian medicine. Although the Canadians lead Americans in the delivery of health care, American medicine furnishes scientific leadership to the world.

There are, however, still many problems and areas in which change seems imminent. One of the most noticeable changes in American nursing is in the marital status of the women involved. Before World War II, marriage usually, though not always, meant that a nurse retired. Nursing leaders were therefore generally unmarried older women, while much of the actual nursing was done by younger unmarried women who would soon leave nursing. In some countries this is still true. For example, in Australia in 1967 an estimated 60 per cent of nursing graduates from 1957 to 1966 were no longer in practice.[21] Such a drain from the profession made it difficult for nurses to organize effectively or to demand any radical changes in nursing education. It also meant that the married women who did pursue a nursing career worked under considerable handicaps, since many of the key nursing leaders were either spinsters or lesbians, although only a small minority were as open and accepting of their lesbianism as Lillian Wald.[22]

The first major change came during World War II when the demand for nurses encouraged large numbers of married women to return to work. The Cadet Corps was also important in changing traditional patterns since it admitted married students, a group previously excluded from most of the hospital schools. Undoubtedly, the opportunity to continue her profession has opened up possibilities for a fuller life for the married nurse, but at the same time it has posed problems to nursing. Since many married nurses, during at least part of their childbearing years, prefer not to work full-time, hospitals hired them for part-time work, and thus could operate without having to make the job more attractive in order to recruit full-time nurses. Part time nurses often did not identify with nursing organizations, and a much smaller percentage of them joined professional associations or took an active part in organizational duties. This helped explain the gap between the nursing organization and the general duty nurse, a gap that in some areas made it difficult for nursing organizations to represent nurses effectively. Even when the married nurse worked full-time, she often lacked the time or energy to take over either organizational or administrative positions. These positions came to be occupied by those nurses who were able to devote most of their time and energy to nursing. These nurses gradually rose to positions of responsibility. Because of these factors, leadership in the field has accrued to unmarried nurses. In a recent study Gwendolyn Safier interviewed seventeen major figures who represented the leadership in nursing education, administration, and practice. Eight had never been married, and five others had delayed marriage until after the age of 30. Only two of the seventeen had children.[23]

In a sense nursing is like any other profession whose leaders are also those who devote time and energy to their work. In nursing, however, the social sanctions associated with the roles of women eliminated many married women who might have sought to be leaders. This has begun to change as the feminist movement has become more militant, and fewer young women feel they are neglecting their families if they work full-time. Higher salaries for general duty nurses will also help change the situation because it will enable mothers to hire baby sitters and housekeepers in order to devote more time to nursing duties and professional activities. But the married nurse does not yet hold the key organizational and leadership positions, and there is still a dichotomy between the rank and file and the leadership, which is accentuated by the differing marital statuses of the two groups. Undoubtedly, the ability of the schools, the health care institutions, and the nursing organizations to absorb married nurses will significantly determine the future direction of nursing.

Even without this dichotomy, organized nursing still faces other difficulties. There are more than a million registered nurses in the country, but only fifteen per cent belong to the ANA. When only the 800,000 employed nurses are considered, the ANA membership is higher, approximately 21 per cent, but that is still low for controlling working conditions or dealing with state and federal governments.[24] Organizational leaders had hoped in 1952 that cutting the number of nursing organizations to two would strengthen the position of the ANA and the NLN vis-a-vis their members and the public. In retrospect this may not have been a wise decision. Any organization of potentially a million members can no longer be a volunteer organization; increasingly, the ANA, and particularly the NLN is run by paid professionals. If volunteer nursing leaders are accused of not representing the general duty nurse, it follows that paid professionals are even further removed.

Moreover, one of the effects of the 1952 reorganization was to lessen the impact of special interest groups. For example, the National Organization for Public Health Nursing was able to speak effectively for public health nurses and to stimulate the growth of the specialty. While supposedly the NLN assumed this role, many public health nurses have felt lost in the NLN. Others have looked to the American Public Health Association, but it has been dominated by its physician members. As a result it has also failed to fill the shoes of the NOPHN.[25] While the ANA, in its reorganization plan, provided for sections for specialties, this has not developed as well as anticipated. Inevitably, some of the more vital groups within nursing have organized outside of the ANA structure; these include the Association of Operating Room Nurses, The American Association of Colleges of Nursing, The American Association of Critical Care Nurses, The National Association of Pediatric Nurse Practitioners and Associates, and other groups. Though the National Association of Colored Graduate Nurses merged with the ANA, Black nurses have more recently wanted a unique platform and have organized the Council of Black Nurses. It seems that these smaller groups give members a feeling of comradery, of common action that is missing in larger organizations. It may be that the time has come for a federation of nursing organizations to unite the various groups rather than trying to sustain only one or two organizations.

The present situation is problematic because nurses are not exercising their potential power to influence decisions that affect them. For example, nurses have very little power to decide how hospitals are operated and little effective say in what constitutes good nursing service within the hospitals. The Joint Commission on Accreditation of Hospitals, established in 1951, officially accredits health care institutions. Sixteen of its commissioners are physicians, three are hospital executives, and one is an executive involved in health affairs. As the *American Journal of Nursing* pointed out in 1977, nineteen of the 20 commissioners at that time were male, and no ethnic minorities were represented. Thirteen of the sixteen physician members were in private practice, while the other three were hospital executives.[26] Though nurses have officially requested representation with full voting rights on the Joint Commission and on the National Professional Standards Review Council, they have been refused, even though nursing service accounts for an estimated 60 per cent of a hospital's budget.

The same discrimination exists in the Professional Standards Review Organization which was established by Congressional action to provide for the review of health care for beneficiaries of Medicare, Medicaid, and Maternal and Child Health funds. Though nurses are now members on utilization review groups or committees, the law until 1976 stipulated that only physicians can be members of the national organization.[27] Similarly, nurses have been barred from effective participation in the accreditation of long-term care facilities. In some states accredited and licensed nursing homes did not even have to have professional nurses on their staff. The list could go on, but the conclusion is the same. Nursing as yet has little political power and is often regulated by outside forces. Potentially, however, nurses have enough clout to demand admission, even to sue if the JCAH does not admit them as participating members, and to demand that Congress change the Professional Standards Review Organization. So far, however, nurses have been content to request rather than demand, to be "ladylike" rather than to fight with the men who control these organizations.

One of the difficulties brought on by the stratification of nursing within the institutional setting is the status hierarchy that has developed among the various levels of nursing personnel. The higher the position of the nurse in this hierarchy, the less actual patient contact. Practical nurses or nurses aids who work like practical nurses can spend most of their time with patients, while registered nurses have had to assume more responsibility for the highly technical nursing functions, the supervision of the care given by other nurses, and the proliferation of paper work. Nurses with additional educational preparation at the baccalaureate level or beyond are likely to advance and have more administrative and educational duties and even less patient contact. In fact there is seemingly an inverse ratio between the educational requirements, pay, and status of the position and the amount of patient contact. These hierarchical differences are not quite so solid in the public health setting, but even here they are developing.

In the language of business management, this is sometimes called the "rationalization of the system" because a complex role has been broken into component parts and allocated to individual workers for maximum efficiency. Maximum efficiency, however, does not necessarily provide the most humane patient care. Moreover, many, nurses feel personally deprived because the resultant fragmentation is less satisfying to them, and many decry that the role of the nurse has changed from that of providing direct patient care to being a coordinator, administrator, and/or technician.[28] There is considerable literature on "bringing nurses back to the bedside,"[29] trying to counter the trend toward stratifying nursing.

Three related movements of the mid-sixties sought to deal with this problem: (1) the development of the clinical specialist; (2) the emergence of the nurse practitioner; and (3) the utilization of the hospital-based primary care nurse. Clinical specialists are nurses who have obtained educational preparation beyond the baccalaureate, usually at the masters degree level; their advanced study is designed to enable them to give expert care to seriously ill patients, to act as role models, and to spend time with patients who need emotional support.[30] Since the clinical specialty in psychiatric nursing was an early development, financed largely by the federal government,[31] it has been a model for many of the other specialities, and the importance of the psychological aspects of care has been emphasized. Since the movement started in the educational system rather than within health care institutions, with nurse educators trying to reform practice by preparing graduates to fill a new role, there have been problems establishing that role. Much of the difficulty has arisen because hospital and nursing administrators were the authors of the original stratification of nursing which was in part the result of economic necessity. To turn the clock back with the clinical specialist might well be desirable from the patient's point of view, but most administrators are unwilling to pay the salaries necessary to attract clinical specialists. Some administrators have indicated this willingness to accept them if they also had administrative functions, while others have suggested that clinical specialists should be willing to work for the same wages as basic registered nurses. Still, there is a slowly growing use of clinical specialists, particularly in the more up-to-date medical centers.

The nurse practitioner movement also allows nurses with advanced education and new skills to participate in patient care. Its emphasis on diagnosis and treatment distinguishes it from the clinical specialist, but the two roles are both directed toward patient care.

A third effort to combat the fragmentation of care has been the development of primary nursing units. On these units the nursing team is replaced with registered or practical nurses who give total care on their shift to a group of patients and plan for those patients' care on other shifts. This gives the patient someone to whom he can relate.[32] While this system, if carried to its logical conclusion, puts a considerable burden on the individual nurse without corresponding financial rewards, it does return nurses to the bedside and improves patient care. The primary care movement is related to the clinical specialist effort, and an early successful trial of clinical specialists used an administrative structure similar to the primary nursing model.[33] While the primary nursing approach sounds in many ways like a return to traditional nursing care, it does have some differences. Probably the key element in its success is not simply the use of registered nurses in place of aides, but the power given to the nurse when she is made accountable for a small group of patients. Research indicates that patients' outcomes are most favorable when nurses are given the greatest responsibility over patient care.[34]

Research

An important development within nursing itself has been the growing emphasis on research. During much of the modern period, nurses depended on others for the research that helped to develop the profession. Florence Nightingale was one of the chief exceptions. She did intensive, interesting, and significant work in health care. However, throughout most of the history of nursing, research about the profession and its problems has been done by outsiders. Since World War II, there has been a growth in nursing research. Although that development was painfully slow at first, it is now gaining momentum and is helping to give nurses a stronger voice in the decisions that affect them. The foundation of the journal *Nursing Research* 1952 indicates this growing emphasis in nursing. Also important was the establishment in 1955 of the American Nurses' Foundation to encourage research. In 1963 the Foundation initiated a small grants program to assist nurses in specific research projects. More important, at least in terms of monetary aid, was the willingness of the various government agencies to support nursing research, a move also followed by some of the private foundations. Though there is probably less research in nursing than in other professions, the quality equals that in any other field, and nurses publish in all kinds of scholarly journals.

Other Trends and Problems

One of the difficulties nurses have recently faced is that some of their potential allies in the feminist movement have in fact been their worst enemies. Feminists have agitated over why women become nurses instead of physicians and have demanded that girl children be given doctor kits instead of nurse hats. While we firmly believe that more women should become physicians and more men become nurses, we think that the feminist rhetoric has been misplaced. What should be emphasized is how far a group of women have come on their own, fighting all the way. Nursing is what people make it. Though they have had many male allies, they also have had to make their way in a world that has historically been dominated by masculine values and masculine professions. Instead of attacking nursing for being subordinate to medicine—and it has been in the past—the feminists should be encouraging its struggle.

Throughout this book we have tried to emphasize that the development of the modern nurse has been closely allied with the rising status of women. Wherever women have had very little freedom, nursing has had difficulty developing as a profession. Where respectable women do not leave their homes, where educational opportunities for women have been limited, where actual nursing care is regarded as a low status occupation, nursing still remains in its infancy. Modern nursing has depended on the development of modern medicine and the hospital; this development has often been told, but the reverse dependence of modern medicine and the development of the hospital on modern nursing has not. We believe that the individual most responsible for the development of modern medicine is the nurse.

Nursing still has many unsolved difficulties; it is still a changing profession. In some of our other books we have tried to portray some of the possibilities, but there are still many options. Part of the answer to its future development must be given in terms of what is best for the patient. This is an area in which nurses are contributing significant research, and here nursing research itself might help to decide which direction the profession should take. Part of the answer must also involve future developments in medicine. Early ambulation, intensive-care centers, electronic monitoring devices, antibiotics, and modern surgery—all have radically changed the hospital and with it the duties of the nurse. Future discoveries and innovation will probably cause changes that will be every bit as radical, and within the American context the whole nature of nursing will change with adoption of national health insurance. We hope that nursing will be able to take advantage of the opportunities afforded by government-supported medical care. Obviously, much of nursing's future depends on the decisions which nurses themselves will make.

Future decisions will depend on the ability of nurses to achieve better education, to earn more money for their services, and to offer more effective patient care. We have attempted to show the development of modern nursing, indicating how it arrived at its present position, some of the obstacles it had to overcome, and some of the difficulties that still remain. Nursing has a long and important history, but its future is in part for the nurses of today (and tomorrow) to decide. We hope that the information given here will help them make better decisions.

Notes

Chapter 1

1 Herodotus, *History*, A. D. Godley, ed. and trans., 4 vols. (London: William Heinemann, 1920–1924), II, p. 84.

2 *Edwin Smith Surgical Papyrus*, J. H. Breasted, ed. and trans., 2 vols. (Chicago: University of Chicago Press, 1930).

3 *Ebers Papyrus*, B. Ebbel, ed. and trans. (Copenhagen: Levin and Munksgaard, 1937). A popular edition of the same papyrus entitled *The Papyrus Ebers* (New York: D. Appleton & Company, 1931) is also available.

4 *Edwin Smith Surgical Papyrus*, I, pp. 54–55.

5 The letter can be found in a selection of the epistolary literature of Mesopotamia by R. H. Pfeiffer, *State Letters of Assyria* (New Haven: Yale University Press, 1935), No. 290, p. 202.

6 The quotation is from R. Campbell Thompson, *The Devils and Evil Spirits of Babylonia* (London: Luzac & Company, 1903), p. 201.

7 *Sushruta Samhita*, K. K. Bhishagratna, ed. and trans., second edition, 3 vols. (India: Chowkhamba Sanscrit Series, 1963), vol. I, chap. xxxiv, pp. 305–307.

8 *Carka Samhita*, A. Kaviratna, ed. and trans. (Calcutta: 1899), I, pp. 102–103. There is another translation in six volumes by the Shree Gulabkunverba Ayurvedic Society (Jamnagar, India: S.G.A.S., 1949), but it is more difficult to use.

9 See Ilza Veith, *The Yellow Emperor's Classic of Internal Medicine*, new edition (Berkeley: University of California Press, 1972). This is a translation of part of Hung Ti, *Nei Ching su Wën*.

10 Hippocrates, *The Art*, W. H. S. Jones, vol. 2, in *Hippocrates*, 4 vols., rep. (London: William Heinemann, 1967), W. H. S. Jones and E. T. Withington, eds. and trans.

11 There are numerous editions of the *Odyssey* and the *Iliad*. The references in Homer occur in the *Odyssey*, ii, 349, 361, 372; xvii, 499; xix, 15, 21, 489; *Iliad*, vi, 389, xxii, 503. For a discussion see Sister Mary Rosaria, *The Nurse in Greek Life* (Boston: n.p., 1917), pp. 7–8. Sister Rosaria's work was a doctoral dissertation at the Catholic University of America.

12 Xenophon, *Oeconomicus*, vii, 37, E. C. Marchant, ed. and trans. (London: William Heinemann, 1953).

13 Hippocrates, *Regimen in Acute Diseases*, LXV, LXVI, vol. 2, W. H. S. Jones, *op. cit.*

14 Xenophon, *Anabasis*, III, iv, pp. 30–32, C. L. Brownson and O. J. Todd, eds. and trans., 2 vols. (London: William Heinemann, 1947–1953).

15 Hippocrates, *Epidemics*, vol. I, W. H. S. Jones, *op. cit.*

16 Hippocrates, *Decorum*, XVII, vol. 2, W. H. S. Jones, *op. cit.*

17 Hippocrates, *In the Surgery*, vol. 3, E. T. Withington, *op. cit.*

18 Ludwig Edelstein, *Asclepius*, 2 vols. (Baltimore: The Johns Hopkins Press, 1945).

19 See Louis Cohn-Haft, *The Public Physicians of Ancient Greece* (Northampton, Massachusetts: Smith College, 1956).

20 Cato, *De agricultura*, chaps. CXXII, CXXIII, CXXVI, CXXVII, CLVI,

CLVIII, CLX, W. D. Hooper and H. B. Ash, eds. and trans. (London: William Heinemann, 1934).

21 Pliny, *Natural History*, 10 vols., H. Rackham, W. H. S. Jones, and D. E. Eichholz, eds. and trans. (London: William Heinemann, 1947–1963), *passim.*

22 Plutarch, "Cato Maior, xxiii, 3–4," *Parallel Lives*, vol. 2 (11 vols.), B. Perrin, ed. and trans. (London: William Heinemann, 1954–1962).

23 Celsus, *De medicina*, 3 vols., W. G. Spencer, ed. and trans. (London: William Heinemann, 1935–1938).

24 Livy, *History*, II, xlvii, 13 vols., B. O. Foster *et al.*, ed. and trans. (London: William Heinemann, 1919–1951).

25 Vegetius, *Military Institutions of the Romans*, Bk. III, ch. 2, John Clark, trans. (Harrisburg, Pennsylvania: The Military Service Publishing Company, 1944).

26 Columella, *De Re Rustica*, Book XI, chap. 1, paras. 18–19 (3 vols.), H. B. Ash, E. S. Forster, and E. Heffner, eds. and trans. (London: William Heinemann, 1960).

27 *Ibid.*, XI, chap. 3, paras. 7–8.

28 Tacitus, *Dialogus*, chapter 21, Sir William Peterson, ed. and trans. (London: William Heinemann, 1946).

29 Celsus, *De medicina*, "Prooemium," 65–66.

30 Marcus Valerius Martial, *Epigrams*, V, 9, Walter C. A. Ker, ed. and trans. (London: William Heinemann, 1925).

31 Seneca, *De Constantia*, xii, 3, in vol. I *Moral Essays*, John W. Basore, ed. and trans. (London: William Heinemann, 1951–1958).

32 Plautus, *Two Menaechmuses*, Act 5, Scene 5, verses 947–955, Paul Nixon, ed. and trans., in vol. 2 in the Loeb, *Plautus*, 5 vols. (London: William Heinemann, 1959–1963).

33 It should be noted that G. E. Gask and J. Todd, "The Origins of Hospitals," in *Science, Medicine and History*, 2 vols. E. A. Underwood, ed. (Oxford: Oxford University Press, 1953), I, pp. 122–130, claim that the concept of the hospital did not appear in Roman society as a whole until Christian times.

34 Soranus, *Gynecology*, translated with an introduction by Owsei Temkin (Baltimore: Johns Hopkins Press, 1956), II, 12–13, pp. 82–84.

35 Galen, *On the Natural Faculties*, III, iii (152), Arthur John Brock, ed. and trans. (London: William Heinemann, 1963).

36 Galen, *Hygiene*, vii, Robert M. Green, trans. (Springfield, Illinois: Charles C. Thomas, 1951), p. 21.

Chapter 2

1 Tacitus, *Germania*, 7, Maurice Hutton, ed. and trans. (London: William Heinemann, 1924).

2 Snorri Sturluson, *Heimskringla*, 4 vols., translated from the Icelandic by William Morris and E. Magnusson (London: Bernard Quaritch, 1893–1905), "The Story of Magnus the Good," chap. xxix.

3 Herbert Thurston, "Deaconesses," *Catholic Encylopedia* (New York: Apple-
tone, 1908–1914), IV p. 651. The new edition of the *Catholic Encyclopedia*
devotes somewhat less space to the subject.

4 *Romans*, 16: 1–2. The quotation is from the Authorized Version.

5 *I Timothy*, 5: 9–10 (Douay Version).

6 *Constitutions*, I, 1, 5, translated in the *Ante Nicene Fathers*, vol. VII
Alexander Roberts and James Donaldson, eds., revised by A. Cleveland Coxe
(Buffalo: Christian Literature Company, 1886).

7 See some of the discussion in Burton Scott Easton, *The Apostolic Tradition of
Hippolytus*, (Cambridge: University Press, 1934), and also *La Didascalia*, trans-
lated into French by F. Nau (Paris: P. Lethilleux, 1912), specially pp. 123–133.
There is an English version *Didascalia Apostolorum*, translated by Margaret
Dunlop Gibson (London: Clay, 1903), III, pp. i–xvi.

8 See *Decrees and Canons of the Seven Ecumenical Councils, Nicene and Post
Nicene Fathers*, Series 2, XIV (reprinted) (Grand Rapids, Michigan: Eerdmans,
1956), 50, canon No. 70.

9 For general discussion see Léon Lallemand, *Histoire de la Charité*, 4 vols.
(Paris: Alphonse Picard et Fils, 1902–1908), and Jean Imbert, *Les Hôpitaux en
Droit Canonique* (Paris: J. Vrin, 1947).

10 For a discussion of some of these see Demetrios J. Constantelos, *Byzantine
Philanthropy and Social Welfare* (New Brunswick: Rutgers University Press,
1968), pp. 154–158.

11 Theodoretos of Cyrrhus, *Ecclesiastical History*, V, 19, 314, Leon Parmentier,
ed., under the title of *Theodoret Kirchengeschichte*, second edition, (Berlin:
Akademie-Verlag, 1954).

12 St. Jerome, *Letters*, LXXVII, par. 6, in *Select Letters of St. Jerome*, F. A.
Wright, ed. and trans. (London: W. Heinemann, 1933).

13 St. Benedict, *Regula, cap.* xxxvi, "De Infirmia Fratibus." There are many
editions. An English translation can be found in Dom Paul DeLatte, *The Rule of
St. Benedict*, Dom Justin McCann, trans. (Latrobe, Pennsylvania: The Archabbey Press, 1950), pp. 258–264.

14 *The Letters of Abelard and Heloise*, Letter VII, Abelard to Heloise, Betty
Radice, trans. (Hammondsworth, England: Penguin Books, 1974), p. 215.

15 Anna Comnena, *Alexiad*, Bk. XV, 7, Elizabeth A. S. Dawes, trans. (London:
Kegan Paul, Trench Trubner, 1928).

16 Pan S. Codellas, "The Pantocrator, the Imperial Byzantine Medical Center
of the XIIth Century A.D. in Constantinople," *Bulletin of the History of Medicine*
XII (1942), pp. 392–410.

17 Quoted by A. A. Vasiliev, *History of the Byzantine Empire*, second edition,
(Madison: University of Wisconsin, 1952), p. 472.

18 "Description of the Holy Land by John of Würzburg," Aubrey Stewart,
trans., in *Palestine Pilgrims' Text Society* (London: 1896), V, 44, and quoted by
Edgar Erskine Hume, *Medical Work of the Knights Hospitallers of Saint John of
Jerusalem* (Baltimore: Johns Hopkins University Press, 1940), pp. 14–15. His
book is invaluable for an account of the Order.

19 Many of the stories about St. Francis were written down by his contemporary, Brother Thomas (i.e., Thomas de Celano), who wrote two lives of the saint,

Vita Prima and *Vita Secundo,* 2 vols. (Florence: College of St. Bonaventura, 1926–1927).

20 A good description of hospitals is available in Rotha Mary Clay, *The Medieval Hospitals of England* (London: Methuen & Company, 1909), and Norman Moore, *The History of St. Bartholomew's Hospitals,* 2 vols. (London: C. Arthur Pearson, Ltd., 1918).

21 For a description of the system as it became more fully developed see Carlo M. Cipolla, *Cristofano and the Plague* (Berkeley: University of California Press, 1973).

22 G. G. Coulton, trans., from St. Bernardine's *Sermons,* printed in *Life in the Middle Ages,* 4 vols. (Cambridge: University Press, 1954), I, p. 225.

23 Anna Comnena, *op. cit.,* Bk XV, ch. 11.

Chapter 3

1 Dordrecht Confession of Anabaptists (April, 1632), Art. 9, sect. 5, quoted by Lena Mae Smith, "Deaconess," *Mennonite Encyclopedia* (Scottdale, Pennsylvania: Mennonite Publishing House, 1955–1959), vol. 2, pp. 22–25.

2 *Memoranda, References and Comments Relating to the Royal Hospitals of the City of London* (London: 1836), and quoted in Norman Moore, *The History of St. Bartholomew's Hospital,* 2 vols. (London: C. Arthur Pearson, Ltd., 1918), II, p. 150.

3 *The Ordre of the Hospital of S. Bartholomew in West Smythfielde in London* (London: Richard Grafton, 1552), as quoted in Moore, *op. ct.,* II, p. 171. The account is from 1552.

4 Moore, *op. cit.,* vol. 2, pp. 759–760.

5 *Ibid.,* II, pp. 757–758.

6 *Ibid.,* II, p. 762.

7 Ireland, *Acts and Statutes Made in Parliament* Dublin, 1716, Reign of George I, 1715. First session beginning Nov. 12, 1715, and also in Moore, *op. cit.,* II, p. 764.

8 Thomas Fuller, *Exantematologia: or, An Attempt to Give a Rational Account of Eruptive Fevers, especially of the Small Pox* (London: Charles Rivington and Stephen Austen, 1730), pp. 208–209.

9 Moore, *op. cit.,* II, p. 765.

10 *Ibid.,* II, p. 764.

11 *Ibid.,* II, pp. 766–768.

12 *Ibid.,* II, p. 770. There was some variation in wages in the period. In 1814, for example, wages were somewhat higher if only because each sister received one shilling on admission. The most marked change was in the four men's foul wards in which each sister received two shillings on the admission of a patient and 52 pounds a year. Moore, *op. cit.,* II, p. 382.

13 *Ibid.,* II, p. 344. For an account of an Italian Hospital in the sixteenth

century see Bernice J. Trexler, "Hospital Patients in Florence," *Bulletin of the History of Medicine* 48 (1974), pp. 41–58.

14 *Conférènces de S. Paul aux Filles de la Charité* (Paris, 1881), I, p. 76. See also Pierre Coste, *The Life and Works of Saint Vincent de Paul,* 3 vols. (London: Burns, 1934), and Cyprian W. Emanuel, *The Charities of St. Vincent de Paul* (Ph.D. dissertation, Washington, D.C.: Catholic University of America, 1923).

15 W. H. Lewis, *The Splendid Century* (London: Eyre and Spottiswoode, 1953), pp. 204–205.

16 The incident is recounted by Charlotte Carmichael Stopes, *The Life of Henry, Third Earl of Southampton* (Cambridge: University Press, 1922), p. 90, and reported on by Lu Emily Pearson, *Elizabethans at Home* (Palo Alto, California: Stanford University, 1957), pp. 404–405.

17 William Bradford, *History of Plymouth Plantation* (Boston: Wright & Potter, 1898), Bk II (1620), p. 111.

18 *Diary* of Mary Stockly.

19 Carlo M. Cipolla, *Cristofano and the Plague: A Study in the History of Public Health in the Age of Galileo* (Berkeley: University of California, 1973); Geoffrey Marks, *The Medieval Plague* (New York: Garden City, 1971); William M. Bowsky, *The Black Death A Turning Point in History* (New York: Holt Rinehart and Winston, 1971).

20 Article, "Infirmier," in *Encyclopédie où Dictionnaire des sciences, des Arts et des Métiers,* Denis Diderot, ed., 17 vols. (Paris: Briasson *et al.,* 1751–1765), VIII, pp. 707–708.

21 John Howard, *An Account of the Principal Lazarettoes in Europe: with Various Papers Relative to the Plague, Together with Further Observations on Some Foreign Prisons and Hospitals, and Additional Remarks on the Present State of those in Great Britain and Ireland* (Warrington: Printed by William Eyres, 1789), p. 86.

22 J. Tenon, *Memoires sur les hôpitaux de Paris* (Paris: Pierres, 1788), and particularly, Dora B. Weiner, "The French Revolution, Napoleon, and the Nursing Profession," *Bulletin of the History of Medicine* 46 (1972), pp. 274–305.

23 Tenon, *op. cit.,* pp. 306–309, states there were 528 paid male servants, 98 unpaid male servants, 66 paid female servants, and 67 unpaid female (convalescents). There were also 40 nurse's aides, i.e., "filles brunes," and "filles noires." Weiner, *op. cit.,* pp. 279–280, note 16.

24 M. Möring, C. Quentin, and L. Briele, eds., *Collection de documents pour servir à l'histoire des hôpitaux de Paris,* 4 vols. (Paris: Imprimerie nationale, 1881–1887), II, p. 2.

25 *Ibid.,* II, p. 288.

26 See A. Berman, "The Scientific Tradition in French Hospital Pharmacy," *American Journal of Hospital Pharmacy* 18 (1961), pp. 110–119; "The Pharmaceutical Component of 19th-Century French Public Health and Hygiene," *Pharmacy in History* 11 (1969), pp. 5–10; and "Conflict and anomaly in the scientific orientation of French pharmacy, 1800–1873," *Bulletin of the History of Medicine,* 37 (1963), pp. 440–462.

27 Weiner, *op. cit.,* pp. 286–287.

28 Quoted by Weiner, *op. cit.,* p. 289.

29 *Notes et souvenirs,* p. 312, in-folio Mss., 742, Archives, Religeuses Augustines hôspitalières de l'Hôtel de Paris, and in Weiner, *op. cit.,* pp. 295–296.
30 *Moniteur Universal,* February 7, 1808, and Weiner, *op. cit.,* p. 299.

Chapter 4

1 See Robert Gooch, "Protestant Sisters of Charity," *Blackwood's Edinburgh Magazine* (November, 1825), pp. 732–735, and Robert Gooch, *The London Medical Gazette,* I (1827), pp. 55–58. Extracts of the letters are printed by Anne L. Austin, *History of Nursing Source Book* (New York: G. P. Putnam's Sons, 1957), pp. 176–177.
2 See Robert Southey, *Sir Thomas Moore; or Colloquies on the Progress and Prospects of Society* (London: Murray, 1829), II, 318, and appendix, and also *The Life and Correspondence of the Late Robert Southey,* ed. Charles Cuthbert Southey, 6 vols. (London: Longmans, 1850), IV, p. 156; V, pp. 25, 237; VI, pp. 52, 71–72.
3 See Emma Pöel, *Life of Amelia Wilhelmina Sieveking,* Catherine Winkworth, trans. (London: Longmans, 1863).
4 See *Life of Pastor Fliedner of Kaiserswerth,* Catherine Winkworth, trans. (London: Longmans, 1867), and also Marie Gallison, *The Ministry of Women: 100 years of Women's Work at Kaiserswerth 1836–1936* (London: Lutterworth Press, 1936). Fliedner wrote a brief autobiography, *Kurzer Abriss Seines Lebens* (Kaiserswerth, 1866), which is cited in the English version of the life, but we have not seen it.
5 See D. Disselhoff, "The Deaconesses of Kaiserswerth: A Hundred Years' Work," *International Nursing Review* I (1934), pp. 19–28. Disselhoff was a granddaughter of Fredericke Münster Fliedner. Extracts are given in Austin, *op. cit.,* pp. 190–192.
6 In addition to the references cited in footnotes 4 and 5, Florence Nightingale also wrote about Kaiserswerth. See Florence Nightingale, *The Institution of Kaiserswerth on the Rhine, for the Practical Training of Deaconesses* (London: Printed by the Inmates of the Ragged Colonial Training School, 1851). This is a 32-page pamphlet. See Edward Cook, *The Life of Florence Nightingale,* 2 vols. (London: Macmillan, 1913), II, p. 437.
7 Edward Ryder, published a compendium of her journal under the title of *Memoirs of the Life of Elizabeth Fry: Life and Labors of the Eminent Philanthropist, Preacher, and Prison Reformer* (New York: E. Walker's Sons, 1884); two of her daughters, Katherine Fry and R. E. Cresswell, edited *Memoirs of the Life of Elizabeth Fry* (London: J. Hatchard, 1847). See also Janet Whitney, *Elizabeth Fry* (Boston: Little Brown & Company, 1936).
8 H. P. Liddon, *Life of Edward Bouverie Pusey,* 4 vols., fourth edition (London: Longmans, 1894–1897), III, chap. 1, "The Early Days of Anglican Sisterhoods," and for amalgamation, pp. 192–200. See also [Mary Stanley] *Hospitals and Sisterhoods* (London: Murray, 1854).

9   See M. Adelaide Nutting and Lavinia L. Dock, *A History of Nursing* (New York: G. P. Putnam's Sons, 1907–1912), II, pp. 79–94.

10   Charles Dickens, *The Life and Adventures of Martin Chuzzlewit*, many editions. Chap. XXV. See also Chap. XXIX. The novel was written in 1843–1844. In the preface to his novel, Dickens wrote that Sarah Gamp represented the hired attendant on the poor in sickness, while Betsy Prig was a fair specimen of a hospital nurse.

11   Many physicians were convinced. A good example was Sir Edward Parry, superintendent of Haslar Hospital, as well as other physicians associated with the hospital. Some of the letters and other materials were collected by Austin, *op. cit.*, pp. 181–187. Bence Jones, another physician, had urged the formation of a training school for London and was perhaps influential in directing the energies of Florence Nightingale. See Zachary Cope, *Florence Nightingale and the Doctors*, (London Museum Press, 1958) pp. 21–23.

12   Nightingale is one of the most written about women in history. There are numerous biographies of her, including the more or less authorized one by Edward Cook mentioned above. This section relies, however, more on Cecil Woodham-Smith, *Florence Nightingale 1820–1910* (New York: McGraw-Hill, 1951), then on Cook. A rather unorthodox picture of her is given by Lytton Strachey, *Eminent Victorians* (New York: G. P. Putnam's Sons, 1918). W. J. Bishop and Sue Goldie, with the International Council of Nurses, issued a *Bio-bibliography of Florence Nightingale* (London: International Council of Nurses, 1962).

13   She spent two weeks at Kaiserswerth in 1850 and an additional three months in 1851, and as a result wrote a short account, cited in footnote 6.

14   The quarterly reports which she made as superintendent have been preserved and published. See *Florence Nightingale at Harley Street: Her Reports to the Governors of Her Nursing Home, 1853–1854*, with an introduction by Sir Harry Verney (London: J. M. Dent & Sons, 1970).

15   See for example, "Who is Mrs. Nightingale?" *London Times*, October 30, 1854.

16   Several women and others who were at Scutari later wrote memoirs. Several of them are summarized in Cook, *op. cit.*; others can be found in Austin, *op. cit.*, pp. 239–248. Austin includes extracts from Mary Stanley, Fanny M. Taylor, Sister Mary Aloysius, and Margaret Goodman.

17   London: Privately printed for Nightingale by Harrison and Sons, 1858.

18   In 1858 she had also written *Subsidiary Notes as to the Introduction of Female Nursing into Military Hospitals in Peace and War* (London: Privately printed by Harrison and Sons, 1858).

19   (London: Harrison and Sons, 1859, second edition, 1860.) The American edition appeared in 1860. It was reprinted in 1946 (Philadelphia: J. B. Lippincott, 1946).

20   London: John W. Parker and Sons, 1859. The third edition was almost completely rewritten (London: Longmans, Green and Co., 1863).

21   A training school had been suggested to her in 1855 by the physician, Bence Jones. See Cope, *op. cit.*, pp. 21–22.

22   *The Nightingale Training School: St. Thomas' Hospital, 1860–1910* (privately printed for the Nightingale Training School for Nurses, 1960), and

hereafter cited as *The Nightingale Training School*. See also Florence Nightingale, "The Reform of Sick Nursing and the Late Mrs. Wardroper, The Extinction of Mrs. Gamp," *British Medical Journal* (December 31, 1892), p. 1448.
23   *The Nightingale Training School.*
24   Woodham-Smith, *op. cit.*, p. 352.
25   Isabel Maitland Stewart, *The Education of Nurses: Historical Foundations and Modern Trends* (New York: Macmillan, 1945), pp. 59–62, and the *Nightingale Training School*, pp. 40–82.
26   See The Florence Nightingale Letter to Dr. Wylie, reprinted in Nutting and Dock, *op. cit.*, II, pp. 388–393.
27   See William Rathbone, *Sketch of the History and Progress of District Nursing From Its Commencement in the Year 1859 to the Present Date* (New York: Macmillan, 1890), and Eleanor F. Rathbone, *William Rathbone, A Memoir* (New York: Macmillan, 1905).
28   See *"Una and Her Paupers;" Memorials of Agnes Elizabeth Jones* by her sister (New York: Routledge, 1872).
29   Nightingale's official suggestions for the training and organizing of nurses for the sick poor in workhouse infirmaries can be found in the *Report of the Committee Appointed to Consider the Cubic Space of Metropolitan Workhouses*, Paper No. XVI (pp. 64–79), and this was reprinted in Lucy Ridgely Seymer, *Selected Writings of Florence Nightingale* (New York: Macmillan Company, 1954), pp. 271–309.
30   In 1876 she wrote and signed a letter to the London *Times* which was reprinted as a pamphlet, Florence Nightingale, *On Trained Nursing for the Sick Poor* (London: Metropolitan and National Nursing Association, 1876). This can also be found in Seymer, *op. cit.*, pp. 311–318.
31   Woodham-Smith, *op. cit.*, pp. 182 ff.

Chapter 5

1   Joseph Warrington, *The Nurses Guide* (Philadelphia: Thomas Cowperwaite, 1893), and excerpted in Anne L. Austin, *History of Nursing Source Book* (New York: G. P. Putnam's Sons, 1949), pp. 255–256.
2   Joseph Dirvan, *Mrs. Seton, Foundress of the American Sisters of Charity* (New York: Farrar, Straus & Cudahy, 1963). See also R. Seton, *Memoirs, Letters and Journals of Elizabeth Seton*, 2 vols. (New York: 1869).
3   See James J. Walsh, *These Splendid Sisters* (New York: J. H. Sears, 1927), and the articles on various nursing orders in the *New Catholic Encyclopedia* (Washington, D. C.: Catholic University, 1967).
4   A good account of Muhlenberg is in Alvin W. Skardon, *Church Leader in the Cities: William Augustus Muhlenberg* (Philadelphia University of Pennsylvania Press, 1971), *passim*, and pp. 125–137. See also Anne Ayres, *The Life and Work of William Augustus Muhlenberg* (New York: Randolph, 1880), and [Malvina W. Keller], *History of the St. Luke's Hospital Training School for Nurses* (New York: St. Luke's Hospital, 1938).

5   See Anne Ayres, *Evangelical Sisterhoods, In Two Letters to a Friend*, W. A. Muhlenberg, ed. (New York: T. Whittaker, 1867). See also *Two Letters on Protestant Sisterhoods*, third edition (New York: R. Craighead, printer, 1856), and *Practical Thoughts on Sisterhoods* (New York: T. Whittaker, 1864).

6   Skardon, *op. cit.*, pp. 132–133.

7   G. H. Herberding, *Life and Letters of W. A. Passavant*, third edition (Greenville, Pennsylvania: Young Lutheran Company, 1906). Fliedner accompanied the first group of nurses to Pittsburgh where they served more or less as public health nurses. They did not associate with a hospital until 1853.

8   Passavant Hospital in Pittsburgh, which originally was called the Pittsburgh Infirmary. The hospital opened for use in 1852.

9   Skardon, *op. cit.*, p. 136, and "Beginnings of Some Famous Schools," *Trained Nurse and Hospital Review* 101 (August, 1938), pp. 115–122.

10   Skardon, *op. cit.*, pp. 133–135.

11   Eleanor Flexner, *Century of Struggle: The Woman's Rights Movement in the United States* (Cambridge: Harvard University Press, 1959).

12   Elizabeth Blackwell, *Pioneer Work in Opening the Medical Profession to Women* (London: Longmans, Green and Co., 1895). See also John B. Blake, "Women and Medicine in Ante-Bellum America," *Bulletin of the History of Medicine* 39 (1965), pp. 99–123. A good overview is in Mary Roth Walsh, *Doctors Wanted: No Women Need Apply* (New Haven: Yale University Press, 1977).

13   Elinor Rice Hays, *Those Extraordinary Blackwells* (New York: Harcourt, Brace and World, 1967).

14   Blackwell, *op. cit.*, and Ishbel Ross, *Child of Destiny* (London: Victor Gollancz, 1950).

15   "Beginnings of Some Famous Schools," *op. cit.*, pp. 115–122.

16   M. Adelaide Nutting and Lavinia L. Dock, *A History of Nursing* (4 vols., New York: Putnam, 1907–1912), II, pp. 347–354. See also Linda Richards, *Reminiscences of Linda Richards: America's First Trained Nurse* (Boston: Whitcomb and Barrows, 1911).

17   See Martin Kaufman, "The Admission of Women to 19th-Century American Medical Societies," *Bulletin of the History of Medicine* 50 (1976), pp. 251–260; Mary Roth Walsh, *op. cit.*, and Walsh, "Feminism: A Support System for Women Physicians," *Journal of the American Medical Women's Association* 31 (June 1976), pp. 247–250. For earlier accounts see Kate Campbell Hurd-Mead, *Medical Women of America* (New York: Froben Press, 1933), and also her *A History of Women in Medicine* (Haddam, Connecticut: Haddam Press, 1938).

18   Henry Wadsworth Longfellow, *The Complete Poetical Works of Longfellow* (Boston: Houghton-Mifflin Company, 1922), p. 197.

19   Florence Nigtingale, *Notes on Nursing* (New York: D. Appleton, 1860).

20   Marjorie Barstow Greenbie, *Lincoln's Daughters of Mercy* (New York: G. P. Putnam's Sons, 1944), pp. 37–53.

21   Greenbie, *op. cit.*, pp. 54–56; Blackwell, *op. cit.*, pp. 235–236; see also George Worthington Adams, *Doctors in Blue* (New York: Henry Schuman, 1952); *The Documents of the United States Sanitary Commission*, 2 vols. (New York: 1871), henceforth cited as *Documents*, and Henry Whitney Bellows, *Report Concerning the Woman's Central Association of Relief at New York to the United States*

Sanitary Commission (New York: Bryant, 1861), and also included in *Documents,* Document 32.

22   William Quentin Maxwell, *Lincoln's Fifth Wheel: The Political History of the United States Sanitary Commission* (New York: Longmans, Green & Co., 1956).

23   Helen E. Marshall, *Dorothea Dix* (Chapel Hill: University of North Carolina, 1937), pp. 200–203.

24   Mary A. Gardiner Holland, *Our Army Nurses* (Boston: B. Wilkins & Co., 1895), p. 19.

25   *Ibid.*

26   John H. Brinton, *Personal Memoirs* (New York: Neale Publishing Company, 1914), pp. 42–43.

27   Walt Whitman, *Complete Writings,* 10 vols. (New York: G. P. Putnam's Sons, 1902), and the more scholarly edition *The Collected Writings of Walt Whitman* (New York: New York University, 1961 ff).

28   Louisa May Alcott, *Hospital Sketches* (New York: Sagamore Press, 1957).

29   Florence Shaw Kellogg, *Mother Bickerdyke* (Chicago: Unity Publishing Company), and Nina Brown Baker, *Cyclone in Calico: The Story of Mary Ann Bickerdyke* (Boston: Little Brown, 1952).

30   Matthew Page Andrews, *The Women of the South in War Times,* new edition (Baltimore: Norman Remington, 1927), pp. 127–130; Bonnie and Vern Bullough, "The Origins of Modern American Nursing: The Civil War Era," *Nursing Forum* II, No. 2 (1963), pp. 13–27.

31   Anne L. Austin, *The Woolsey Sisters of New York: 1860–1900* (Philadelphia: American Philosophical Society, 1971).

32   Quoted in *Noble Women of the North,* compiled and edited by Sylvia G. L. Dannett (New York: Thomas Yoseloff, 1959), p. 88.

33   *Ibid.,* pp. 98–99.

34   In addition to the works cited above, see, for example, L. P. Brockett and Mary C. Vaughan, *Woman's Work in the Civil War: A Record of Heroism, Patriotism and Patience* (Philadelphia: Zeigler, McCurdy and Co., 1868) which is more propaganda than history, since so many of the biographical facts about its heroines are wrong. Still, it is symbolic. S. Emma E. Edmonds, *Nurse and Spy in the Union Army* (Hartford, Connecticut: W. S. Williams & Company, 1865). Edmonds had served for two years as Franklin Thompson before she was unmasked. Mary A. Livermore, *My Story of the War: A Woman's Narrative of Four Years Personal Experience as Nurse* (Hartford, Connecticut: A. D. Worthington and Company, 1889); Frank Moore, *Women of the War: Their Heroism and Self-Sacrifice* (Hartford, Connecticut: S. S. Scranton & Company, 1866); Belle Boyd, *Belle Boyd in Camp and Prison* (New York: Blelock & Co., 1865); Sophronia E. Bucklin, *In Hospital and Camp* (Philadelphia: J. E. Potter, 1869); Katherine M. Jones, *Heroines of Dixie* (Indianapolis: Bobbs-Merrill, 1955); James Welch Patton and Francis Butler Simkins, *The Women of the Confederacy* (Richmond: Garrett and Massie, 1936); James Phinney Munroe, *Adventures of an Army Nurse in Two Wars,* edited from the diary and correspondence of Mary Phinney, Baroness von Olnhausen (Boston: Little, Brown & Co., 1904); Ishbel Ross, *Angel of the Battlefield* (New York: Harper, 1956), and W. E. Barton, *Life*

of Clara Barton, 2 vols. (Boston: Houghton Mifflin, 1922); Mary Elizabeth Massey, *Bonnet Brigade* (New York: Alfred A. Knopf, 1966); Kate Cumming, *Kate: The Journal of a Confederate Nurse,* Richard Barksdale Harwell, ed. (Baton Rouge: Louisiana State University, 1959); Adelaide W. Smith, *Reminiscences of an Army Nurse During the Great War* (New York: 1911); Madeleine Stern, "Civil War Nurse," *Americana* XXXVII (1943), pp. 296-325; C. Edward Trenchard, *The Services and Sacrifices of the Daughters of the Republic During the Civil War* (New York: 1912); Annie T. Wittmeyer, *Under the Guns: A Women's Reminiscences of the Civil War* (Boston: 1895); Jane Stuart Woolsey, *Hospital Days* (New York: 1870); Katharine Prescott Wormeley, *The Other Side of the War With the Army of the Potomac* (Boston: Ticknor, 1889), later published as *The Cruel Side of War* (Boston: Roberts, 1898); C. G. Worthington, *The Woman in Battle* (Hartford, Connecticut: 1876). There are many more, plus a host of journal and magazine articles too numerous to mention. See also H. H. Cunningham, *Doctors in Gray,* (Baton Rouge: Louisiana State University, 1958).

35   Morris Fishbein, *A History of the American Medical Association, 1847-1947* (Philadelphia: W. B. Saunders, 1947), p. 78.

36   "Report of Committee on the Training of Nurses," *Transactions of the American Medical Association,* 1869, pp. 161-174. See also Samuel D. Gross, *Autobiography of Samuel D. Gross* (Philadelphia: G. Barrie, 1887).

37   See, for example, "Lady Nurses," *Godey's Lady's Book and Magazine* LXXXII (1871), pp. 188-189, and reprinted in Austin, *Source Book,* pp. 431-432.

38   Elizabeth Christophers Hobson, *Founding of the Bellevue Training School for Nurses* (New York: G. P. Putnam's Sons, 1916), and reprinted in *A Century of Nursing* (New York: G. P. Putnam's Sons, 1951).

39   Mrs. Curtis and Miss Denny, "Early History of the Boston Training School," *American Journal of Nursing* 2 (February, 1902), pp. 331-335.

40   Josephine Doland, "Nurses in American History: Three Schools—1873," *American Journal of Nursing* 75 (June, 1975), pp. 989-992.

41   Hobson, *op. cit.,* p. 153; Helen Jamieson Jordon, *Cornell University—New York Hospital School of Nursing 1877-1952* (New York: New York Hospital, 1952), pp. 15-22; Agnes Deans and Anne L. Austin, *The History of the Farrand Training School for Nurses* (Detroit: Alumnae Association of the Farrand School for Nurses, 1936), p. 34.

42   Mary Adelaide Nutting, *A Sound Economic Basis for Schools of Nursing and Other Addresses* (New York: G. P. Putnam, 1926), pp. 3-17.

43   Linda Richards, "Recollections of a Pioneer Nurse," *American Journal of Nursing* 3 (January, 1903), pp. 245-252; Linda Richards, "Early Days in the First American Training School for Nurses," *American Journal of Nursing* 73 (September, 1973), pp. 574-575; Isabel Maitland Stewart, *The Education of Nurses: Historical Foundations and Modern Trends* (New York: Macmillan, 1945), p. 106; Nutting, *op. cit.,* p. 295.

44   Grace Fay Schryver, *History of the Illinois Training School for Nurses 1880-1929* (Chicago: Board of Directors of the Illinois Training School for Nurses, 1930) p. 22; Nolie Mumey, *Cap, Pin and Diploma; A History of the Colorado Training School,* (Boulder, Colorado: Johnson Publishing Co. 1968), p. 72; Ruth Chamberlin, *The School of Nursing of the Medical College of South Carolina: Its Story* (Columbia, South Carolina: 1970), p. 7.

45   Ethel Johns and Blanche Pfefferkorn, *The Johns Hopkins Hospital School of Nursing 1889–1949* (Baltimore: The Johns Hopkins Press, 1954), p. 110; Abby Howland Woolsey, *Hospitals and Training Schools Report of the Standing Committee on Hospitals of the State Charities Aid Association*, New York, May 24, 1876, reprinted in *A Century of Nursing* (New York: G. P. Putnam's Sons, 1950), p. 129.

46   Giles, *op. cit.*, p. 142; Maria D. Andrea Loftus, *A History of St. Vincent's Hospital School of Nursing, Indianapolis, Indiana: 1896–1970* (Indianapolis: Litho Press, 1972), p. 15.

47   Mary Adelaide Nutting, "The Evolution of Nursing Education from Hospital to University," in Nutting, *A Sound Economic Basis for Schools of Nursing, op. cit.*, p. 298.

48   *Ibid.*

49   Stewart, *op. cit.*, p. 125; Alfred Worcester, *Nurses and Nursing* (Cambridge: Harvard University, 1927), pp. 103–104.

50   Johns and Pfefferkorn, *op. cit.*, p. 53.

51   Jane Hodson (Editor) *How to Become a Trained Nurse* (New York: William Abbatt, 1898), p. 256.

52   Anne A. Hintz, "The Probationary Term," in Hodson, *op. cit.*, pp. 15–19.

53   *Ibid.*, p. 19.

54   Anne A. Hintz, "The Training Term," in Hodson, *op. cit.*, pp. 20–24.

55   Hodson, *op. cit.*, pp. 110–227.

56   E. L. Hobson, *op. cit.*

57   Mrs. Curtis and Miss Denny, *op. cit.*

58   Woolsey, *op. cit.*, pp. 118–119; Jordon, *op. cit.*, p. 23.

59   Hodson, *op. cit.*, pp. 239–240.

60   Vern L. Bullough (with a final chapter by Bonnie Bullough), *The Subordinate Sex: A History of Attitudes Towards Women* (Urbana, Illinois: University of Illinois Press, 1973).

61   Vern and Bonnie Bullough, "Nursing and History," *Nursing Outlook*, 12 October 1964, pp. 41–46.

62   Jessamine S. Whitney, "Tuberculosis Among Young Women—With Special Reference to Tuberculosis Among Nurses," *American Journal of Nursing* 28, (August, 1928), pp. 766–768; Mumey, *op. cit.*, p. 91; Hodson, *op. cit.*, p. 106; James Gray, *Education for Nursing: A History of the University of Minnesota School* (Minneapolis: University of Minnesota Press, 1960) p. 91.

63   Harriet Berger Koch, *Militant Angel* (New York: Macmillan, 1951), p. 14.

64   Grace Whiting Myers, *A History of the Massachusetts General Hospital, June 1872, to December 1900* (Boston: Griffith-Stilling Press, 1930), p. 80.

65   M. Adelaide Nutting, *Educational Status of Nursing*, United States Bureau of Education, Bulletin 1912, No. 7 (Washington, D.C.: U.S. Government Printing Office, 1912), p. 24; Margene O. Faddis, *A School of Nursing Comes of Age: A History of the Frances Payne Bolton School of Nursing, Case Western University* (Cleveland: The Alumnae of the Frances Payne Bolton School of Nursing, 1973), pp. 94–96.

66   Martin Gumpert, *Dunant: The Story of the Red Cross* (New York: Oxford University Press, 1938).

67 Henri Dunant, *A Memory of Solferino* (Washington, D.C.: American National Red Cross, 1939).
68 Foster Rhea Dulles, *The American Red Cross: A History* (New York: Harper, 1950).
69 Nutting and Dock, *op. cit.*, III, pp. 287ff., have a good account of this.
70 A. Hamilton, *Les gardes malades congréganistes, mercenaires, professionelles, amateurs* (Paris: Vigot, 1901).
71 See X. Xeclainche, "La profession d'infirmière," in *Quatre novelles années d'action hospitalière sociale et médico-sociale, 1956 à 1960* (Paris: Imprimerie municipale, 1960), and G. Recordon, "Le cinquantenaire de l'école des infirmières de l'assistance publique," *Revue de l'assistance publique à Paris,* 8, 1957, pp. 423–428.
72 See Margaret Breay and Ethel G. Fenwick, *The History of the International Council of Nurses 1899–1925* (Geneva: International Council of Nurses, 1931), and D. C. Bridges, *A History of the International Council of Nurses, 1899–1964* (London: Pitman, 1967). For Cavell see A. A. Hoehling, *A Whisper of Eternity: The Mystery of Edith Cavell* (New York: Thomas Yoseloff, 1957), and Rowland Ryder, *Edith Cavell* (New York: Stein and Day, 1975).
73 See Lavinia Dock, Sarah Pickett, Clara Noyes, *et al., History of American Red Cross Nursing* (New York: Macmillan, 1922), and the more recent Portia B. Kernodle, *The Red Cross Nurse in Action* (New York: Harper, 1949).
74 M. Eugenie Hibbard, "The Establishment of Schools for Nurses in Cuba," *American Journal of Nursing* 2 (1902), p. 985.
75 See Mary M. Roberts, *American Nursing* (New York: Macmillan, 1961), pp. 35–38.
76 Sarah A. Tooley, *The History of Nursing in the British Empire* (London: S. H. Bousfield & Co., 1906); John Murray Gibson and Mary S. Mathewson, *Three Centuries of Canadian Nursing* (Toronto: Macmillan, 1947).
77 Floyd Keeler, *Catholic Medical Missions* (New York: Macmillan, 1925). For a Protestant group see Harold Walton and Kathryn Jensen Nelson, *Historical Sketches of the Medical Work of Seventh Day Adventists* (Washington, D.C.: Review & Herald Publishing Co., 1948).
78 Gordon Seagrave, *Burma Surgeon* (New York: W. W. Norton, 1943).
79 See Edward H. Hume, *Doctors Courageous* (New York: Harper & Brothers, 1950), and *International Nursing Review* (July, 1930), pp. 334–342.
80 See Richards, *op. cit.*, p. 81.
81 Nutting and Dock, *op. cit.*, IV, pp. 229–255, and *International Nursing Review* (May, 1930), pp. 228–235.
82 Breay and Fenwich, *op. cit.*, and Bridges, *op. cit., passim.*
83 *International Nursing Review,* October 1927, pp. 292–303.
84 Walton and Nelson, *op. cit., passim.*
85 See *The American Journal of Nursing* 28 (November 1928). Part of this was based upon personal visitation by the authors.
86 Breay and Fenwick, *op. cit.*, and D. C. Bridges, *op. cit., passim.* See also various issues of the *International Nursing Review,* published by the International Council of Nurses.

Chapter 6

1   Michael M. Davis, *Clinics, Hospitals and Health Centers* (New York: Harper & Brothers, 1 27), pp. 4–5. E. H. L. Corwin, *The American Hospital* (New York: Commonwealth Fund, 1946), however, wrote that there were 178 institutions providing in-patient care of the sick, 88 of which were located in New York, Pennsylvania, and Massachusetts.

2   Arthur E. Hertzler, *The Horse and Buggy Doctor* (New York: Paul B. Hoeber, 1938), p. 250.

3   *Ibid.,* p. 260.

4   See Vern L. Bullough and Bonnie Bullough, *The Subordinate Sex* (Urbana: University of Illinois, 1973, and Penguin Books, 1974).

5   Mary M. Roberts, *American Nursing: History and Interpretation* (New York: Macmillan, 1961), pp. 20–31.

6   All the papers delivered at the Congress were published in *Nursing of the Sick: 1893* (reprinted for NLN, New York: McGraw-Hill, 1949).

7   Roberts, *op. cit.,* pp. 20–31.

8   S. Tooley, *The History of Nursing in the British Empire* (London: Bousfield, 1906), p. 363.

9   M. Adelaide Nutting and Lavinia L. Dock, *A History of Nursing*, 4 vols. (New York: G. P. Putnam's Sons, 1907–1912), III, p. 144.

10   Lavinia L. Dock, "What We May Expect from the Law," *American Journal of Nursing* 1 (1900), pp. 8–12.

11   "Address of the President, Isabel Hampton Robb, Before the Third Annual Convention of the Associated Alumnae of Trained Nurses in the United States," *American Journal of Nursing* 1 (1900), pp. 97–104.

12   Dent *v* West Virginia, *United States Reports: Cases Adjudged in the Supreme Court*, 129 (1888), pp. 114–128.

13   Robb, *op. cit.,* and Roberta Mayhew West, *History of Nursing in Pennsylvania* (Pennsylvania State Nurses' Association, 1933), pp. 41–58.

14   Lucy Ridgely Seymer, *A General History of Nursing* (New York: Macmillan, 1933), p. 250.

15   Milton J. Lesnik and Bernice E. Anderson, *Legal Aspects of Nursing* (Philadelphia: J. B. Lippincott, 1947), pp. 306–314.

16   *Ibid.,* pp. 312–314.

17   *Ibid.,* pp. 306–307.

18   "The Biennial," *American Journal of Nursing* 34 (1934), pp. 603–627.

19   West, *op. cit.,* p. 98, and "Nursing Legislation, 1939: What the State Nurses' Association Accomplished," *American Journal of Nursing* 39 (1939), pp. 974–981.

20   Bonnie Bullough, *The Law and the Expanding Nursing Role* (New York: Century-Crofts, 1975), pp. 7–21.

21   *Nursing of the Sick, 1893,* pp. 4ff.

22   Ethel Johns and Blanche Pfefferkorn, *The Johns Hopkins Hospital School of*

Nursing 1889-1949 (Baltimore: Johns Hopkins Press, 1954), p. 108, and West, *op. cit.*, p. 799.

23   Agnes Deans and Anne L. Austin, *The History of the Farrand Training School for Nurses* (Detroit: Alumnae Association of the Farrand School for Nurses, 1936), p. 39.

24   Martha P. Parker, "Preparatory Work at the Waltham Training School," *American Journal of Nursing* 3 (1903), pp. 264–266.

25   "Miss Nutting's Report," *American Journal of Nursing* 3 (1903), pp. 272–273, and Helen E. Marshall, *Mary Adelaide Nutting: Pioneer of Modern Nursing* (Baltimore: Johns Hopkins Press, 1972), p. 108.

26   Margene O. Faddis, *A School of Nursing Comes of Age: A History of the Frances Payne Bolton School of Nursing, Case Western University* (Cleveland: Alumnae of the Frances Payne Bolton School of Nursing, 1973), p. 70.

27   Teresa E. Christy, *Cornerstone for Nursing Education: A History of the Division of Nursing Education of Teachers College, Columbia University, 1899-1947* (New York: Teachers College Press, 1969), pp. 1-18.

28   Elizabeth V. Cunningham, "Education for Leadership in Nursing 1899-1959," *Nursing Outlook,* 7 (May, 1959), pp. 268-272.

29   Christy, *op. cit.,* pp. 19–41.

30   Mary Ellis Chayer, "The Trail of the Nursing Textbook," *American Journal of Nursing* 50 (1950), pp. 606–607.

31   Roberts, *op. cit.,* pp. 40–41.

32   See Katherine DeWitt and Helen Munson, "The Journal's First Fifty Years," *American Journal of Nursing* 50 (1950), pp. 590-595, and Margaret E. Kerr, "Fifty Years Young," *American Journal of Nursing* 55 (1955), p. 302.

33   Mary M. Roberts, "Lavinia Lloyd Dock—Nurse, Feminist, Internationalist," *American Journal of Nursing* 56 (1956), pp. 176-179.

34   Lavinia L. Dock, "Some Urgent Social Claims," *American Journal of Nursing* 7 (1907), p. 895.

35   "Journal's Attitude on the Suffrage Question," *American Journal of Nursing* 8 (1908), pp. 956-957.

36   Lavinia L. Dock, "Self Portrait," *Nursing Outlook* 25 (January 1977), pp. 23-26; Teresa Christy, "Equal Rights for Women: Voice From the Past," *American Journal of Nursing* 71 (1971), pp. 288-293; and Teresa Christy, "Portrait of a Leader: Lavinia L. Dock," *Nursing Outlook* 17 (June, 1969), pp. 72-75.

37   Mary S. Gardner, *Public Health Nursing,* third edition (New York: Macmillan, 1936), p. 39.

38   A. M. Brainard, *The Evolution of Public Health Nursing* (Philadelphia: W. B. Saunders, 1922), pp. 130-148.

39   S. Tooley, *The History of Nursing in the British Empire* (London: Bousfield, 1906), chaps. 17 and 18.

40   Brainard, *op. cit.*

41   See Lillian D. Wald, *The House on Henry Street* (New York: Henry Holt, 1915); *Windows on Henry Street* (Boston: Little, Brown & Company, 1933): R. L. Duffus, *Lillian Wald, Neighbor and Crusader* (New York: Macmillan, 1938); Mary S. Gardner, *op. cit.*

42   Theodore B. Sachs, "The Tuberculosis Nurse," *American Journal of Nursing* 8 (1908), 597.

43   Roberts, *op. cit.,* pp. 87–88.

44   Ysabella Waters, *"Vistiting Nursing in the United States"* (New York: Charities Publication Committee, 1909); C. E. A. Winslow, "The Role of the Visiting Nurse in the Campaign for Public Health," *American Journal of Nursing* 11 (1911), pp. 909–920; Harriet Fulmer, "History of Visiting Nurse Work in America," *American Journal of Nursing* 2 (1902), p. 411; Brainard, *op. cit., passim*; and George Rosen, *History of Public Health* (New York: M.D. Publications, 1958), pp. 358–360.

45   See Lavinia L. Dock and Fannie F. Clement, "From Rural Nursing to the Public Health Service," in Lavinia L. Dock, Sarah Elizabeth Pickett, Clara D. Noyes, Fannie F. Clement, Elizabeth G. Fox, and Anna R. Van Meter, *History of American Red Cross Nursing* (New York: Macmillan, 1922), pp. 1211–1292; Elizabeth G. Fox, "Red Cross Public Health Nursing After the War," in *op. cit.,* pp. 1293–1351; Fannie F. Clement, "History of Rural Nursing," *American Journal of Nursing* 13 (1913); and Portia B. Kernodle, *The Red Cross Nurse in Action, 1882–1948* (New York: Harper & Brothers, 1949), pp. 256–305. See also Louis I. Dublin and Alfred J. Lotka, *Twenty-five Years of Health Progress* (New York: Metropolitan Life Insurance Company, 1937).

46   See Lucy A. Bannister, "A New Field, The Nurse's Opportunity in Factory Work," *Fourteenth Annual Report of the American Society of Superintendents of Training Schools for Nurses,* 1908, p. 104; Bethel J. McGrath, *Nursing in Commerce and Industry* (New York: Commonwealth Fund, 1946); Irene Charley, *The Birth of Industrial Nursing: Its History and Development in Great Britain* (London: Baillière, Tindall and Cox, 1954) has an occasional reference to the United States; Ada Stewart Markolf, "Industrial Nursing Begins in Vermont," *Public Health Nursing* 37 (1945), p. 125; "A Study of Industrial Nursing Services," *Public Health Nursing* 32 (1940), pp. 631–636.

47   Roberts, *op. cit.,* pp. 119–120.

48   For Minneapolis see Bertha Estelle Merrill, *The Trek from Yesterday—A History of Organized Nursing in Minneapolis, 1883–1936* (Minneapolis: Nurses' Association, 1944).

49   West, *op. cit.,* p. 87.

50   Theophilus Parvin, *Lectures on Obstetric Nursing* (Philadelphia: Blakiston, Son, 1889), pp. 42–43.

51   West *op. cit.* pp. 86–96.

52   Emily Oatway Bosswall, "Development of Private Duty Nursing," *American Journal of Nursing* 25 (1925), pp. 848–850.

53   Janet M. Geister, "Hearsay and Facts in Private Duty," *American Journal of Nursing* 26 (1926), pp. 515–528.

54   See, for example, E. D., *Recollections of a Nurse* (London and New York: Macmillan and Company, 1889), who went off to Africa.

55   Vern and Bonnie Bullough, "How Rough Red Hands Led to Rubber Gloves," *American Journal of Nursing* 70 (1970), p. 777. See also W. S. Halsted, "Ligature and Suture Material," *Journal of the American Medical Association* 60 (May 13, 1913), p. 1123.

Chapter 7

1 See Isabel Hampton Robb, "The Three Years' Course of Training in Connection with the Eight Hours System," *First and Second Annual Reports of the American Society of Superintendents of Training Schools for Nurses* (1897); see also Mary Roberts, *American Nursing: History and Interpretation* (New York: Macmillan, 1961).

2 There is a list of nursing schools with their requirements for admission, the course of study, and other information as of 1897 in Jane Hodson, *How To Become a Trained Nurse* (New York: William Abbatt, 1898). The Farrand school is listed as having a three-year curriculum and an eight-hour day, *op. cit.,* p. 151.

3 *Ibid.,* pp. 131–132.

4 See, for example, Ethel Johns and Blanche Pfefferkorn, *The Johns Hopkins Hospital School of Nursing 1889–1949* (Baltimore: Johns Hopkins Press, 1954), and Anges Deans and Anne L. Austin, *The History of the Farrand Training School for Nurses* (Detroit: Alumnae Association of the Farrand School for Nurses, 1936).

5 Hodson, *op. cit.,* lists the number of applicants, of acceptances, and of those who completed the course in her book. The dropout rate varied widely from school to school with some reporting a 100 per cent completion compared to others of less than a 50 percent rate. Jo Ann Ashley, *Hospitals, Paternalism, and the Role of the Nurse* (New York: Teacher's College, 1976) discussed the exploitation of student nurses.

6 Roberts, *op. cit.,* pp. 62–63.

7 Vern and Bonnie Bullough, "Nursing and History," *Nursing Outlook* 12 (October, 1964), pp. 41–46.

8 See Genevieve Parkhurst, "Wanted—100,000 Girls for Sub-Nurses," *Pictorial Review* (October, 1921), pp. 15, 182; interview with Charles H. Mayo reprinted in Vern and Bonnie Bullough, *New Directions for Nurses* (New York: Springer, 1971), pp. 87–94. Mayo himself summarized some of his ideas in "Do you Covet Distinction," *American Journal of Nursing* 22 (1922), p. 251.

9 See Abraham Flexner, *Medical Education in the United States and Canada* (New York: Carnegie Foundation for Advancement of Teaching, 1910), and Richard H. Shryock, *Medicine in America: Historical Essays* (Baltimore: Johns Hopkins Press, 1966). For an earlier account see W. F. Norwood, *Medical Education in the U.S. before the Civil War* (Philadelphia: University of Pennsylvania Press, 1944). For requirements at the turn of the century see Henry L. Taylor, *Professional Education in the United States* (Albany: University of the State of New York, 1900).

10 For an account of these, see William G. Rothstein, *American Physicians in the 19th Century: From Sects to Science* (Baltimore: Johns Hopkins University, 1972).

11 Flexner, *op. cit.,* p. 291.

12 *Ibid.*

13 See "Medical Education in the United States," *Journal of the American Medical Association* 79 (1922), pp. 629-633, for some figures; see also the Richard

H. Shryock, *Medical Licensing in America* 1645–1695 (Baltimore: Johns Hopkins, Press, 1967). Also Flexner, *op. cit., passim.*

14 Brenda L. H. Davis, *The Origin and Growth of Three Nursing Programs at Howard University, 1893–1973* (unpublished dissertation, Teachers College, Columbia University).

15 Richard Olding Beard, "The Social, Economic and Educational Status of the Nurse," *American Journal of Nursing* 20 (1920), pp. 874–876, 955–962. For his answer to Mayo see Richard Olding Beard, "Fair Play for the Trained Nurse," *Pictorial Review* (1922), pp. 28, 95–96.

16 James Gray, *Education for Nursing: History of the University of Minnesota School of Nursing* (Minneapolis: University of Minnesota, 1960), pp. 15–37.

17 Gwendoline MacDonald, *Development of Standards and Accreditation in Collegiate Nursing Education* (New York: Teachers College Press, Columbia University, 1965) p. 53.

18 Mary M. Roberts, *American Nursing; History and Interpretation* (New York: Macmillan, 1961). Stewart, *op. cit.,* p. 226.

19 Eleanor Lee, *Neighbors 1892–1967: A History of the Department of Nursing, Faculty of Medicine, Columbia University 1937–1967 and its Predecessor, the School of Nursing of the Presbyterian Hospital New York, 1892–1937* (New York: Columbia University, Presbyterian Hospital School of Nursing Alumnae Association, 1967), p. 7; Christy, *op. cit.,* p. 56. (Many sources give the starting date of this program as 1916, but 1917 seems to be the more accurate date.)

20 School of Nursing, University of California, San Francisco, *Announcement,* April 1975, p. 5.

21 Lee, *op. cit.,* p. 7.

22 Committee for the Study of Nursing Education (Josephine Goldmark, Secretary), *Nursing and Nursing Education in the United States.* (New York: Macmillan, 1923), p. 486; *Proceedings of Conference on Nursing Schools Connected with Colleges and Universities,* Under the Auspices of the Department of Nursing Education of Teachers College, and the Committee on University Relations of the National League of Nursing Education (New York: National LVEAGUE OF Nursing Education, 1928), p. 7.

23 Helen W. Munson with Katharine Stevens, *The Story of the National League of Nursing Education* (Philadelphia: W. B. Saunders, 1934).

24 *Standard Curriculum for Schools of Nursing* (New York: National League of Nursing Education, 1917).

25 *A Curriculum for Schools of Nursing* (New York: National League of Nursing Education, 1927).

26 *A Curriculum Guide for Schools of Nursing* (New York: National League of Nursing Education, 1937).

27 Anne C. Jamme, "The California Eight-Hour Law for Women," *American Journal of Nursing* 19 (1919), pp. 525–530; Isabel M. Stewart, "The Movement for Shorter Hours in Nurses' Training Schools," *American Journal of Nursing* 19 (1919), pp. 439–443.

28 Committee for the Study of Nursing Education, *op. cit.,* p. 500.

29 *Ibid.,* pp. 499–560.

30 Mary Adelaide Nutting, *A Sound Economic Basis for Schools of Nursing* (New York: G. P. Putnam, 1926); M. Adelaide Nutting, *Educational Status of*

Nursing, United States Bureau of Education, Bulletin, 1912, No. 7 (Washington, D.C.: U.S. Govt. Printing Office, 1912).

31 Committee for the Study of Nursing Education, *op. cit.,* pp. 7–30.

32 *Ibid.,* p. 26.

33 Isabel Maitland Stewart, *The Education of Nurses: Historical Foundations and Modern Trends* (New York: Macmillan, 1945), p. 204. Esther H. Werminghous, *Annie W. Goodrich: Her Journey to Yale* (New York: Macmillan, 1950), pp. 69–73. See also Harriet Berger Koch, *Military Angel* (New York: Macmillan, 1951).

34 Koch, *op. cit.,* p. 122.

35 *Ibid.,* p. 119.

36 Margene O. Faddis, *A School of Nursing Comes of Age: A History of the Frances Payne Bolton School of Nursing, Case Western University* (Cleveland: The Alumnae of the Frances Payne Bolton School of Nursing, 1973).

37 Stewart, *The Education of Nurses, op. cit., passim.*

38 May Ayres Burgess, *Nurses Patients and Pocketbooks* (New York: Committee on the Grading of Nursing Schools, 1928).

39 The Committee on the Grading of Nursing Schools, *Results of the First Grading Study of Nursing Schools* (New York: 1930).

40 The Committee on the Grading of Nursing Schools, *The Second Grading of Nursing Schools* (New York: 1932).

41 The Committee on the Grading of Nursing Schools, *Nursing Schools Today and Tomorrow: Final Report* (New York: 1934), pp. 197–213.

42 Marie L. Rose, "What about Our Own Catastrophe," *American Journal of Nursing* 32 (1932), pp. 62–63; Alphonse M. Schwitalla, "Present Economic Objectives of the Nursing Profession," *American Journal of Nursing* 33 (1933), pp. 1135–1142; Ellen S. Woodward, "Federal Aspects of Unemployment Among Professional Women," *American Journal of Nursing* 34 (1934), pp. 534–538.

43 Stewart, *Education of Nurses,* p. 209.

44 *Facts About Nursing,* 1941 (Nursing Information Bureau of the American Nurses' Association, 1941), p. 21.

45 Some indication of a change appears in an article, Graham Lee Davis, "$33,000 Loss in 12 Hospitals Due to Nursing Schools," *Hospital Management* (August, 1931).

46 Mary Roberts, *American Nursing* (New York: Macmillan, 1961), pp. 230–231; see Miriam Ames, "Hourly Nursing Service," *American Journal of Nursing* 33 (1933), pp. 113, 215, and Michael M. Davis, "The Meaning of the Hourly Nursing Experiment in Chicago," *American Journal of Nursing* 33 (1933), p. 111.

47 The ANA distributed a pamphlet, *The NRA and Nursing* (New York: American Nurses' Association, 1933), and backed it with editorial support, "Notes from Headquarters, American Nurses Association," *American Journal of Nursing* 33 (1933), p. 1001.

48 M. Louise Fitzpatrick, "Nurses in American History: Nursing and the Great Depression," *American Journal of Nursing* 75 (1975), pp. 2188–2190.

49 Ella S. Woodward, "The WPA and Nursing," *American Journal of Nursing* 37 (1937), pp. 994–997, and "WPA Nursing," *American Journal of Nursing* 38 (1938), p. 733.

50   Pearl McIver, "Public Health Nursing in the United States Public Health Service," *American Journal of Nursing* 40 (1940), pp. 996-1000; Thomas Parran, "Public Health Nursing Marches on," *Public Health Nursing* 29 (1937), pp. 617-622.

51   *Facts About Nursing* (The Nursing Information Bureau of the American Nurses Association, 1938), p. 5.

52   *Facts About Nursing* (The Nursing Information Bureau of the American Nurses Association, 1946), p. 13.

53   *Manual of Essentials of Good Hospital Nursing* (American Hospital Association and National League of Nursing Education, 1926). There were several revisions.

54   See Nathan Sinai, Odin W. Anderson, and Melvin L. Dollar, *Health Insurance in the United States* (New York: The Commonwealth Fund, 1946); American Medical Association, *Voluntary Prepayment Medical Benefit Plans* (Chicago: American Medical Association, 1953); O. D. Dickerson, Health Insurance (Homewood, Ill.: Richard D. Irwin, Inc., 1959).

55   Herman Miles Somers and Anne Ramsay Somers, *Doctors, Patients and Health Insurance* (Washington, D.C.: The Brookings Institution, 1961).

Chapter 8

1   See Ellwynne M. Vreeland, "Fifty Years of Nursing in the Federal Government Nursing Services," *American Journal of Nursing* 50 (1950), pp. 626-631; Portia B. Kernodle, *The Red Cross Nurse in Action* (New York: Harper, 1949), pp. 15-20; and Lavinia L. Dock, "The Episode of the Spanish-American War," *History of American Red Cross Nursing,* Lavinia L. Dock, Sarah Elizabeth Pickett, Clara D. Noyes, Fannie F. Clement, Elizabeth G. Fox, and Anna R. Van Meter, eds. (New York: Macmillan, 1922), pp. 25-66. For numbers see *Facts About Nursing, 1941* "Military Nursing" (New York Nursing Information Bureau and American Nurses Association, 1941).

2   Lavinia L. Dock, "Affiliation of the American Red Cross with the Nurses' Association," *History of American Red Cross Nursing, op. cit.,* pp. 67-139.

3   Lavinia L. Dock and Sarah Elizabeth Pickett, "Mobilization," in *History of American Red Cross Nursing,* p. 305.

4   Vreeland, *op. cit., passim.*

5   "Vassar Preparatory Course: A New Experiment in Nursing Education," *American Journal of Nursing* 18 (1918), p. 1155. See also Gladys Bonner Clappison, *Vassar's Rainbow Division* (Lake Mills, Iowa: The Graphic Publishing Company, 1964). For numbers see *Facts About Nursing, 1941, op. cit.*

6   Lavinia L. Dock and Sarah Elizabeth Pickett, *op. cit.,* pp. 273-282.

7   See Annie W. Goodrich, "The Plan for the Army School of Nursing," *Twenty-fifth Annual Report of the National League of Nursing Education* (1918), p. 171. See Harriet Berger Koch, *Militant Angel: Annie W. Goodrich* (New York: Macmillan, 1951), pp. 81-112.

8 Vreeland, *op. cit., passim.*

9 Federal Government section (Report of the Biennial), *American Journal of Nursing,* 38 (1938), pp. 686–687.

10 Hope Newell, *The History of the National Nursing Council* (National Organization for Public Health Nursing, 1951); "Nursing Council on National Defense," *American Journal of Nursing* 40 (1940), p. 1013.

11 "The National Survey," *American Journal of Nursing* 41 (August, 1941), pp. 929–930.

12 Teresa Christy, "Equal Rights for Women: Voices From the Past," *American Journal of Nursing* 71 (1971), pp. 289–293.

13 Edith A. Aynes, *From Nightingale to Eagle: An Army Nurse's History* (Englewood Cliffs, New Jersey: Prentice Hall, 1973); Julia O. Flikke, *Nurses in Action* (Philadelphia: J. B. Lippincott, 1943); U.S. Army Nurse Corps, *The Army Nurse* (Washington, D.C.: 1944); U.S. Navy Nurse Corps, *White Task Force* (Washington, D.C.: 1943).

14 Bonnie Bullough, "Nurses in American History: The Lasting Impact of World War II on Nursing," *American Journal of Nursing* 76 (January, 1976), pp. 118–120.

15 "The Nurses' Contribution to American Victory: Facts and Figures from Pearl Harbor to VJ Day," *American Journal of Nursing* 45 (September, 1945), pp. 683–686. Juanita Redmond, *I Served on Bataan* (Philadelphia: J. B. Lippincott, 1943).

16 Alice R. Clarke, "Thirty-Seven Months as Prisoners of War," *American Journal of Nursing,* 45 (May, 1945), pp. 342–345.

17 "Army Nurses in ETO," *American Journal of Nursing* 45 (May, 1945), pp. 386–387; Mary M. Roberts, *American Nursing: History and Interpretation* (New York: Macmillan, 1954), pp. 342–351; George Korson, *At His Side: The Story of the American Red Cross Overseas in World War II* (New York: Coward-McCann, 1948).

18 Lucile Petry, "The U.S. Cadet Nurse Corps: A Summing Up," *American Journal of Nursing* 45 (December, 1945), pp. 1027–1028; U.S. Public Health Service, *The U.S. Cadet Nurse Corps and Other Federal Nurse Training Programs, 1943–1948* (Washington, D.C.: U.S. Government Printing Office, 1950).

19 Beatrice J. Kalish and Philip A. Kalish, "Nurses in American History: The Cadet Nurse Corps-In World War II," *American Journal of Nursing* 76 (February, 1976), pp. 240–242.

20 Helen Byrne Lippman, "The Future of the Red Cross Volunteer Nurses, Nurses' Aid Corps," *American Journal of Nursing* 45 (October, 1945), pp. 811–812; Dorothy Demings, *The Practical Nurse* (New York: The Commonwealth Fund, 1947); Federal Security Agency, *Practical Nursing* (Washington, D.C.: 1947); Dorothy F. Johnston, *History and Trends of Practical Nursing* (St. Louis: C. V. Mosby, 1966).

21 Mary Roberts, *American Nursing: History and Interpretation* (New York: Macmillan, 1961), pp. 319–322.

22 "News Highlights," *American Journal of Nursing,* 55 (1955), p. 1440. Commissioned Oct. 6, 1955.

23 For new figures see Walter L. Johnson, "Educational Preparation for

Nursing, *"Nursing Outlook,* 24 (September, 1976), pp. 568–577, and for additional information see chapter 10 in this book.

24 Most of the newspapers and news magazines of the time carried news of her adventures. For official American nursing reaction see, "ANA Pays Tribute to French Nurse," *American Journal of Nursing* 54 (1954), p. 999.

25 Jessie M. Scott, "Federal Support for Nursing Education 1964 to 1972," *American Journal of Nursing* 72 (1972), pp. 1855–1861.

26 Susan R. Gortner, "Research in Nursing: The Federal Interest and Grant Program," *American Journal of Nursing* 73 (1973), pp. 1052–1055.

27 Peter A. Corning, *The Evolution of Medicare: From Idea to Law,* U.S. Department of Health, Education, and Welfare, Social Security Administration, Research Report No. 29 (Washington, D.C.: U.S. Government Printing Office, 1969).

28 *The Size and Shape of the Medical Care Dollar,* U.S. Department of Health, Education, and Welfare, Social Security Administration (Washington D.C.: U.S. Government Printing Office, 1970). For nursing support of federal legislation see "The ANA and the Wagner-Murray-Dingell Bill, S1606," *American Journal of Nursing* 46 (1946), pp. 375–376. As early as 1944 the House of Delegates of the American Nurses' Association recommended the expansion of health insurance plans and more intervention by the U.S. government. Earlier accounts are Donald W. Smith, "The Wagner-Murray-Dingell Bill, Senate Bill 1050 H.R. 3293," *American Journal of Nursing* 45 (1945), pp. 933–936 and *passim.*

29 Bonnie Bullough, "The Medicare-Medicaid Amendments," *American Journal of Nursing* 73 (1973), pp. 1926–1929.

30 Gregg W. Downey, "Healthcare Planning Gets Muscles," *Modern Health Care* (March, 1975), pp. 32–37; Donald F. Phillips, "Health Planning: New Hope for a Fresh Start," *Hospitals: Journal of the American Hospital Association* 49 (March 16, 1975), pp. 35–38.

Chapter 9

1 "A Comprehensive Program for Nationwide Action in the Field of Nursing," *American Journal of Nursing* 45 (1945), p. 707.

2 Esther Lucile Brown, *Nursing for the Future: A Report Prepared for the National Nursing Council* (New York: Russell Sage Foundation, 1948).

3 Sister M. Olivia Gowan, ed., *The Nursing Program in the General College* (Washington, D.C.: The Catholic University of America, 1954); see also Committee on the Function of Nursing, *A Program for the Nursing Profession* (New York: Macmillan, 1948).

4 Brown, *op. cit.*

5 Committee on the Function of Nursing, *A Program for the Nursing Profession* (New York: Macmillan, 1948). The report is commonly known as the Ginzberg Report.

6   *American Journal of Nursing* 18 (1918), p. 929.

7   *American Journal of Nursing* 39 (1939), pp. 275–277.

8   See "Trained Attendants and Practical Nurses," *American Journal of Nursing* 44 (1944), pp. 7–8; N. Stevenson, "Curriculum Development in Practical Nurse Education," *American Journal of Nursing* 64 (1964), pp. 81–86; Dorothy Demings, *The Practical Nurse* (New York: Commonwealth Fund, 1947); Federal Security Agency, Practical Nursing (Washington, D.C.: U.S. Government Printing Office, 1947); and especially Dorothy F. Johnston, *History and Trends of Practical Nursing* (St. Louis: C. V. Mosby, 1966). See also Lucile Petry Leone, "Trends and Problems in Practical Nurse Education," *American Journal of Nursing* 56 (1956), pp. 51–53, and Mildred Montag, *The Education of Nursing Technicians* (New York: G. P. Putnam's Sons, 1951).

9   National Center for Health Statistics, U.S. Department of Health, Education, and Welfare, *State Licensing of Health Occupations,* PHS Publication, No. 1758 (Washington, D.C.: U.S. Government Printing Office, 1968), pp. 9–10.

10   Leone, *op. cit.,* pp. 51–53, and Johnston, *op. cit., passim.*

11   The original recommendation was made by the consulting firm of Raymond Rich Associates; see Raymond Rich Associates, "Report on the Structure of Organized Nursing," *American Journal of Nursing* 46 (1946), p. 648. See also "A Tentative Plan for One National Nursing Organization," *American Journal of Nursing* 48 (1948), p. 321; *Handbook on the Structure of Organized Nursing,* second edition, prepared by the Committee on Structure of the National Nursing Organizations (New York, 1949); *New Horizons in Nursing,* compiled by Josephine Nelson (New York: Macmillan, 1950); and for some detail see both the pertinent issues of the *American Journal of Nursing,* and Mary Roberts, *American Nursing* (New York: Macmillan, 1961), pp. 575–596. For the final result see *Proceedings of the Thirty-eighth Convention of the American Nurses Association,* vol. I, House of Delegates, 1952.

12   For the NACGN and Black nurses in general in the period discussed in this section, see Mabel K. Staupers, "Story of the National Association of Colored Graduate Nurses," *American Journal of Nursing* 51 (1951), pp. 222–223, and particularly Staupers, *No Time for Prejudice* (New York: Macmillan, 1961). An earlier account of the Black nurse is Adah M. Thomas, *Pathfinders—A History of the Progress of Colored Graduate Nurses* (New York: Kay, 1929).

13   *Facts About Nursing* (New York: American Nurses Association, 1951), pp. 43–44; *Facts About Nursing* (New York: American Nurses Association 1967), p. 107; "Educational Preparation for Nursing-1975," *Nursing Outlook* 24 (1976), pp. 568–573.

14   National Committee for the Improvement of Nursing Services, *Interim Classification of Schools of Nursing Offering Basic Programs* (New York: NCINS, 1949), and *Nursing Schools at the Mid-Century* (New York: NCINS, 1950), prepared by Margaret West and Christy Hawkins.

15   Mildred Montag, *The Education of Nursing Technicians* (New York: Putnam, 1951), and Jessie Parker Bogue, *The Community College* (New York: McGraw Hill, 1950).

16   Mildred L. Montag and Lassar G. Gotkin, *Community College Education for Nursing* (New York: McGraw Hill, 1959).

17 *Ibid.,* and Mildred L. Montag, *Evaluation of Graduates of Associate Degree Nursing Programs* (New York: Teachers College Press, 1972).

18 Bernice E. Anderson, *Nursing Education in Community Junior Colleges* (Philadelphia: J. B. Lippincott, 1966).

19 Walter L. Johnson, "Educational Preparation for Nursing—1973," *Nursing Outlook* 22 (September 1974), pp. 587–589.

20 *Facts About Nursing,* 1972–1973 (Kansas City: American Nurses Association, 1973), p. 77.

21 National Committee for the Improvement of Nursing Services, *op. cit.,* p. 7, 14.

22 Margaret Bridgman, *Collegiate Education for Nursing* (New York: Russell Sage Foundation, 1953), p. 16.

23 *Ibid., passim.*

24 Helen Nahm, "The Accreditation Program in Nursing," in Sister M. Olivia Gowan, *The Nursing Program in the General College* (Washington, D.C.: The Catholic University of America, 1954) pp. 83–91; Gwendoline McDonald, *Development of Standards and Accreditation in Collegiate Nursing Education* (New York: Teachers College Press, 1965), pp. 59–93.

25 *Facts About Nursing: A Statistical Summary, 1961* (New York: American Nurses' Association, 1961), p. 98; *Facts About Nursing; A Statistical Summary, 1970–1971,* p. 95.

26 Montag and Godkin, *op. cit.,* p. 344.

27 Martha E. Rogers, *Educational Revolution in Nursing* (New York: Macmillan, 1961), pp. 1–15; Lulu Hassenplug, "Preparation of the Nurse Practitioner," *Journal of Nursing Education* 4 (January 1964), pp. 29–42; Dorothy Johnson "Competence in Practice: Technical and Professional," *Nursing Outlook* 14 (October 1966), pp. 30–33; Verle Walters, Shirley Chater, Mary Louise Vivier, Judith H. Urrea, and Holly Skodal Wilson, "Technical and Professional Nursing: An Exploratory Study," *Nursing Research* 21 (March/April, 1972), pp. 124–131.

28 American Nurses' Association, "First Position Paper on Education for Nursing," *American Journal of Nursing* 65 (1965), pp. 106–111; the quotation is from p. 108.

29 Bonnie Bullough, "You Can't Get There from Here," *Journal of Nursing Education* 11 (November 1972), pp. 4–10, reprinted in Jerome P. Lysaught, *Action in Nursing: Progress in Professional Purpose* (New York: McGraw Hill, 1974), pp. 227–233; Purdue University Department of Nursing Baccalaureate Degree Program, "First Annual Report to the W. K. Kellogg Foundation," April 1, 1970 to March 31, 1971, cited in Jerome Lysaught, *From Abstract Into Action* (New York: McGraw-Hill, 1973), p. 155.

30 Bernice E. Anderson *Nursing Education in Community Junior Colleges* (Philadelphia: J. B. Lippincott, 1966).

31 Bonnie Bullough, "Public Legal and Social Pressures for a Career Ladder in Nursing," *Proceedings: Council of Baccalaureate and Higher Degree Programs,* March 22–24, 1972; and Bonnie and Vern Bullough, "A Career Ladder in Nursing: Problems and Prospects," *American Journal of Nursing* 71 (1971), pp. 1938–1943.

32 National Commission for the Study of Nursing and Nursing Education,

Jerome P. Lysaught, Director, *An Abstract for Action* (New York: McGraw-Hill, 1970), p. 116.

33 Carrie B. Lenburg, Walter Johnson, and JoAnn T. Vahey, *Directory of Career Opportunities in Nursing* (New York: National League for Nursing, 1973).

34 Lucille Notter, ed., *Proceedings: Open Curriculum Conference I* (New York: National League for Nursing, 1974).

35 Fred Davis, Virginia L. Olesen, and Elvi Waik Whittaker, "Problems and Issues in Collegiate Nursing Education," in *The Nursing Profession: Five Sociological Essays,* Fred Davis, ed. (New York: John Wiley, 1966), pp. 138-175.

36 Lysaught, *An Abstract for Action,* pp. 162-168; Davis, Olesen, and Whittaker, *op. cit.*

37 Diane McGivern, "Baccalaureate Preparation of the Nurse Practioner," *Nursing Outlook* 22 (February, 1974), pp. 94-98; *Proceedings: Issues in Family Nurse Practitioner Education at the Baccalaureate Level,* Conference held at California State College, Sonoma, June 16-17, 1975; Rose Marie Chioni and Eugenia Schoen, "Preparing Tomorrow's Nurse Practitioner," *Nursing Outlook* 18 (October, 1970), pp. 50-56.

38 Gabrielle D. Martel and Marilyn Winterton Edmunds, "Nurse-Internship in Chicago," *American Journal of Nursing* 72 (1972), pp. 940-943.

39 Mildred E. Schwier, Lena R. Paskewita, Frances K. Peterson, and Florence E. Elliot, *Ten Thousand Nurse Faculty Members in Basic Professional Schools of Nursing* (New York: National League for Nursing, 1953), p. 48.

40 Teresa E. Christy, *Cornerstone for Nursing Education: A History of the Division of Nursing Education of Teachers College, Columbia University 1899-1947* (New York: Teachers College, 1969), pp. 1-18.

41 Margene O. Faddis, *A School of Nursing Comes of Age: A History of the Frances Paye Bolton School of Nursing, Case Western University* (Cleveland: The Alumnae of the Frances Payne Bolton School of Nursing, 1973); Harriet Berger Koch, *Militant Angel* (New York: Macmillan, 1951), p. 132.

42 Joseph D. Matarazzo, "Perspective," in *Future Directions of Doctoral Education for Nurses,* report of a conference in Bethesda, Maryland, January 20, 1971, pp. 64-67.

43 U.S. Department of Health, Education, and Welfare, Division of Nursing, *Health Manpower Source Book, 2, Nursing Personnel* (Washington D.C.: U.S. Government Printing Office, Public Health Publication No. 263, Section 2, revised, 1969), p. 53.

44 *Facts About Nursing,* 1972-1973, pp. 108-122; Walter L. Johnson, *op. cit.*

45 *International Director of Nurses with Doctoral Degrees* (New York: American Nurses Foundation, 1973).

46 National Commission for the Study of Nursing and Nursing Education, *op. cit.*

47 Frances E. Kobrin, "The American Midwife Controversy: A Crisis of Professionalization," *Bulletin of the History of Medicine* XL (1966), pp. 350-363.

48 L. Olsen, "The Expanded Role of the Nurse in Maternity Practice," *Nurs. Clin. North America* 9 (1974), pp. 459-466.

49 See Sister M. Thophane Shoemaker, *History of Nurse-Midwifery in the United States* (Washington, D.C.: The Catholic University of America, 1947); Maternity Center Association, *Twenty Years of Nurse Midwifery* (New York: The

Maternity Center Association, 1953). Mary Breckinridge wrote the standard account of the Kentucky experiment, *Wide Neighborhood: A Study of Frontier Nursing Service* (New York: Harper, 1952).

50 Olsen, *op. cit.*

51 E. H. Fogotson, R. J. Roemer, and R. W. Newman, "Legal Regulation of Health Personnel in the United States," *Report of the National Advisory Commission on Health Manpower,* vol. 2 (Washington, D.C.: U.S. Government Printing Office, 1967), pp. 416–418.

52 Ruth Roemer, "The Nurse Practitioner in Family Planning Services: Law and Practice," *Family Planning Population Reporter,* Vol. 6, No. 3 (June, 1977), pp. 28–34; A. M. Forman and E. M. Cooper, "Legislation and Nurse-Midwifery Practice in USA," *Journal of Nurse-Midwifery,* Vol. 21, No. 2 (Summer, 1976).

53 Helen Clapesattle, *The Doctors Mayo* (reprinted) (New York: Garden City Publishing Co., 1943), pp. 259–260.

54 *Ibid.,* pp. 362–363, 429.

55 Virginia S. Thatcher, *A History of Anesthesia: With Emphasis on the Nurse Specialist* (Philadelphia: J. B. Lippincott, 1952), p. 5; Alice Magaw, "A Review of Over 14,000 Surgical Anesthetics," *Surgery, Gynecology, and Obstetrics* 3 (1906), pp. 795–799.

56 Gertrude L. Fife, "The Nurse As Anesthetist," *American Journal of Nursing* 47 (1947), p. 308.

57 Thatcher, *op. cit.,* pp. 132–152.

58 Bonnie Bullough, *The Law and the Expanding Nursing Role* (New York: Appleton, Century Crofts, 1975), pp. 167–168.

59 B. Tighe, *Review of the Training Programs and Utilization of Paraprofessionals in Medicine and Dentistry,* Institute for the Study of Health and Society (1972), pp. 34–35.

60 L. Meltzer and J. Roderick, "The Development and Current Status of Coronary Care," in L. Meltzer and A. Dunning, eds., *Textbook of Coronary Care* (1972).

61 William B. Kouwenhoven, James R. Jude, and G. Guy Knickerbocker, "Closed Chest Cardiac Massage," *Journal of the American Medical Association* 173: 10 (1960), pp. 1064–1067; James W. Jude, W. B. Kouwenhoven, and G. Guy Knickerbocker, "Cardiac Resuscitation Without Thoracotomy," *Maryland State Medical Journal* 9 (1960), pp. 712–713; and William B. Kouwenhoven, James R. Jude, and G. Guy Knickerbocker, "Heart Activation in Cardiac Arrest," *Modern Concepts in Cardiovascular Disease* 30 (1961), pp. 639–643.

62 Bernard Lown, Raghavan Amarasingham, and Barouk V. Berkovits, "New Method of Terminating Cardiac Arrhythmias: Use of Synchronized Capacitor Discharge," *Journal of the American Medical Association* 182:5 (1962), pp. 548–555.

63 For a good discussion see Anita Berwind, "The Nurse in the Coronary Care Unit," in Bullough, *op. cit.,* pp. 82–94.

64 H. Silver and L. Ford, "The Pediatric Nurse Practitioner at Colorado," *American Journal of Nursing* 67 (1967), pp. 1143–1144, and H. Silver, L. Ford, and S. Stearly, "A Program to Increase Health Care for Children: The Pediatric Nurse Practitioner Program," *Pediatrics* 39 (1967), pp. 756–760.

65 G. E. Siegel and S. Bryson, "Redefinition of the Role of the Public Health

Nurse in Child Health Supervision," *American Journal of Public Health* 53 (1972), pp. 1015-1024.

66 B. Noonan, "Eight Years in a Medical Nurse Clinic," *American Journal of Nursing* 72 (1972), pp. 1128-1130.

67 E. A. Stead, Jr., "Training and Use of Paramedical Personnel," *New England Journal of Medicine* 277 (October 12, 1967), pp. 800-801; and Duke University, *Physician's Assistant Program, Duke University Bulletin, 1969-1970,* pp. 1-4.

68 Bullough, *op. cit.*, p. 57.

69 Lucie Young Kelly, *Dimensions of Professional Nursing* (New York: Macmillan, 1975) pp. 101-103, 142-143; American Medical Association, *Accredited Educational Programs for the Assistant to the Primary Care Physician* (March 1974).

70 "Executive Board Initiates Child Health Manpower Training Program in a Major Effort to Improve Pediatric Care," *Newsletter, American Academy of Pediatrics* 20 (July 1, 1969), pp. 1, 4.

71 Committee on Nursing, "Medicine and Nursing in the 1970's: A Position Statement," *Journal of the American Medical Association* 21 (September 14, 1970), pp. 1881-1883. See also A. Bergman, "Physicians Assistants Belong in the Nursing Profession," *American Journal of Nursing* 71 (1971), pp. 975-977.

Chapter 10

1 *ISR Newsletter,* Institute for Social Research, The University of Michigan (Summer, 1977), p. 8.

2 *The Economic Status of Registered Professional Nurses, 1946-47,* Bulletin 931, Department of Labor, Bureau of Labor Statistics (Washington, D.C.: U.S. Government Printing Office, 1947).

3 "Nurse Membership in Union" (editorial), *American Journal of Nursing* 37 (1937), pp. 766-767; and Mary M. Roberts, *American Nursing: History and Interpretation* (New York: Macmillan, 1954), p. 405.

4 *C.S.N.A. and the Economic Security of Its Members,* (California State Nurses' Association, 1943).

5 William Scott, "Shall Professional Nurses Associations Become Collective Bargaining Agents for Their Members?" *American Journal of Nursing* 44 (1944), pp. 231-232.

6 "Employment Conditions for Registered Nurses" (editorial), *American Journal of Nursing* 46 (1946), pp. 437-438.

7 Anne Zimmerman, "The ANA Economic Security Program in Retrospect," *Nursing Forum* 10, No. 3 (1971), pp. 313-321.

8 "The Biennial," *American Journal of Nursing* 46 (1946), pp. 728-746.

9 William G. Scott, Elizabeth K. Porter and Donald W. Smith, "The Long Shadow," *American Journal of Nursing* 66 (1966), pp. 538-554; and Archie Kleingarnter, "Nurses, Collective Bargaining and Labor Legislation," *Labor Law Journal* 18 (April, 1967), pp. 236-245.

10 Barbara Carter, "Medicine's Forgotten Women," *Issues in Nursing,* Bonnie and Vern Bullough, eds. (New York: Springer, 1966), pp. 171–177.

11 Roberts, *op. cit.,* p. 569.

12 Shirley Titus, "Economic Facts of Life for Nurses," *American Journal of Nursing* 52 (1952), pp. 1109–1112.

13 Martha Belote, "Nurses Are Making It Happen," *American Journal of Nursing* 67 (1967), pp. 285–289.

14 Dorothy Peters, "The Kewanee Story," *American Journal of Nursing* 61 (1961), pp. 74–79.

15 "The Bradenton Story: A Community Crisis," *American Journal of Nursing* 62 (1962), pp. 58–63.

16 Jon D. Miller and Stephen M. Shortell, "Hospital Unionization: A Study of Trends," *Hospitals* 43 (August 16, 1969), pp. 67–72.

17 *Facts About Nursing, 1962–1963* (New York: American Nurses' Association, 1963), p. 57.

18 *Facts About Nursing, 1966–1967* (New York: American Nurses' Association, 1967), p. 137.

19 Belote, *op. cit.,* p. 386.

20 Edith P. Lewis, "The New York City Hospital Story," *American Journal of Nursing* 66 (1966), pp. 1526–1533.

21 Ben Mittman and Beatrice Bumgarner, "What Happened in San Francisco," *American Journal of Nursing* 67 (1967), pp. 80–84.

22 Ada Jacox, "Collective Action and Control of Practice by Professionals," *Nursing Forum* 10, No. 3 (1971), pp. 239–257.

23 Ingeborg Mauksch, "How Did It Come to Pass," *Nursing Forum* 10, No. 3 (1971), pp. 258–272.

24 Belote, *op. cit.*

25 Kleingarnter, *op. cit.*

26 Barbara G. Schutt, "The Right to Strike" (editorial), *American Journal of Nursing* 68 (1968), p. 1455.

27 "L.V.N. Group Asks More Pay, Rescinds No Strike Policy," *Hospitals* 43 (November 16, 1969), p. 107.

28 Anne Zimmerman, "Taft-Hartley Amended; Implications for Nursing: The Industrial Model," *American Journal of Nursing* 75 (1975), pp. 284–288.

29 Bonnie Bullough, "The New Militancy in Nursing," *Nursing Forum* 10, No. 3 (1971), pp. 273–288.

30 Norman E. Amundson, "Will the Supervisor Issue Destroy the Nurses Association as a Professional Organization?" *The Journal of Nursing Administration* (July/August, 1973), pp. 6, 61.

31 "ILO/WHO Group Draws Up Instrument on Personnel Practices Recommended for Adoption for Nurses Worldwide," *American Journal of Nursing* 74 (1974), p. 89.

32 Leonard Stein, "The Doctor-Nurse Game," *American Journal of Nursing* 68 (1968), pp. 101–105, also *New Directions for Nurses,* Bonnie and Vern Bullough, eds. (New York: Springer, 1971), pp. 129–137.

33 "Editorial," *American Journal of Nursing,* 39 (1939), pp. 275–277; "Trained Attendants and Practical Nurses," *American Journal of Nursing* 44 (1944), pp. 7–8; "Statutory Status of Six Professions," *Research Bulletin of the National*

Educational Association 16 (September, 1938), pp. 184–223; Elizabeth M. Jamieson and Mary Sewell, *Trends in Nursing History* (Philadelphia: W. B. Saunders, 1944), pp. 533–534.

34 "A.N.A. Board Approves a Definition of Nursing Practice," *American Journal of Nursing* 55 (1955), p. 1474.

35 Edward Fogotson, Ruth Roemer, Roger W. Newman and John L. Cook, "Licensure of Other Medical Personnel," *Report of the National Advisory Commission on Health Manpower* vol. 2 (Washington, D.C.: U.S. Government Printing Office, 1967), pp. 407–492.

36 Bonnie Bullough, *The Law and the Expanding Nursing Role* (New York: Appleton-Century-Croft, 1975), pp. 15–17.

37 Grace G. Barbee, "Special Procedures: I.V.s, Blood Transfusions and Skin Testing," *Proceedings: Institute on Medico-Legal Aspects of Nursing Practice* (Santa Monica, California: California Nurses' Association, 1961), pp. 41–44.

38 Nathan Hershey, "Legal Issues in Nursing Practice," *Professional Nursing: Foundations, Perspectives and Relationships,* Eugenia K. Spalding and Lucile E. Notter, eds. (Philadelphia: J. B. Lippincott, 1970), pp. 110–127.

39 Harvey Sarner, *The Nurse and the Law* (Philadelphia: W. B. Saunders, 1968), pp. 89–90.

40 National Commission for the Study of Nursing and Nursing Education, *An Abstract for Action* (New York: McGraw-Hill, 1970).

41 *Extending the Scope of Nursing Practice: A Report of the Secretary's Committee to Study Extended Roles for Nurses,* U.S. Department of Health, Education, and Welfare (November, 1971).

42 Arizona Attorney General, *Opinion,* No. 71-30, August 6, 1971, cited in Alfred M. Sadler, Jr. and Blair L. Sadler, "Recent Developments in the Law Relating to Physicians' Assistants," *Vanderbilt Law Review* 24 (November, 1971), p. 1205. See also "Amendment of the Arizona Nursing Practice Law Broadens Definition of Professional Nursing," *American Journal of Nursing* 72 (July, 1972), p. 1203.

43 California Attorney General, *Opinion,* No. CV 72/187, February 15, 1973; and Indexed Letter from the California Attorney General, October 4, 1972.

44 Bullough, *op. cit.,* pp. 153–170, and also Bonnie Bullough, "The Law and the Expanding Nursing Role," *American Journal of Public Health* 66 (March, 1976), pp. 249–254.

45 *Idaho Code,* Section 54-1413.

46 *Minimum Standards, Rules and Regulations for Nurse Practitioners (Expanding Role) and Guidelines for Nurses Writing Prescriptions,* jointly promulgated by the Idaho State Board of Nursing and the Idaho State Board of Medicine as authorized by Section 54-1413 (e), *Idaho Code.*

47 New York State Education Law, Title 8, Article 139, Section 6902.

48 Mrs. Cadwalader Jones, "Looking Back Through Fifty Years," *The Alumnae Journal of New York City Hospital School of Nursing,* Golden Anniversary Number, 1875–1925 (July, 1925), p. 11.

49 Mary Roberts, *op. cit.,* p. 312; and *Facts About Nursing, 1942* (New York: ANA, 1942), p. 6.

50 See Kenneth T. Crummer, "Men Nurses—A Survey of the Present-Day Situation of Graduate Men Nurses," *American Journal of Nursing* 28 (1928), p.

467; Mary Elizabeth May, "Nurse Training Schools of New York State Hospitals," *American Journal of Nursing* 8 (1907), p. 18; George O'Hanlon, "Men Nurses in General Hospitals," *American Journal of Nursing* 34 (1934), p. 16; and William L. Russell, "Men Nurses in Psychiatric Hospitals," *American Journal of Nursing* 34 (1934), p. 19; Frances W. Witte, "Opportunities in Graduate Education for Men Nurses," *American Journal of Nursing* 34 (1934), p. 133.

51 See Herbert J. Nash, "Men Nurses in New York State," *Trained Nurse and Hospital Review* (August, 1936), p. 123; and Roberts, *op. cit.,* p. 318.

52 *Facts About Nursing, 1946* (New York: American Nurses' Association, 1946), p. 35.

53 "Educational Preparation for Nursing—1975," *Nursing Outlook* 24 (September, 1976), pp. 568–573.

54 Bonnie and Vern Bullough, "Sex Segregation in Health Care," *Nursing Outlook* 23 (January, 1975), pp. 40–45.

55 See a brief popular study by Patricia J. Bush, "The Male Nurse: A Challenge to Traditional Role Identities," *Nursing Forum* XV (1976), pp. 390–405. See also Adrian Schoenmaker, "Nursing's Dilemna: Male Versus Female Admissions Choice," *Nursing Forum* XV (1976), pp. 406–412.

56 David J. Boorer, "Men Nurses in Britian," *New Directions in Nursing,* Bonnie and Vern Bullough, eds. (New York: Springer Publishing Company, 1971), pp. 318–323.

Chapter 11

1 Lavinia L. Dock, Sarah Elizabeth Pickett, Clara D. Noyes, Fannie F. Clement, Elizabeth G. Fox, and Anna R. Van Meter, *History of Red Cross Nursing* (New York: Macmillan, 1922), pp. 1140–1147.

2 *Ibid.,* pp. 1144–1145.

3 Portia B. Kernodle, *The Red Cross in Action, 1882–1948* (New York: Harper and Brothers, 1949), pp. 180 ff.; and Yvonne Hentsch, "Influence of the Red Cross on Professional Nursing," *Information Bulletin for Red Cross Nurses,* (Geneva: May-August, 1947). See also Mary Roberts, *American Nursing* (New York: Macmillan, 1961), pp. 607–609.

4 Daisy C. Bridges, "Events in the History of the International Council of Nurses," *American Journal of Nursing* 49 (1949), p. 594; "The ICN and Nursing Education," *American Journal of Nursing* 50 (1950), p. 385; and Margaret Brey and Ethel Gordon Fenwich, *The History of the ICN, 1899–1925* (Geneva: The International Council of Nurses, 1931).

5 "ICN Statement of Nursing Education, Nursing Practice and Service and the Social and Economic Welfare of Nurses," *American Journal of Nursing* 69 (1969), pp. 2177–2179. See also the International Council of Nurses, *Constitution and Regulations.*

6 See Lyle Creelman, Agnes Chagas, and Virginia Arnold, "WHO and Profes-

sional Nursing," *American Journal of Nursing* 54 (1954), pp. 448–449; and *The First Ten Years of WHO* (Geneva: 1958).

7 Much of this information, as well as that in succeeding sections, is based upon our own personal experience and our travels throughout the world.

8 Committee on Nursing, *Report,* Asa Briggs, Chairman (London: Her Majesty's Stationery Office, October, 1972); Sister Mary Hubert Reinkemeyer, "An Inherited Pathology," *Nursing Outlook* 15 (November, 1967), pp. 51–53; Sister Agnes M. Reinkemeyer, "It Won't Be Hospital Nursing," *American Journal of Nursing* 68 (September, 1968), pp. 1936–1940; Cynthia D. Sculco, "An American Nurse at the London Hospital," *Nursing Outlook* 24 (August, 1976), pp. 504–508.

9 For a brief account of her activities see John Shelton Curtis, "Russian Nightingale," *American Journal of Nursing* 68 (1968), pp. 1029–1031; and Curtiss, "Russian Sisters of Mercy in the Crimea, 1854–1855," *Slavic Review* XXV (March, 1966), pp. 84–100.

10 Faye Abdellah, "Nursing and Health Care in the U.S.S.R.," *American Journal of Nursing* 73 (1973), pp. 2096–2099; *Hospital Services in the U.S.S.R.* (Washington, D.C.: U.S. Department of Health, Education, and Welfare, 1966); Mark J. Field, *Soviet Socialized Medicine: An Introduction* (New York: Free Press, 1967), and J. E. Muller, *et al.,* "The Soviet Health System—Aspects of Relevance for Medicine in the United States," *New England Journal of Medicine* 286 (March 30, 1972), pp. 693–702; Victor W. Sidel, "Feldshers and Feldsherism: The Role and Training of the Feldsher in the U.S.S.R.," in Bonnie and Vern Bullough, eds., *New Directions for Nurses* (New York: Springer, 1971), pp. 40–50.

11 Teresa Maria Molina, *Historia de la Enfermeria* (Buenos Aires, Argentina: Intermedica, 1973).

12 For an account of the pioneering efforts of the Rockefeller Foundation see Raymond B. Fosdick, *The Story of the Rockefeller Foundation* (New York: Harper, 1952).

13 For a somewhat hostile account of the relationship of midwifery to nursing in Japan see Mary W. Standlee, *The Great Pulse: Japanese Midwifery and Obstetrics through the Ages* (Rutland, Vermont: Charles E. Tuttle, 1959).

14 For a summary of developments in Australia see Ruth Roemer, "Nursing Functions and the Law: Some Perspectives from Australia and Canada," in Bonnie Bullough, ed., *The Law and the Expanding Nursing* (New York: Appleton-Century-Crofts, 1975), pp. 38–50, especially pp. 41–44. See also *Expansion of Medical Education,* Report of the Committee on Medical Education to the Australian Universities Commission, Peter Karmel, Chairman, (1973).

15 D. Morgan, "The Future Expanded Role of the Nurse," *Canadian Hospital,* 75 (May 1972), and Roemer, *op. cit.,* p. 44. For an earlier account see "Nursing in Canada: From Pioneering History to a Modern Federation," *International Nursing Review* 15 (1968), pp. 1–29.

16 Ministry of National Health and Welfare, National Conference on the Assistance to the Physician, *The Complementary Roles of Physician and the Nurse* (1972).

17 Roemer, *op. cit.,* p. 45.

18 "The Expanded Role of the Nurse: A Joint Statement of CNA/CMA," *Canadian Nurse* (May, 1973), pp. 23–25.

19   David L. Sackett, *et al.,* "The Burlington Randomized Trial of the Nurse Practitioner: Health Outcomes of Patients," *Annals of Internal Medicine* 80 (February, 1974), pp. 137–142. Reprinted in Bonnie and Vern Bullough, eds. *Expanding Horizons for Nurses,* (New York: Springer, 1977), pp. 55–66.

20   Roemer, *op. cit.,* pp. 39–40.

21   Royal Australian Nursing Federation and the National Florence Nightingale Committee of Australia, *Survey Report on the Wastage of General Trained Nurses from Nursing in Australia* (Canberra, 1967)); Roemer, *op. cit.,* p. 42.

22   For Lillian Wald see Allan E. Reznick, *Lillian D. Wald: The Years at Henry Street* (unpublished PhD dissertation: University of Wisconsin, 1973), pp. 147–153, but more especially her correspondence now stored at Columbia University, New York.

23   Gwendolyn Safier, *Contemporary American Leaders: An Oral History* (New York: McGraw-Hill, 1977).

24   *Facts About Nursing, 72–73* (Kansas City: American Nurses Association, 1974), pp. 6–7, 64.

25   M. Louise Fitzpatrick, *National Organization for Public Health Nursing 1912–1952: Development of a Practice Field* (New York: National League for Nursing, 1975), pp. 207–209.

26   "ANA is Denied Place on JCAH Council for Long-Term Care: News," *American Journal of Nursing* 77 (January, 1977), pp. 7–8.

27   Marjorie Ramphal, "Peer Review," *American Journal of Nursing* 74 (1974), pp. 63–67.

28   Marlene Kramer, *Reality Shock: Why Nurses Leave Nursing* (Saint Louis: C. V. Mosby Co., 1974); M. Louise Fitzpatrick, "Nursing," *Signs* 2 (Summer, 1977), pp. 818–834.

29   Frances R. Kreuter, "What is Good Nursing Care?" *Nursing Outlook* 5 (1957), pp. 302–304; Dorothy Johnson, "A Philosophy of Nursing" *Nursing Outlook* 7 (1959), pp. 198–200; Martha Rogers, *Reveille in Nursing* (Philadelphia: F. A. Davis, 1964).

30   Joan P. Riehl and Joan Wilcox McVay, eds., *The Clinical Nurse Specialist; Interpretations* (New York: Appleton-Century-Crofts, 1973).

31   Grayce M. Sills, "Historical Developments in Psychiatric and Mental Health Nursing," in Madeleine Leininger, ed., *Contemporary Issues in Mental Health Nursing* (Boston: Little Brown & Co., 1973).

32   G. D. Marram, M. W. Schlegel, and E. O. Bevis, *Primary Nursing: A Model for Individualized Care* (St. Louis: Mosby, 1974).

33   Basil S. Georgopoulas and Luther Christman, "The Clinical Nurse Specialist: A Role Mode," in *The Clinical Nurse Specialist; Interpretations, op. cit.*

34   Gayle Lorain Brault, *Primary Care Nursing* (unpublished thesis: California State University, Long Beach, 1976).

Bibliography

Abdellah, Faye, "Nursing and Health Care in the USSR," *American Journal of Nursing* 73 (1973), pp. 2096–2099

Abdellah, Faye; Beland, Irene; Martin, Almeda; and Matheney, Ruth, *Patient-Centered Approaches to Nursing* (New York: Macmillan, 1960)

Abel-Smith, Brian, *A History of the Nursing Profession* (London: William Heinemann, 1960)

Ackerknecht, Erwin H., *A Short History of Medicine* (New York: Ronald Press, 1955)

Ackerknecht, Erwin H., *History and Geography of the Most Important Diseases* (New York: Hafner, 1965)

Adams, George Worthington, *Doctors in Blue* (New York: Henry Schuman, 1952)

Alcott, Louisa May, *Hospital Sketches* (reprinted (New York: Sagamore Press, 1957)

Alexander, Franz G. and Selesnicic, Sheldon T., *The History of Psychiatry* (New York: Harper and Row, 1966)

Allbutt, Sir Thomas Clifford, *Greek Medicine in Rome* (London: Macmillan, 1921)

"Amendment of the Arizona Nursing Practice Law Broadens Definition of Professional Nursing," *American Journal of Nursing* 72 (1972), p. 1203

American Medical Association, *Accredited Educational Programs for the Assistant to the Primary Care Physician* (Chicago: American Medical Association, March 1974)

American Medical Association, *Voluntary Prepayment Medical Benefit Plans* (Chicago: American Medical Association, 1953)

The American Nation: A History from Original Sources, edited by A. B. Hart, 28 vols. (New York: Harper, 1906–1918)

American Nurses' Association, "First Position Paper on Education for Nursing," *American Journal of Nursing* 66 (1966), pp. 106–111

Ames, Miriam, "Hourly Nursing Service," *American Journal of Nursing* 33 (1833), pp. 113, 215

Amundson, Norman E., "Will the Supervisor Issue Destroy the Nurses Association as a Professional Organization?" *The Journal of Nursing Administration* (July/August 1973), pp. 6, 61

An American Woman, *Suggestions for the Sick Room* (New York: Anson D. F. Randolph, 1876)

"The ANA and the Wagner-Murray-Dingell Bill, S1606," *American Journal of Nursing* 46 (1946), pp. 375–376

"ANA Board Approves a Definition of Nursing Practice," *American Journal of Nursing* 55 (1955), p. 1474

"ANA is Denied Place on JCAH Council for Long-Term Care: News." *American Journal of Nursing* 77 (1977), pp. 7–8

"ANA Pays Tribute to French Nurse," *American Journal of Nursing* 54 (1954), p. 999

Anderson, Bernice E., *Nursing Education in Community Junior Colleges* (Philadelphia: J. P. Lippincott, 1966)

Andrews, Matthew Page, *The Women of the South in War Times,* new edition (Baltimore: Norman, Remington, 1927)

Arderne, John, *Treatises of Fistula in Ano, Haemorrhoids and Clysters,* edited by Sir D'Arcy Power (London: Kegan Paul, Trench, Trubner & Co., Ltd., 1910) (Middle English Edition)

Arizona Attorney General, *Opinion* No. 71-30 (August 6, 1971)

"Army Nurses in ETO," *American Journal of Nursing* 45 (1945), pp. 386–387

Ashley, Jo Ann, *Hospitals, Paternalism, and the Role of the Nurse* (New York: Teacher's College, 1976)

Ashley, Jo Ann, "Nurses in American History: Nursing and Early Feminism," *American Journal of Nursing* 75 (1975), pp. 1465–1467

Ashton, T. S., *The Industrial Revolution* (Oxford: Oxford University, 1948)

Aurelianus, Caelius, *On Acute Diseases and on Chronic Diseases,* translated by I. E. Drabkin (Chicago: University of Chicago, 1950)

Austin, Anne L., *History of Nursing Source Book* (New York: G. P. Putnam's Sons, 1957)

Austin, Anne L., *The Woolsey Sisters of New York: 1860–1900* (Philadelphia: American Philosophical Society, 1971)

Aynes, Edith A., *From Nightingale to Eagle: An Army Nurse's History* (Englewood Cliffs, New Jersey: Prentice Hall, 1973)

Ayres, Anne, *Evangelical Sisterhoods, In Two Letters to a Friend,* edited by W. A. Muhlenberg (New York: T. Whittaker, 1867); reprinted as *The Letters on Protestant Sisterhoods* (New York: R. Craighead, 1856)

Ayres, Anne, *The Life and Work of William Augustus Muhlenberg* (New York: Harper & Bro., 1880)

Baker, Nina Brown, *Cyclone in Calico: The Story of Mary Ann Bickerdyke* (Boston: Little, Brown, 1952)

Bannister, Lucy A., "A New Field: The Nurse's Opportunity in Factory Work," *Fourteenth Annual Report of the American Society of Superintendents of Training Schools for Nurses* (1908), p. 104

Barbee, Grace G., "Special Procedures: I.V.s, Blood Transfusions and Skin Testing," *Proceedings: Institute on Medico-Legal Aspects of Nursing Practice* (Santa Monica, California: California Nurses' Association, 1961), pp. 41–44

Barton, W. E., *Life of Clara Barton,* 2 vols. (Boston: Houghton Mifflin, 1922)

Baumgartner, Leona, *John Howard: Hospital and Prison Reformer* (Baltimore: Johns Hopkins, 1939)

Beard, Richard Olding, 'Fair Play for the Trained Nurse," *Pictorial Review* (February, 1922), pp. 28, 95–96

Beard, Richard Olding, "The Social, Economic, and Educational Status of the Nurse," *American Journal of Nursing* 20 (1920), pp. 874–876

Beck, Flora, *Ten Patients and an Almoner* (London: George Allen and Unwin, 1956)

"Beginnings of Some Famous Schools," *Trained Nurse and Hospital Review* (August, 1938)

Bell, E. Moberly, *The Story of the Hospital Almoners* (London: Faber & Faber, 1961)

Bellows, Henry Whitney, *Report Concerning the Women's Central Association of Relief at New York to the United States Sanitary Commission* (New York: Bryant, 1861)

Belote, Martha, "Nurses are Making it Happen," *American Journal of Nursing* 67 (1967), pp. 185-189

Benedict St., *Regula.* English translation in Dom Paul Delatte, *The Rule of St. Benedict,* translated by Dom Justin McCann (Latrobe, Pennsylvania: The Archabbey Press, 1950)

Benne, Kenneth D. and Bennis, Warren, "Role Conflict in Nursing," *American Journal of Nursing* 59 (1959), pp. 196-198, 380-383

Bergman, A., "Physicians Assistants Belong in the Nursing Profession," *American Journal of Nursing* 71 (1971), pp. 975-977

Berman, A., "Conflict and Anomaly in the Scientific Orientation of French Pharmacy, 1800-1873," *Bulletin of the History of Medicine* 37 (1963), pp. 1440-1462

Berman, A., "The Pharmaceutical Component of 19th-Century French Public Health and Hygiene," *Pharmacy in History* 11 (1969), pp. 5-10

Berman, A., "The Scientific Tradition in French Hospital Pharmacy," *American Journal of Hospital Pharmacy* 18 (1961), pp. 110-119

Bernardine St., *Sermons,* translated by G. G. Coulton, printed in *Life in the Middle Ages,* 4 vols. (Cambridge: University Press, 1954)

Berwind, Anita, "The Nurse in the Coronary Care Unit," in Bonnie Bullough: *The Law and the Expanding Nursing Role* (New York: Appleton-Century-Crofts, 1975)

Bettmann, Otto L., *A Pictorial History of Medicine* (Springfield, Illinois: Charles C. Thomas, 1956)

"The Biennial," *American Journal of Nursing* 34 (1934), pp. 603-627

"The Biennial," *American Journal of Nursing* 38 (1938), pp. 686-687

"The Biennial," *American Journal of Nursing* 46 (1946), pp. 728-746

Bio-Bibliography of Florence Nightingale, issued by W. J. Bishop and Sue Goldie with the International Council of Nurses (London: International Council of Nurses, 1962)

Blackwell, Elizabeth, *Pioneer Work in Opening the Medical Profession to Women* (London: Longmans, Green, 1895)

Blake, John B., "Women and Medicine in Ante-Bellum America," *Bulletin of the History of Medicine* 39 (1965), pp. 99-123

Bogue, Jessie Parker, *The Community College* (New York: McGraw Hill, 1950)

Bonser, Wilfrid, *The Medical Background of Anglo-Saxon England* (London: Wellcome Historical Medical Library, 1963)

Boorer, David J., "Men Nurses in Britain," *New Directions in Nursing,* edited by Bonnie and Vern Bullough (New York: Springer, 1971), pp. 318-323

Bordley, James and McGehee, A. Harvey, *Two Centuries of American Medicine* (Philadelphia: W. B. Saunders, 1976)

Boswall, Emily Oatway, "Development of Private Duty Nursing," *American Journal of Nursing* 25 (1925), pp. 848-850

Bowsky, William M., *The Black Death, A Turning Point in History* (New York: Holt Rinehart and Winston, 1971)

Bowman, Gerald, *The Lamp and the Book: The Story of the RCN, 1916-1966* (London: Queen Anne Press, 1967)

Boyd. Belle, *Belle Boyd in Camp and Prison* (New York: Blelock, 1865)

"The Bradenton Story: A Community Crisis," *American Journal of Nursing* 62 (1962), pp. 58-63

Bradford, William, *History of Plymouth Plantation* (New York: Charles Scribner's Sons, 1923)

Brainard, A. M., *The Evolution of Public Health Nursing* (Philadelphia: W. B. Saunders, 1922)

Breasted, J. H., *The Edwin Smith Surgical Papyrus,* 2 vols. (Chicago: University of Chicago Press Oriental Institute Publication, 1930)

Breay, Margaret, and Fenwick, Ethel G., *The History of the International Council of Nurses, 1899–1925* (Geneva: International Council of Nurses, 1931)

Breckinridge, Mary, *Wide Neighborhood: A Study of Frontier Nursing Service* (New York: Harper, 1952)

Breckinridge, Sophonisba, *Women in the Twentieth Century* (New York: McGraw-Hill, 1933)

Bridges, Daisy C., "Events in the History of the International Council of Nurses," *American Journal of Nursing* 49 (1949), p. 594

Bridges, Daisy C., *A History of the International Council of Nurses, 1899–1964* (Philadelphia: J. P. Lippincott, 1967)

Bridges, Daisy C., *Outstanding Events in the History of the I.C.N.* (Stockholm: International Council of Nurses, 1949)

Bridgman, Margaret, *Collegiate Education for Nursing* (New York: Russell Sage Foundation, 1953)

Briele, L., *Collection de documents pour servir à l'histoire des hôpitaux de Paris,* 4 vols. (Paris: Imprimerie nationale, 1881–1887)

Briggs, Asa, Chairman, Committee on Nursing, *Report* (London: Her Majesty's Stationery Office, October 1972)

Brinton, John H., *Personal Memoirs* (New York: Neale, 1914)

Brock, A. J., *Greek Medicine* (London: J. M. Dent & Sons, Ltd., 1929)

Brockett, L. P., and Vaughan, Mary C., *Women's Work in the Civil War: A Record of Heroism, Patriotism and Patience* (Philadelphia: Zeigler, McCurdy, 1867)

Brown, Esther Lucille, *Nursing as a Profession* (New York: Russell Sage Foundation, 1936)

Brown, Esther Lucille, *Nursing for the Future: A Report Prepared for the National Nursing Council* (New York: Russell Sage Foundation, 1948)

Bryan, Cyril, the *Papyrus Ebers* (New York: D. Appleton & Co., 1931)

Bucklin, Sophronia E., *In Hospital and Camp* (Philadelphia: J. E. Potter, 1869)

The Bulletin of the History of Medicine, published by the Institute of Medical History at The Johns Hopkins University, and the American Association for the History of Medicine

Bulloch, W., *The History of Bacteriology* (London: Oxford University, 1938)

Bullough, Bonnie, *The Law and the Expanding Nursing Role* (New York: Appleton-Century-Croft, 1975)

Bullough, Bonnie, "The Law and the Expanding Nursing Role," *American Journal of Public Health* 66 (March 1976), pp. 249–254

Bullough, Bonnie, "The Medicare-Medicaid Amendments," *American Journal of Nursing* 73 (1973), pp. 1926–1929

Bullough, Bonnie, "The New Militancy in Nursing," *Nursing Forum* 10 No. 3 (1971), pp. 273–288

Bullough, Bonnie, "Nurses in American History: The Lasting Impact of World War II on Nursing," *American Journal of Nursing* 76, (1976), pp. 118–120

Bullough, Bonnie, "Public, Legal and Social Pressures for a Career Ladder in Nursing," *Proceedings: Council of Baccalaureate and Higher Degree Programs, March 22-24, 1972*

Bullough, Bonnie, "You Can't Get There from Here," Journal of *Nursing Education* 11 (November, 1972), pp. 4-10

Bullough, Bonnie and Vern, "A Career Ladder in Nursing: Problems and Prospects," *American Journal of Nursing* 71 (1971), pp. 1938-1943

Bullough, Bonnie and Vern, "Collegiate Nursing in the United States—A Historical Review," *International Nursing Review* 10 (1963), pp. 41-47

Bullough, Bonnie and Vern, *Issues in Nursing* (New York: Springer, 1966)

Bullough, Bonnie and Vern, "The Origins of Modern American Nursing: The Civil War Era," *Nursing Forum* II No. 2 (1963), pp. 13-27

Bullough, Bonnie and Vern, "The Problem of Goal Changes," *Nursing Forum* 4 (1965), pp. 79-92

Bullough, Bonnie and Vern, "Sex Segregation in Health Care," *Nursing Outlook* 23 (January, 1975), pp. 40-45

Bullough, Vern, *The Development of Medicine as a Profession* (Basle: S. Karger; New York: Hafner, 1966)

Bullough, Vern (with a final chapter by Bonnie Bullough), *The Subordinate Sex: A History of Attitudes Towards Women* (Urbana, Illinois: University of Illinois, 1973). See also Penguin Books, 1974

Bullough, Vern and Bonnie, "How Rough Red Hands Led to Rubber Gloves," *American Journal of Nursing* 70 (1970)

Bullough, Vern and Bonnie, "Nursing and History," *Nursing Outlook* 12 (October, 1964), pp. 41-46

Burgess, May Ayres, *Nurses, Patients and Pocketbooks* (New York: Committee on the Grading of Nursing Schools, 1928)

Burosh, Phyllis, "Physician's Attitudes Towards Nurse-Midwives," *Nursing Outlook* 23 (7) (July, 1975), pp. 452-456

Bush, Patricia J., "The Male Nurse: A Challenge to Traditional Role Identities," *Nursing Forum* XV (1976), pp. 390-405

Calder, Jean McKinley, *The Story of Nursing* (London: Methuen, 1954)

California Attorney General, Indexed Letter, October 4, 1972

California Attorney General, *Opinion* No. CV 72/187, February 15, 1973

California State Nurses' Association and the Economic Security of its Members (California State Nurses' Association, 1943)

California, University of, San Francisco, School of Nursing, *Announcement,* April, 1975

The Cambridge Ancient History, 12 vols. (Cambridge: Cambridge University, 1928-1939)

The Cambridge Medieval History, 8 vols. (Cambridge: Cambridge University, 1922-1930)

The Cambridge Modern History, 14 vols. (Cambridge: Cambridge University, 1902-1912, now being revised)

Campbell, Donald, *Arabian Medicine and Its Influence on the Middle Ages,* 2 vols. (London: Kegan Paul, Trench, Trubner & Co., Ltd., 1926)

Carka Samhita, translated and edited by A. Kaviratna (Calcutta: 1899)

Carka Samhita, translation in six volumes by the Shree Gulabkunverba Ayurvedic Society (Jamnagar, India: S.G.A.S., 1949)

Carter, Barbara, "Medicine's Forgotten Women," *The Reporter* (March 1, 1962), reprinted in *Issues in Nursing,* edited by Bonnie and Vern Bullough (New York: Springer, 1966), pp. 171–177

Castiglioni, Arturo, *A History of Medicine,* translated by E. B. Krumbhaar, 2nd edition (New York: Alfred A. Knopf, 1947)

The Catholic Encyclopedia (New York: Robert Appleton, 1908–1914)

Cato, *De agricultura,* edited and translated by W. D. Hooper and H. B. Ash (London: William Heinemamn, 1934)

Caudill, William, *The Psychiatric Hospital as a Small Society* (Cambridge: Harvard University, 1958)

Celsus, *De medicina,* edited and translated by W. G. Spencer, 3 vols. (London: William Heinemann, 1935–1938)

Chamberlin, Ruth, *The School of Nursing of the Medical College of South Carolina: Its Story* (Columbia, South Carolina: 1970)

Chance, Burton, *Ophthalmology* (New York: Hafner, 1962)

Charley, Irene, *The Birth of Industrial Nursing: Its History and Development in Great Britain* (London: Baillière, Tindall and Cox, 1954)

Chauliac, Guy de, *La Grande Chirurgie,* edited by E. Nicaise (Paris: Felix Alcan, 1890)

Chauliac, Guy de, *On Wounds and Fractures,* translated by W. A. Brennan (Chicago: privately printed, 1923)

Chayer, Mary E., *Nursing in Modern Society* (New York: G. P. Putnam's Sons, 1947)

Chayer, Mary E., "The Trail of the Nursing Textbook," *American Journal of Nursing* 50 (1950), pp. 606–607

Chioni, Rose Marie, and Schoen, Eugenie, "Preparing Tomorrow's Nurse Practitioner," *Nursing Outlook* 18 (October 1970), pp. 50–53

Christy, Teresa, *Cornerstone for Nursing Education: A History of the Division of Nursing Education of Teachers College, Columbia University, 1899–1947* (New York: Teachers College, 1969), pp. 1–18

Christy, Teresa, "Equal Rights for Women: Voices from the Past," *American Journal of Nursing* 71 (1971), pp. 288–293

Christy, Teresa, "The First 50 Years," *American Journal of Nursing* 71 (1971), pp. 1778–1784

Christy, Teresa, "Portrait of a Leader: Lavinia L. Dock," *Nursing Outlook* 17 (June 1969), pp. 72–75

Cipolla, Carlo M., *Cristofano and the Plague: A Study in the History of Public Health in the Age of Galileo* (Berkeley: University of California, 1973)

Cipolla, Carlo M., *Public Health and the Medical Profession in the Renaissance* (Cambridge University Press, 1976)

Clapesattle, Helen, *The Doctors Mayo,* reprinted (Garden City, N.Y.: Garden City, 1943)

Clappison, Gladys Bonner, *Vassar's Rainbow Division* (Lake Mills, Iowa: The Graphic Publishing Company, 1964)

Clarke, Alice R., "Thirty-Seven Months as Prisoners of War," *American Journal of Nursing* 45 (1945), pp. 342–345

Clay, Rotha Mary, *The Medieval Hospitals of England* (London: Methuen, 1909)

Clement, Fannie F., "History of Rural Nursing," *American Journal of Nursing* 13 (1913)

Clendening, Logan, *Source Book of Medical History* (New York: Hoeber, 1942)

Cockayne, Thomas Oswald, *Leechdoms, Wortcunning, and Starcraft of Early England,* 3 vols. (London: Longman, Green, 1864–1866)

Codellas, Pan S., "The Pantocrator, the Imperial Byzantine Medical Center of the XIIth Century A.D. in Constantinople," *Bulletin of the History of Medicine* XII (1942), pp. 392–410

Cohen, M. R., and Drabkin, I. E., *A Source Book in Greek Science* (New York: McGraw-Hill, 1948)

Cohn-Haft, Louis, *The Public Physicians of Ancient Greece* (Northampton, Massachusetts: Smith College, 1956)

The Collected Writings of Walt Whitman (New York: New York University, 1961)

Columella, *De Re Rustica,* edited and translated by H. B. Ash, E. S. Forster, and E. Heffner, 3 vols. (London: William Heinemann, 1960)

Commission on Hospital Care, *Hospital Care in the United States* (New York: The Commonwealth Fund, 1947)

Committee for the Study of Nursing Education, *Nursing and Nursing Education in the United States* (New York: Macmillan, 1923)

Committee on Nursing, Asa Briggs, Chairman, *Report* (London: Her Majesty's Stationery Office, October 1972)

Committee on Nursing, "Medicine and Nursing in the 1970's: A Position Statement," *Journal of the American Medical Association* 21 (September 14, 1970), pp. 1881–1883

Committee on the Function of Nursing, *A Program for the Nursing Profession* (New York: Macmillan, 1948)

The Committee on the Grading of Nursing Schools, *Results of the First Grading Study of Nursing Schools* (New York: 1930)

The Committee on the Grading of Nursing Schools, *The Second Grading of Nursing Schools* (New York: 1932)

The Committee on the Grading of Nursing Schools, *Nursing Schools Today and Tomorrow: Final Report* (New York: 1934)

Comnena, Anna, *Alexiad,* translated by Elizabeth A. S. Dawes (London: Kegan Paul, Trench, Trubner, 1928)

"A Comprehensive Program for Nationwide Action in the Field of Nursing," *American Journal of Nursing* 45 (1945), p. 707

Conferences de S. Paul aux Filles de la Charité (Paris, 1881)

Constantelos, Demetrios J., *Byzantine Philanthropy and Social Welfare* (New Brunswick: Rutgers University, 1968)

Cook, Edward, *The Life of Florence Nightingale,* 2 vols. (London: Macmillan, 1913 and 1914)

Cooper, Page, *The Bellevue Story* (New York: Thomas Y. Crowell, 1948)

Cope, Zachary, *Florence Nightingale and the Doctors* (London: Museum Press, 1958), pp. 21–23

Corner, G. W., *Anatomy* (New York: Hafner, 1964)

Corning, Peter, A., *The Evolution of Medicare: From Idea to Law,* U.S. Department of Health, Education and Welfare, Social Security Administration, Research Report No. 29 (Washington, D.C.: U.S. Government Printing Office, 1969)

Corwin, E. H. L., *The American Hospital* (New York: The Commonwealth Fund, 1946)

Coser, Rose L., *Life in the Ward* (New York: Atheneum, 1964)

Coste, Pierre, *The Life and Works of Saint Vincent de Paul,* 3 vols. (London: Oates and Washbourne, 1934)

Cowan, Cordelia, *The Yearbook of Modern Nursing* (New York: G. P. Putnam's Sons, 1956 and 1958)

Creelman, Lyle; Chagas, Agnes; Arnold, Virginia, "WHO and Professional Nursing," *American Journal of Nursing* 54 (1954), pp. 448–449, and *The First Ten Years of WHO* (Geneva: 1958)

Crosby, Alfred W., *Epidemic and Peace, 1918* (Westport, Connecticut: Greenwood Press, 1976)

Crummer, Kenneth T., "Men Nurses—A Survey of the Present-Day Situation of Graduate Men Nurses," *American Journal of Nursing* 28 (1928), p. 467

Cumming, Kate, *Kate: The Journal of a Confederate Nurse,* edited by Richard Barksdale Harwell (Baton Rouge: Louisiana State University, 1959)

Cunningham, Elizabeth V., "Education for Leadership in Nursing 1899–1959," *Nursing Outlook,* May 7, 1959, pp. 268–272

Cunningham, H. H. *Doctors in Gray* (Baton Rouge: Louisiana State University, 1958)

Current Work in the History of Medicine: An International Bibliography (London: Wellcome Historical Medical Library, published quarterly)

A Curriculum for Schools of Nursing (New York: NLNE, 1927)

A Curriculum Guide for Schools of Nursing (New York: NLNE, 1937)

Curtis, John Shelton, "Russian Nightingale," *American Journal of Nursing* 68 (1968), pp. 1029–1031

Curtis, John Shelton, "Russian Sisters of Mercy in the Crimea, 1854–1855," *Slavic Review* XXV (March, 1966), pp. 84–100

Curtis, Mrs., and Denny, Miss, "Early History of the Boston Training School," *American Journal of Nursing* 2 (1902), pp. 331–335

Dannett, Sylvia G., *Noble Women of the North* (New York: Thomas Yoseloff, 1959)

Davis, Brenda L. H., "The Origin and Growth of Three Nursing Programs at Howard University, 1893–1973 (unpublished dissertation, Teachers College Columbia University, 1976)

Davis, Fred, "Problems and Issues in Collegiate Nursing Education," in *The Nursing Profession: Five Sociological Essays,* (New York: Wiley, 1966)

Davis, Graham Lee, "$33,000 Loss in 12 Hospitals Due to Nursing Schools," *Hospital Management* (August, 1931)

Davis, Michael M., *Clinics, Hospitals and Health Centers* (New York: Harper & Brothers, 1927)

Davis, Michael M., "The Meaning of the Hourly Nursing Experiment in Chicago," *American Journal of Nursing* 33 (1933), p. 111

D. E., *Recollections of a Nurse* (London and New York: Macmillan, 1889)

Deans, Agnes and Austin, Anne L., *The History of the Farrand Training School for Nurses* (Detroit: Alumnae Association of the Farrand School for Nurses, 1936)

Defoe, Daniel, *A Journal of the Plague Year* (many editions)

Delatte, Paul, *The Rule of Saint Benedict,* translated by Dom Justin McCann (Latrobe, Pennsylvania: The Archabbey Press, 1950)

Deming, Dorothy, *The Practical Nurse* (New York: The Commonwealth Fund, 1947)

Dent *v* West Virginia, *United States Reports: Cases Adjudged in the Supreme Court* 129 (1888), pp. 114–128

DeWitt, Katherine and Munson, Helen, "The Journal's First Fifty Years," *American Journal of Nursing* 50 (1950), pp. 590–595

Dickens, Charles, *The Life and Adventures of Martin Chuzzlewit* (many editions)

Dickerson, O. D., *Health Insurance* (Homewood, Illinois: Richard D. Irwin, Inc., 1959)

Didascalia Apostolorum, translated by Margaret Dunlop Gibson (London: Clay, 1903)

Didascalia, La, translated into French by F. Nau (Paris: P. Lethilleux, 1912)

Dietz, Lena Dixon, *History and Modern Nursing* (Philadelphia: F. A. Davis, 1963)

Dietz, Lena Dixon and Lehozky, Aurelia R., *History and Modern Nursing* (Philadelphia: F. A. Davis, 1967)

Dirvin, Joseph, *Mrs. Seton, Foundress of the American Sisters of Charity* (New York: Farrar, Straus & Cudahy, 1962)

Disselhoff, D., "The Deaconesses of Kaiserswerth: A Hundred Years' Work," *International Nursing Review,* I (1934), pp. 19–28

Dock, Lavinia L., "Affiliation of the American Red Cross with the Nurses' Association," *History of the American Red Cross Nursing,* pp. 67–139

Dock Lavinia L., "The Episode of the Spanish-American War," *History of the American Red Cross Nursing* (New York: Macmillan, 1922)

Dock, Lavinia L., "Self Portrait," *Nursing Outlook* 25 (January, 1977), pp. 23–26

Dock, Lavinia L., "Some Urgent Social Claims," *American Journal of Nursing* 7 (1907), p. 895

Dock, Lavinia L., "What We May Expect from the Law," *American Journal of Nursing* 1 (1900), pp. 8–12

Dock, Lavinia L. and Clement, Fannie F., "From Rural Nursing to the Public Health Service," in *History of the American Red Cross Nursing* (New York: Macmillan, 1922), pp. 1211–1292

Dock Lavinia L.; Pickett, Sarah; Noyes, Clara, *History of American Red Cross Nursing* (New York: Macmillan, 1922)

Dock, Lavinia L. and Stewart, Isabel M., *A Short History of Nursing* (New York: G. P. Putnam's Sons, 1920)

The Documents of the United States Sanitary Commission, 2 vols. (New York: 1871)

Dolan, Josephine, A., *Goodnow's History of Nursing* (Philadelphia: W. B. Saunders, 1963)

Dolan, Josephine A., "Nurses in American History: Three Schools—1873," *American Journal of Nursing* 75 (1975), pp. 989–992

Dolan, Josephine A., *Nursing in Society: A Historical Perspective,* 13th edition (Philadelphia: W. B. Saunders, 1973)

Downey, Gregg W., "Healthcare Planning Gets Muscles," *Modern Health Care* 3 (March, 1975), pp. 32–37

Dublin, Louis I. and Lotka, Alfred J., *Twenty-five Years of Health Progress* (New York: Metropolitan Life Insurance Company, 1937)

Duffus, R. L., *Lillian Wald, Neighbor and Crusader* (New York: Macmillan, 1938)

Duffy, John, *The Healers: The Rise of the Medical Establishment* (New York: McGraw-Hill, 1976)

Duke University, *Physician's Assistant Program, Duke University Bulletin,* 1969-1970, pp. 1-4

Dulles, Foster Rhea, *The American Red Cross: A History* (New York: Harper, 1950)

Dunant, Henri, *A Memory of Solferino* (Washington, D.C.: American National Red Cross, 1939)

Dunham, A. Warren, *Community and Schizophrenia: An Epidemiological Analysis* (Detroit: Wayne State University, 1965)

Easton, Burton Scott, *The Apostolic Tradition of Hippolytus,* translated into English by Burton Scott Easton (Cambridge: Cambridge University, 1934)

Ebers Papyrus, edited and translated by Bendix Ebbel (London: H. Milford, Oxford University, 1937)

The Economic Status of Registered Professional Nurses, 1946-47, Bulletin 931, Department of Labor, Bureau of Labor Statistics (Washington, D.C.: U.S. Government Printing Office, 1947)

E. D., *Recollections of a Nurse* (London: Macmillan, 1889)

Edelstein, Emma J. and Ludwig, *Asclepius,* 2 vols. (Baltimore: Johns Hopkins, 1945)

Edelstein, Ludwig, *The Hippocratic Oath* (Baltimore: Johns Hopkins, 1943)

"Editorial" *American Journal of Nursing* 39 (1939), pp. 275-277

Edmonds, S. Emma E., *Nurse and Spy in the Union Army* (Hartford: W. S. Williams, 1865)

"Educational Preparation for Nursing—1975," *Nursing Outlook* 24 (September, 1976), pp. 568-573

Edwin Smith Surgical Papyrus, edited and translated by J. H. Breasted, 2 vols. (Chicago: University of Chicago, 1930)

Emanuel, Cyprian W., *The Charities of St. Vincent de Paul* (Ph.D. dissertation, Washington, D.C., Catholic University of America, 1923)

"Employment Conditions for Registered Nurses" (editorial), *American Journal of Nursing* 46 (1946), pp. 437-438

"Executive Board Initiates Child Health Manpower Training Program in a Major Effort to Improve Pediatric Care," *Newsletter, American Academy of Pediatrics* 20 (July 1, 1969), pp. 1, 4

"The Expanded Role of the Nurse: A Joint Statement of CNA/CMA," *Canadian Nurse* (May, 1973), pp. 23-25

Expansion of Medical Education, Report of the Committee on Medical Education to the Australian Universities Commission, Peter Karmel, Chairman, 1973

Faber, Knud, *Nosography in Modern Internal Medicine* (New York: P. B. Hoeber, Inc., 1923); and *Nosography, the Evolution of Clinical Medicine in Modern Times* (New York: Hoeber, 1930)

Facts About Nursing (New York: American Nurses' Association, 1938, 1942, 1946, 1951, 1961, 1967, 1970-1971)

Facts About Nursing, 72-73 (Kansas City: American Nurses' Association, 1974)

Faddis, Margene O., *A School of Nursing Comes of Age: A History of the Frances Payne Bolton School of Nursing, Case Western University* (Cleveland: Alumnae of the Frances Payne Bolton School of Nursing, 1973)

Franklin, Alfred, *La Vie Privée D'Autrefois: Variétés Chirurgicales* (Paris: Librarie Plon, 1894)

Framborough, Florence, *Nurse at the Russian Front, A Diary 1914-1918* (London: Constable, 1974)

Federal Security Agency, *Practical Nursing* (Washington, D.C.: 1947)

Field, Mark G., *Soviet Socialized Medicine: An Introduction* (New York: Free Press, 1967)

Fife, Gertrude L., "The Nurse as Anesthetist," *American Journal of Nursing* 47 (1947), p. 308

Fishbein, Morris, *A History of the American Medical Association, 1847-1947* (Philadelphia: W. B. Saunders, 1947)

Fitzpatrick, M. Louise, *National Organization for Public Health Nursing 1912-1952: Development of a Practice Field* (New York: National League for Nursing, 1975)

Fitzpatrick, M. Louise, "Nurses in American History: Nursing and the Great Depression," *American Journal of Nursing* 75 (1975), pp. 2188-2190

Fitzpatrick, M. Louise, "Nursing," *Signs* 2 (Summer 1977), pp. 818-834

Flanagan, Lydia, *One Strong Voice: The Story of the American Nurses' Association* (The American Nurses' Association, 1976)

Flexner, Abraham, *Medical Education in the United States and Canada* (New York: Carnegie Foundation for Advancement of Teaching, 1910)

Flexner, Eleanor, *Century of Struggle: The Women's Rights Movement in the United States* (Cambridge: Harvard University, 1959)

Fliedner, *Life of Pastor Fliedner of Kaiserswerth*, translated from the German by Catherine Winkworth (London: Longmans, Green, 1867), *Kurzer Abriss seines Lebens* (Kaiserswerth: 1859)

Flikke, Julia O., *Nurses in Action* (Philadelphia: J. B. Lippincott, 1943)

Fogotson, Edward H.; Roemer, Ruth J.; Newman, Roger W., "Legal Regulation of Health Personnel in the United States," *Report of the National Advisory Commission on Health Manpower*, Vol. 2 (Washington, D.C.: U.S. Government Printing Office, 1967), pp. 416-418

Fogotson, Edward H.; Roemer, Ruth J.; Newman, Roger W.; Cook, John L., *Report of the National Advisory Commission on Health Manpower*, Vol. 2 (Washington, D.C.: U.S. Government Printing Office, 1967), pp. 407-492

Forman, A. M. and Cooper, E. M., "Legislation and Nurse-Midwifery Practice in USA," *Journal of Nurse-Midwifery,* American College of Nurse-Midwives, Washington, D.C., Vol. 21, No. 2, Summer 1976

Fort, George F., *Medical Economy During the Middle Ages* (New York: J. W. Bouton, 1883)

Fosdick, Raymond B., *The Story of the Rockefeller Foundation* (New York: Harper, 1952)

Foster, William Derek, *A History of Parasitology* (Baltimore: Williams & Wilkins Co., 1965)

Fox, Elizabeth G., "Red Cross Public Health Nursing After the War," in *History of American Red Cross Nursing* (New York: Macmillan, 1922), pp. 1293-1351

Frank, Sister Charles Marie, *The Historical Development of Nursing* (Philadelphia: W. B. Saunders, 1953)

Freeman, Howard E.; Levine, Sol; Reeder, Leo G., *Handbook of Medical Sociology* (Englewood Cliffs, N.J.: Prentice Hall, 1963)

Freeman, Howard E. and Simmons, Ozzie G., *The Mental Patient Comes Home* (New York: John Wiley, 1963)

Freidson, Eliot, *The Hospital in Modern Society* (New York: The Free Press of Glencoe, 1963)

Fry, *Memoirs of the Life of Elizabeth Fry: Life and Labors of the Eminent Philanthropist, Preacher, and Prison Reformer,* published by Edward Ryder (New York: E. Walker's Sons, 1884), *Memoirs of the Life of Elizabeth Fry,* edited by Katherine Fry and R. E. Cresswell (London: J. Hatchard, 1848)

Fuller, Thomas, *Exantematologia: or, An Attempt to Give a Rational Account of Eruptive Fevers, especially in the Small Pox* (London: Charles Rivington and Stephen Austen, 1730)

Fulmer, Harriet, "History of Visting Nurse Work in America," *American Journal of Nursing* (1902), p. 411

Fulton, J. F., *Physiology* (New York: Hoeber, 1931)

Galen, *Hygiene,* translated by Robert M. Green (Springfield, Illinois: Charles C. Thomas, 1951)

Galen, *On Anatomical Procedures,* translated by Charles Singer (Oxford: Oxford University Press, 1956)

Galen, *On the Natural Faculties,* edited and translated by Arthur John Brock (London: William Heinemann, 1963)

Gallison, Marie, *The Ministry of Women: 100 Years of Women's Work at Kaiserswerth 1836-1936* (London: Lutterworth Press, 1936)

Gardner, Mary S., *Public Health Nursing,* 3rd edition (New York: Macmillan, 1945)

Garrison, F. H., *Introduction to the History of Medicine* (Philadelphia: W. B. Saunders, 1929)

Garrison, F. H. and Morton, L. T., *A Medical Bibliography: A Check-List of Text Illustrating the History of Medical Sciences* (London: Grafton, 1943)

Gask, G. E. and Todd, J., "The Origins of Hospitals," in *Science, Medicine and History,* edited by E. A. Underwood, 2 vols. (Oxford: Oxford University, 1953)

Gately, Sister M. J., *The Sisters of Mercy* (New York: Macmillan, 1931)

Geister, Janet M., "Hearsay and Facts in Private Duty," *American Journal of Nursing* 26 (1926), pp. 515-528

Georgopoulas, Basil S. and Christman, Luther, "The Clinical Nurse Specialist: A Role Model," in *The Clinical Nurse Specialist; Interpretations,* edited by Riehl and McVay (New York: Appleton-Century-Crofts, 1973)

Ghalioungui, Paul, *Magic and Medical Science in Ancient Egypt* (London: Hodder and Stoughton, 1963)

Gibson, John Murray and Mathewson, Mary S., *Three Centuries of Canadian Nursing* (Toronto: Macmillan, 1947)

Gilpin, Fanny, *Scenes from Hospital Life* (London: Drane's, n.d.)

Goffman, Erving, *Asylums* (Garden City, New York: Anchor Books, 1961)

Gooch, Robert, "*Protestant Sisters of Charity,*" *Blackwood's Edinburgh Magazine* (November 1825), pp. 732-735; *The London Medical Gazette,* 1 (1827), pp. 55-58

Good, Harry G., *A History of American Education* (New York: Macmillan, 1956); *A History of Western Education* (New York: Macmillan, 1950)

Goodnow, Minnie, *Nursing History,* revised by Josephine A. Dolan as *Goodnow's History of Nursing* (Philadelphia: W. B. Saunders, 1963)

Goodrich, Annie W., "The Plan for the Army School of Nursing," *Twenty-fifth Annual Report of the National League of Nursing Education* (1918), p. 171

Gordon, Benjamin Lee, *Medieval and Renaissance Medicine* (New York: Philosophical Library, 1959)

Gordon, Maurice B., *Aesculapius Comes to the Colonies* (Ventor, New Jersey: Ventor Publications, 1949)

Gortner, Susan R., "Research in Nursing: The Federal Interest and Grant Program," *American Journal of Nursing* 73 (1973), pp. 1052–1055

Gowan, Sister M. Olivia, editor, *The Nursing Program in the General College* (Washington, D.C.: The Catholic University of America, 1954)

Gowan, Sister M. Olivia and Sheehy, Sister M. Maurice, "Contribution of Religious Communities to Nursing Education," *Trained Nurse and Hospital Review* (1938), Vol. 100, pp. 404–409, 652–655, 700

Gray, James, *Education for Nursing: History of the University of Minnesota School of Nursing* (Minneapolis: University of Minnesota, 1960)

Great Days in New Zealand Nursing (London: George G. Harrap, 1961)

Greenbie, Marjorie Barstow, *Lincoln's Daughters of Mercy* (New York: G. P. Putnam's Sons, 1944)

Griffin, Gerald Joseph and Griffin, Joanne King, *History and Trends of Professional Nursing* (St. Louis: C. V. Mosby, 1973)

Grissum, Marlene and Spengler, Carol, *Womanpower and Health Care* (Boston: Little, Brown, 1976)

Gross, D., *Autobiography of Samuel D. Gross* (Philadelphia: G. Barrie, 1887)

Gumpert, Martin, *Dunant: The Story of the Red Cross* (New York: Oxford University, 1938)

Halsted, W. S., "Ligature and Suture Material," *Journal of the American Medical Association* 60 (May 13, 1913), p. 1123

Hamilton, Anna Emile, *Les gardes malades congréganistes, mercenaires, professionelles, amateurs* (Paris: Vigot, 1901)

Handbook on the Structure of National Nursing Organizations, published by the Committee on the Structure of National Nursing Organizations (New York: 1949)

Harley, G. W., *Native African Medicine* (Cambridge, Massachusetts: Harvard University, 1941)

Hartog, Jan de, *The Hospital* (New York: Atheneum, 1964)

Hassenplug, Lulu Wolf, "Nursing Education in Universities," *Nursing Outlook* 8 (1960), pp. 92–95, 154–155

Hassenplug, Lulu Wolf, "Preparation of the Nurse Practitioner," *Journal of Nursing Education* 4 (January, 1965), pp. 29–42

Hays, Elinor Rice, *Those Extraordinary Blackwells* (New York: Harcourt, Brace and World, 1967)

Heberding, G. H., *Life and Letters of W. A. Passavant,* 3rd edition (Greenville, Pennsylvania: Young Lutheran Company, 1906)

Henry, Frederick P., *Standard History of the Medical Profession in Philadelphia* (Chicago: Goodspeed Brothers, 1897)

Hentsch, Yvonne, "Influence of the Red Cross on Professional Nursing," *Information Bulletin for Red Cross Nurses* (Geneva: May-August 1947)

Herodotus, *History,* edited and translated by A. D. Godley, 4 vols. (London: William Heinemann, 1920–1924)

Hershey, Nathan, "Legal Issues in Nursing Practice," in *Professional Nursing: Foundations, Perspectives and Relationships,* edited by Eugenia K. Spalding and Lucile E. Notter (Philadelphia: J. B. Lippincott, 1970), pp. 110–127

Herskovits, Melville J., *Dahomey, an Ancient West African Kingdom* (New York: J. J. Augustin, 1938)

Hertzler, Arthur E., *The Horse and Buggy Doctor* (New York: Hoeber, 1938)

Hibbard, Eugenie, "The Establishment of Schools for Nurses in Cuba," *American Journal of Nursing* 2 (1902), p. 985

Hintz, Anne A., "The Probationary Term," in Jane Hodson, *How To Become A Trained Nurse* (New York: William Abbatt, 1898), pp. 15–19

Hintz, Anne A., "The Training Term," in Jane Hodson, *How To Become A Trained Nurse* (New York: William Abbatt, 1898), pp. 20–24

Hippocrates, Loeb Classical Library Edition, translated and edited by W. H. S. Jones and E. T. Withington, 4 vols. (London: William Heinemann, 1939–1948)

A History of American Life, edited by A. M. Schlesinger and D. R. Fox, 12 vols. (New York: Macmillan, 1929–1944)

Hobson, Elizabeth Cristophers, *Founding of of the Bellevue Training School for Nurses* (New York: G. P. Putnam's Sons, 1916) reprinted in *A Century of Nursing* (New York: G. P. Putnam's Sons, 1950)

Hodson, Jane, *How To Become A Trained Nurse* (New York: William Abbatt, 1898)

Hoehling, A. A., *The Great Epidemic* (Boston: Little, Brown, 1961)

Hoehling, A. A., *A Whisper of Eternity: The Mystery of Edith Cavell* (New York: Thomas Yoseloff, 1957)

Hole, Christina, *The English Housewife in the Seventeenth Century* (London: Chatto & Windus, 1953)

Holland, Mary A. Gardiner, *Our Army Nurses* (Boston: B. Wilkins & Company, 1895)

Hospital Services in the U.S.S.R. (Washington D.C.: U.S. Department of Health, Education, and Welfare, 1966)

Howard, John, *An Account of the Principal Lazarettoes in Europe: with Various Papers Relative to the Plague, Together with Further Observations on some Foreign Prisons and Hospitals, and Additional Remarjs on the Present State of those in Great Britain and Ireland* (Warrington: Printed by William Eyres, 1789)

Hughes, Everett C.; Hughes, Helen MacGill, and Deutscher, Irwin, *Twenty Thousand Nurses Tell Their Story* (Philadelphia: J. B. Lippincott, 1958)

Hughes, Muriel Joy, *Women Healers in Medieval Life and Literature* (New York: King's Crown Press, 1943)

Hughes, Sister Marie Jeanne d'Arc, *Crimean Diary of Mother M. Francis Bridgman* (doctoral dissertation, available at The Catholic University of America)

Human Relations Area Files

Hume, Edgar Erskine, *Medical Work of the Knights Hospitallers of Saint John of Jerusalem* (Baltimore: Johns Hopkins, 1940)

Hume, Edward H., *Doctors Courageous* (New York: Harper & Brothers, 1950)

Hurd-Mead, Kate Campbell, *A History of Women in Medicine* (Haddam, Connecticut: Haddam Press, 1938)

Hurd-Mead, Kate Campbell, *Medical Women of America* (New York: Froben Press, 1933)

"The ICN and Nursing Education," *American Journal of Nursing* 50 (1950), p. 385

ICN Statement of Nursing Education, Nsrsing Practice and Service and the Social and Econooic Welfare of Nurses," *American Journal of Nursing* 69 (1969), pp. 2177–2179

Idaho Code, Section 54-1413

Idaho State Board of Nursing and Idaho State Board of Medicine, *Minimum Standard, Rules and Regulations for Nurse Practitioners (Expanding Role) and Guidelines for Nurses Writing Prescriptions*

"ILO/WHO Group Draws Up Instrument on Personnel Practices recommended for Adoption for Nurses Worldwide," *American Journal of Nursing* 74 (1974), p. 189

Imbert, Jean, *Les Hôpitaux en Droit Canonique* (Paris: J. Vrin, 1947)

Index-Catalogue of the Library of the Surgeon-General's Office, United States Army (Washington, D.C.: since 1880)

"Infirmier," in *Encyclopédie où Dictionnaire des Sciences, des Arts et des Metiers*, ed. Denis Diderot, 17 vols. (Paris; Briasson et al., 1751-1765), VIII, pp. 707–708

Ingles, Thelma, "The University Medical Center as a Setting for Nursing Education," *The Journal of Medical Education* 37 (1962), pp. 411–420

Instruction pour les fraters et les infirmiers de l'armeé Fédérale (Berne: Haller, 1862)

International Council of Nurses, *Constitution and Regulations International Director of Nurses with Doctoral Degrees* (New York: American Nurses Foundation, 1973)

Ireland, *Acts and Statutes Made in Parliament*, Dublin, 1716

ISR Newsletter, Institute for Social Research, The University of Michigan, Summer 1977, p. 8

Jaco, E. Gartly, *Patients, Physicians and Illness* (Glencoe, Illinois: The Free Press of Glencoe, 1958)

Jacox, Ada, "Collective Action and Control of Practice by Professionals," *Nursing Forum* 10 No. 3 (1971), pp. 239–257

Jameson, E., *Gynecology and Obstetrics* (New York: Hafner, 1962)

Jamieson, Elizabeth and Sewell, Mary, *Trends in Nursing History* (Philadelphia: W. B. Saunders, 1944). Other editions

Jamieson, Elizabeth; Sewell, Mary, and Suhrie, Eleanor, *Trends in Nursing History* (Philadelphia: W. B. Saunders, 1966)

Jamme, Anne C., "The California Eight-Hour Law for Women," *American Journal of Nursing* 19 (1919), pp. 525–530

Jay, Walter Addison, *The Healing Gods of Ancient Civilization* (New Haven: Yale University, 1925)

Jensen, Deborah MacLurg, *History and Trends of Professional Nursing*, revised by Gerald J. and H. Joanne King Griffin under the title of *Jensen's History and Trends of Professional Nursing* (St. Louis: C. V. Mosby, 1965)

Jerome (Hieronymus) St., *Select Letters of St. Jerome*, edited and translated by F. A. Wright (London: William Heinemann, 1933)

John of Wurzburg, "Description of the Holy Land," translated by Aubrey Stewart in *Palestine Pilgrim's Text Society* (London: 1896), Vol. V

Johns, Ethel and Pfefferkorn, Blanche, *The Johns Hopkins Hospital School of Nursing 1889-1949* (Baltimore: Johns Hopkins, 1954)

Johnson, Dorothy, "Competence in Practice: Technical and Professional," *Nursing Outlook* 14 (October 1966), pp. 30–33

Johnson, Dorothy, "The Nature of the Science of Nursing," *Nursing Outlook* 7 (1959), pp. 291–294

Johnson, Dorothy, "A Philosophy of Nursing" *Nursing Outlook* 7 (1959), pp. 198-200

Johnson, Walter L., "Educational Preparation for Nursing—1974," *Nursing Outlook* 23 (September, 1974), pp. 78–82

Johnson, Walter L., "Educational Preparation for Nursing," *Nursing Outlook* 24 (September, 1975), pp. 568–577

Johnston, Dorothy F., *History and Trends of Practical Nursing* (St. Louis: C. V. Mosby, 1966)

Jones, Agnes Elizabeth, "Una and Her Paupers," *Memorials of Agnes Elizabeth Jones* by her sister (New York: Routledge, 1872)

Jones, Cadwalader, Mrs., "Looking Back Through Fifty Years," *The Alumnae Journal of New York City Hospital School of Nursing,* Golden Anniversary Number, 1875–1925 (July, 1925), p. 11

Jones, Katharine M., *Heroines of Dixie* (Indianapolis: Bobbs-Merrill, 1955)

Jones, Maxwell, *The Therapeutic Community* (New York: Basic Books, 1953)

Jordon, Helen Jamieson, *Cornell University—New York Hospital School of Nursing 1877–1952* (New York: New York Hospital, 1952)

"Journal's Attitude on the Suffrage Question," *American Journal of Nursing* 8 (1908), pp. 956–957

Jude, James W.; Kouwenhoven, W. B.; Knickerbocker, G. Guy, "Cardiac Resuscitation Without Thoracotomy," *Maryland State Medical Journal* 9 (1960), pp. 712–713

Kalish, Beatrice J. and Kalish, Philip A., "Nurses in American History: The Cadet Nurse Corps—In World War II," *American Journal of Nursing* 76 (1976), pp. 240–242

Kalish, Philip A. and Kalish, Beatrice J., *The Advance of American Nursing* (Boston: Little, Brown, 1978)

Kaufman, Martin, "The Admission of Women to 19th-Century American Medical Societies," *Bulletin of the History of Medicine* (1976)

Keeler, Floyd, *Catholic Medical Missions* (New York: Macmillan, 1925)

Keller, Malvina W., *History of the St. Luke's Hospital Training School for Nurses* (New York: St. Luke's Hospital, 1938)

Kellogg, Florence Shaw, *Mother Bickerdyke* (Chicago: United Publishing, 1907)

Kelly, Lucie Young, *Dimensions of Professional Nursing,* 3rd ed. (New York: Macmillan, 1975)

Kennedy, Donald Gilbert, *Field Notes on the Culture of Vaitupu* (Memoirs of the Polynesian Society, Vol. IX, New Plymouth, N.Z.: Thomas Avery & Sons, 1931)

Kernodle, Portia B., *The Red Cross Nurse in Action, 1882–1948* (New York: Harper & Brothers, 1949)

Kerr, Margaret E., "Fifty Years Young," *American Journal of Nursing* 55 (1955), p. 302

Keys, Thomas E., *The History of Surgical Anesthesia* (New York: Schuman, 1945)

King-Hall, Magdalen, *The Story of the Nursery* (London: Routledge and Kegan Paul, 1958)

King, Lester S., *The Medical World of the Eighteenth Century* (Chicago: University of Chicago, 1958)

Kleingartner, Archie, "Nurses, Collective Bargaining and Labor Legislation," *Labor Law Journal* 18 (April, 1967), pp. 236–245

Kobrin, Frances E., "The American Midwife Controversy: A Crisis of Professionalization," *Bulletin of the History of Medicine* XL (1966), pp. 350–363

Koch, Harriet Berger, *Militant Angel: Annie W. Goodrich* (New York: Macmillan, 1951)

Korson, George, *At His Side: The Story of the American Red Cross Overseas in World War II* (New York: Coward-McCann, 1945)

Kouwenhoven, William B.; Jude, James R.; Knickerbocker, G. Guy, "Closed Chest Cardiac Massage," *Journal of the American Medical Association* 173 (1960), pp. 1064–1067

Kouwenhoven, William B.; Jude, James R.; Knickerbocker, G. Guy, "Heart Activation in Cardiac Arrest," *Modern Concepts in Cardio-vascular Diseases* 30 (1961), pp. 639–643

Kramer, Marlene, *Reality Shock: Why Nurses Leave Nursing* (St. Louis: C. V. Mosby, 1974)

Kreuter, Frances R., "What is Good Nursing Care?" *Nursing Outlook* 5 (1957), pp. 302–304

Krumbhaar, E. B., *Pathology* (New York: Hafner, 1962)

"Lady Nurses," *Godey's Lady's Book and Magazine,* LXXXII, (1871), pp. 188–189, reprinted in Austin, *Source Book,* pp. 431–432

Lallemand, Leon, *Histoire de la Charité,* 4 vols. (Paris: Alphonse Picard et Fils, 1902–1912)

Lamb, Albert R., *The Presbyterian Hospital and the Columbia-Presbyterian Medical Center 1868–1943* (New York: Columbia University, 1955)

Lambertsen, Eleanor, *Nursing Team Organization and Functioning* (New York: Teachers College, 1953)

Lanfranc, *Science of Cirurgie,* edited by Robert von Fleishhacker (London: Early English Text Society, 1894)

Latourette, K. S., *A History of the Expansion of Christianity,* especially Volume I (New York; London: Harper & Bros., 1937)

Lecky, William E. H., *History of European Morals* (London: Longmans, Green, 1869)

Lee, Eleanor, *Neighbors 1892–1967: A History of the Department of Nursing, Faculty of Medicine, Columbia University 1937–1967 and its Predecessor, the School of Nursing of the Presbyterian Hospital New York, 1892–1937* (New York: Columbia University, Presbyterian Hospital School of Nursing Alumnae Association, 1967)

Lees, Florence S., *Handbook for Hospital Sisters* (London: W. Isbister & Co., 1874)

Lenburg, Carrie B.; Johnson, Walter, and Vahey, JoAnn T., *Directory of Career Opportunities in Nursing* (New York: National League for Nursing, 1973)

Leone, Lucile Petry, "Trends and Problems in Practical Nurse Education," *American Journal of Nursing* 56 (1956), pp. 51–53

Lesnik, Milton J., and Anderson, Bernice E., *Legal Aspects of Nursing* (Philadelphia: J. B. Lippincott, 1947)

Letters of Abelard and Heloise, Letter VII, Abelard to Heloise, translated by Betty Radice (Hammondsworth, England: Penguin, 1974)

Lewis, Edith P., "The New York City Hospital Story," *American Journal of Nursing* 66 (1966), pp. 1526–1533

Lewis, W. H., *The Splendid Century* (London: Eyre and Spottiswoode, 1953)

Liddon, H. P., *Life of Edward Bouverie Pusey,* 4 vols., 4th edition (London: Longmans, Green, 1894–1897), III, chap. I, "The Early Days of Anglican Sisterhoods"

Lippman, Helen Byrne, "The Future of the Red Cross Volunteer Nurses," Nurses' Aid Corps, *American Journal of Nursing* 45 (1945), pp. 811–812

Livermore, Mary A., *My Story of the War: A Woman's Narrative of Four Years Personal Experience as Nurse* (Hartford, Connecticut: A. D. Worthington and Company, 1889)

Livy, *History,* edited and translated by B. O. Foster *et al.,* 13 vols. (London: William Heinemann, 1919–1951)

Loftus, Maria D. Andrea, *A History of St. Vincent's Hospital School of Nursing, Indianapolis, Indiana: 1806–1970* (Indianapolis: Litho Press, 1972)

Long, Esmond R., *A History of Pathology* (Baltimore: Williams & Wilkins, 1928)

Long, Esmond R., (ed.), *Selected Readings in Pathology* (Springfield, Illinois: Charles C. Thomas, 1929)

Longfellow, Henry Wadsworth, *The Complete Poetical Works of Longfellow* (Boston: Houghton-Mifflin, 1922)

Longway, Ina Madge, "Curriculum Concepts: A Historical Analysis," *Nursing Outlook* 20 (February, 1972), pp. 116–120

Lonsdale, Margaret, *Sister Dora: A Biography* (London: Kegan Paul, 1880)

Lown, Bernard; Amarasingham, Raghaven; Berkovits, Barouk V., "New Method of Terminating Cardiac Arrhythmias: Use of Synchronized Capacitor Discharge," *Journal of the American Medical Association* 182 (1962), pp. 548–555

Lückes, Eva C. E., *Hospital Sisters and Their Duties* (London: Scientific Press, 1893)

Lusk, Graham, *Nutrition* (New York: Hafner, 1964)

"L.V.N. Group Asks More Pay, Rescinds No Strike Policy," *Hospitals* 43 (November 16, 1969), p. 107

Lysaught, Jerome P., *Action in Nursing: Progress in Professional Purpose* (New York: McGraw Hill, 1974)

MacDonald, Gwendoline, *Development of Standards and Accreditation in Collegiate Nursing Education* (New York: Teachers College, 1965)

McKinney, Loren C., Early Medieval Medicine (Baltimore: Johns Hopkins, 1937)

MacManus, Emily E. P., *Matron of Guy's* (London: Andrew Melrose, 1956)

Magaw, Alice, "A Review of Over 14,000 Surgical Anesthetics," *Surgery, Gynecology, and Obstetrics* 3 (1906), pp. 79t–799

Magic, Faith and Healing: Studies in Primitive Psychiatry Today, edited by Ari Kiev (New York: The Free Press of Glencoe, 1964)

Major, R. H., *Classic Description of Disease,* 3rd edition (Springfield, Illinois: Charles C. Thomas, 1945)

Manual of Essentials of Good Hospital Nursing (American Hospital Association and National League of Nursing Education, 1926)

Manual of Essentials of Good Hospital Nursing Service, issued by the American Hospital Association and the NLNE in 1936. Several revisions.

Markolf, Ada Stewart, "Industrial Nursing Begins in Vermont," *Public Health Nursing* 37 (1945), p. 125

Marks, Geoffrey, *The Medieval Plague* (Garden City, New York: Doubleday, 1971)

Marram, Gwen D.; Schlegel, M. W., and Bevis, E. O., *Primary Nursing: A Model for Individualized Care* (St. Louis: C. V. Mosby, 1974)

Marshall, Helen E., *Dorothea Dix* (Chapel Hill: University of North Carolina, 1937)

Marshall, Helen E., *Mary Adelaide Nutting: Pioneer of Modern Nursing* (Baltimore: Johns Hopkins, 1972)

Martel, Gabrielle D., and Edmunds, Marilyn Winterton, "Nurse-Internship in Chicago," *American Journal of Nursing* 72 (1972), pp. 940-943

Martial, Marcus Valerius, *Epigrams,* edited and translated by Walter C. A. Ker (London: William Heinemann, 1925)

Massey, Mary Elizabeth, *Bonnet Brigade* (New York: Alfred A. Knopf, 1966)

Matarazzo, Joseph D., "Perspective," in *Future Directions of Doctoral Education for Nurses,* Report of a Conference, Bethesda, Maryland, January 20, 1971, pp. 64-67

Maternity Center Association, *Twenty Years of Nurse Midwifery* (New York: The Maternity Center Association, 1953)

Mauksch, Hans, "Nursing Dilemma in the Organization of Patient Care," *Nursing Outlook* 5 (1957), pp. 31-33

Mauksch, Ingeborg, "How Did It Come To Pass," *Nursing Forum* 10 (1917), pp. 258-272

Maxson, Edwin R., *Hospitals: British, French, and American* (Philadelphia: privately printed, 1868)

Maxwell, William Quentin, *Lincoln's Fifth Wheel: The Political History of the United States Sanitary Commission* (New York: Longmans, Green, 1956)

May, Mary Elizabeth, "Nurse Training Schools of the New York State Hospitals," *American Journal of Nursing* 8 (1907), p. 18

Mayo, Charles H., "Do You Covet Distinction," *American Journal of Nursing* 22 (1922), p. 251

Mayo, Charles H., "Wanted—100,000 Girls for Sub-Nurses: An Answer to the Nursing Problem," *Pictorial Review* (October 1921), pp. 15, 82 reprinted in *New Directions for Nurses,* edited by Bonnie and Vern Bullough (New York: Springer, 1971), pp. 87-94

McDonald, Gwendoline, *Development of Standards and Accreditation in Collegiate Nursing Education* (New York: Teachers College, 1965)

McGivern, Diane, "Baccalaureate Preparation of the Nurse Practitioner," *Nursing Outlook* 22 (February 1974), pp. 94-98

McGrath, Bethel J., *Nursing in Commerce and Industry* (New York: The Commonwealth Fund, 1946)

McIver, Pearl, "Nursing Moves Forward," *American Journal of Nursing* 52 (1952), pp. 821-823

McIver, Pearl, "Public Health Nursing in the United States Public Health Service," *American Journal of Nursing* 40 (1940), pp. 996-1000

McKenzie, Dan, *The Infancy of Medicine* (London: Macmillan, 1927)

Mead, Kate Campbell Hurd, *A History of Women in Medicine* (Haddam, Connecticut: Haddam Press, 1938)

"Medical Education in the United States," *Journal of the American Medical Association* 79 (1922), pp. 629-633

Meltzer, L., and Roderick, J., "The Development and Current Status of Coronary Care," in L. Meltzer and A. Dunning, editors, *Intensive Coronary Care* (Philadelphia: Charles Press, 1970)

Merrill, Bertha Estelle, *The Trek from Yesterday—A History of Organized Nursing in Minneapolis, 1883-1936* (Minneapolis: Nurses' Association, 1944)

Mettler, Cecelia C., *History of Medicine* (Philadelphia: Blakiston, 1947)

Meyer, Burton, and Heidgerken, Loretta, *Introduction to Research in Nursing* (Philadelphia: J. B. Lippincott, 1962)

Miller, Jon D., and Shortell, Stephen M., "Hospital Unionization: A Study of Trends," Hospitals 43 (August 16, 1969), pp. 67-72

"Miss Nutting's Report," *American Journal of Nursing* 3 (1903), pp. 272-273

Mittman, Ben and Bumgarner, Beatrice, "What Happened in San Francisco," *American Journal of Nursing* 67 (1967), pp. 80-84

Molina, Teresa Maria, *Historia de la Enfermeria* (Buenos Aires, Argentina: Intermedica, 1973)

Mondeville, Henry de, *Chirurgie,* edited by E. Nicaise (Paris: Felix Alcan, 1893)

Moniteur Universel, February 7, 1808

Montag, Mildred, *Community College Education* (New York: Blakiston, McGraw-Hill, 1959)

Montag, Mildred, *The Education of Nursing Technicians* (New York: G. P. Putnam's Sons, 1951)

Montag, Mildred, *Evaluation of Graduates of Associate Degree Nursing Programs* (New York: Teachers College, 1972)

Montag, Mildred, and Gotkin, Lassar G., *Community College Education for Nursing* (New York: McGraw-Hill, 1959)

Mooney, James, *The Swimmer Manuscript: Cherokee Sacred Formulas and Medicinal Prescriptions,* revised and edited by Frans M. Olbrechts (Smithsonian Institute, Bureau of American Ethnology, Bulletin No. 99, Washington, D.C., 1932)

Moore, Frank, *Women of the War: The Heroism and Self-sacrifice* (Hartford: S. S. Scranton, 1866)

Moore, Norman, *The History of St. Bartholomew's Hospital* 2 vols. (London: C. Arthur Pearson Ltd., 1918)

Morgan, D., "The Future Expanded Role of the Nurse," *Canadian Hospital* 75 (May, 1972)

Muller, J. E., "The Soviet Health System—Aspects of Relevance for Medicine in the United States," *New England Journal of Medicine* 286 (March 30, 1972), pp. 693-702

Mumey, Nolie, *Cap, Pin and Diploma; A History of the Colorado Training School* (Bolder, Colorado: Johnson, 1968)

Munroe, James Phinney, *Adventures of an Army Nurse in Two Wars,* edited from the diary and correspondence of Mary Phinney, Baroness von Olnhausen (Boston: Little, Brown, 1903)

Munson, Helen W., with Stevens, Katharine, *The Story of the National League of Nursing Education* (Philadelphia: W. B. Saunders, 1934)

Murphy, Denis G., *They Did Not Pass By: The Story of the Early Pioneers of Nursing* (London: Longmans, Green & Co., 1956)

Myers, Grace Whiting, *A History of the Massachusetts General Hospital, June 1872 to December 1900* (Boston: Griffith-Stilling Press, 1929)

Nahm, Helen, "The Accreditation Program in Nursing," in Sister M. Olivia Gowan, *The Nursing Program in the General College* (Washington, D.C.: The Catholic University of America, 1954)

Nash, Herbert J., "Men Nurses in New York State," *Trained Nurse and Hospital Review* (August, 1936), p. 123

National Center for Health Statistics, U.S. Department of Health, Education, and Welfare, *State Licensing of Health Occupations,* PHS Publication No. 1758 (Washington, D.C.: U.S. Government Printing Office, 1968), pp. 9–10

National Commission for the Study of Nursing and Nursing Education, Jerome P. Lysaught, Director, *An Abstract for Action* (New York: McGraw-Hill, 1970)

National Committee for the Improvement of Nursing Services, *Interim Classification of Schools of Nursing Offering Basic Programs* (New York: 1949)

National Committee for the Improvement of Nursing Services, *Nursing Schools at the Mid-Century* (New York: 1950)

National Health and Welfare, Ministry of, National Conference on the Assistance to the Physician, *The Complementary Roles of the Physician and the Nurse* (1972)

National League for Nursing, *Nurses for a Growing Nation* (New York: 1957)

National League of Nursing Education, *A Curriculum for Schools of Nursing* (New York: 1927)

National League of Nursing Education, *A Curriculum Guide for Schools of Nursing* (New York: 1937)

National League of Nursing Education, *Standard Curriculum for Schools of Nursing* (New York: 1917)

National Library of Medicine, *Bibliography of the History of Medicine* (an annual publication since 1964)

"The National Survey," *American Journal of Nursing* 41 (1941), pp. 929–930

Nelson, Josephine, *New Horizons in Nursing* (New York: Macmillan, 1950)

Neuberger, Max, *History of Medicine,* translated by Ernest Playfair (London: Oxford University, 1910)

New Catholic Encyclopedia (Washington, D.C.: The Catholic University of America, 1967)

Newell, Hope, *The History of the National Nursing Council* (New York: National Organization for Public Health Nursing, 1951)

"News Highlights," *American Journal of Nursing* 55 (1955), p. 1440

New York State Education Law, Title 8, Article 139, Section 6902

Nicene and Post Nicene Fathers, Series 2, XIV, reprinted (Grand Rapids, Michigan: Berdmans, 1956)

Nightingale, Florence, *The Institution of Kaiserswerth on the Rhine, for the Practical Training of Deaconesses* (London: Printed by the Inmates of the Ragged Colonial Training School, 1851)

Nightingale, Florence, *Notes on Nursing* (New York: D. Appleton, 1860; reissued, Philadelphia: J. B. Lippincott, 1946)

Nightingale, Florence, *On Trained Nursing for the Sick Poor* (London: Metropolitan and National Nursing Association, 1876)

Nightingale, Florence, "The Reform of Sick Nursing and the Late Mrs. Wardroper, The Extinction of Mrs. Gamp," *British Medical Journal* (December 31, 1892), p. 1448

Nightingale, Florence, *Subsidiary Notes as to the Introduction of Female Nursing into Military Hospitals in Peace and War* (London: Privately printed by Harrison and Sons, 1858)

The Nightingale Training School: St. Thomas' Hospital, 1860-1910, privately printed for the Nightingale Training School for Nurses, 1960

NLN, *Report on the Associate Degree Programs in Nursing* (New York: 1961)

Noonan, B., "Eight Years in a Medical Nurse Clinic," *American Journal of Nursing* 72 (1972), pp. 1128-1130

Norwood, W. F., *Medical Education in the U.S. Before the Civil War* (Philadelphia: University of Pennsylvania, 1944)

Notes et souvenirs, p. 312, in-folio Mss., 742, Archives, Religeuses Augustines hôspitalieres de l'Hôtel de Paris

"Notes from Headquarters, American Nurses Association," *American Journal of Nursing* 33 (1933), p. 1001

Notter, Lucille, editor, *Proceedings: Open Curriculum Conference I* (New York: National League for Nursing, 1974)

Noyes, Clara D., "Sub-Nurses? Why Not Sub-Doctors?" *Pictorial Review* (December, 1921), pp. 28, 79-80

The NRA and Nursing (New York: American Nurses' Association, 1933)

"Nurse Membership in Unions" (editorial), *American Journal of Nursing* 37 (1937), pp. 766-767

"The Nurses' Contribution to American Victory: Facts and Figures From Pearl Harbor to VJ Day," *American Journal of Nursing* 45 (1945), pp. 683-686

Nursing and Nursing Education in the United States, The Committee for the Study of Nursing Education (New York: Macmillan, 1923)

"Nursing Council on National Defense," *American Journal of Nursing* 40 (1940), p. 1013

Nursing Education of Teachers College, Department of, and the Committee on University Relations of the National League of Nursing Education, *Proceedings of Conference on Nursing Schools Connected with Colleges and Universities* (New York: National League of Nursing Education, 1928)

"Nursing in Canada: From Pioneering History to a Modern Federation," *International Nursing Review* 15 (1968), pp. 1-29

"Nursing Legislation, 1939: What the State Nurses' Association Accomplished," *American Journal of Nursing* 39 (1939), pp. 974-981

Nursing of the Sick, 1893, edited by Isabel A. Hampton, reprinted (New York: McGraw-Hill, 1949)

Nursing Schools at the Mid-Century, prepared by Margaret West and Christy Hawkins (New York: NCINS, 1950)

Nursing Schools, Committee on the Grading of, *Results of the First Grading Study of Nursing Schools* (New York: NLNE, 1930)

Nursing Schools, Committee on the Grading of, *Nursing Schools Today and Tomorrow* (New York: NLNE, 1934)

Nutting, M. Adelaide, *Educational Status of Nursing,* United States Bureau of Education, Bulletin 1912, No. 7 (Washington, D.C.: U.S. Government Printing Office, 1912), p. 24

Nutting M., Adelaide, "The Evolution of Nursing Education from Hospital to University," in Nutting, *A Sound Economic Basis for Schools of Nursing,* p. 298

Nutting M. Adelaide, *A Sound Economic Basis for Schools of Nursing and Other Addresses* (New York: G. P. Putnam, 1926)

Nutting M. Adelaide, and Dock, Lavinia L., *A History of Nursing,* 4 vols. (New York: Putnam, 1907-1912)

O'Hanlon, George, "Men Nurses in General Hospitals," *American Journal of Nursing* 34 (1934), p. 16

Olsen, L., "The Expanded Role of the Nurse in Maternity Practice," *Nurs. Clin. North America* 9 (1974), pp. 459–466

Packard, F. R., *History of Medicine in the United States*, 2nd edition, 2 vols. (New York: Hoeber, 1931)

Packard, F. R., *Life and Times of Ambroise Paré* (New York: Hoeber, 1921)

The Papyrus Ebers (New York: D. Appleton, 1931)

Parker, Martha P., "Preparatory Work at the Waltham Training School," *American Journal of Nursing* 3 (1903), pp. 264–266

Parkhurst, Genvieve, "Wanted—100,000 Girls for Sub-Nurses," *Pictorial Review* (October, 1921), pp. 15, 82

Parkhurst, Genvieve, "White Cap Famine," *Pictorial Review* (September 1921), pp. 2, 72–75

Parran, Thomas, "Public Health Nursing Marches On," *Public Health Nursing* 29 (1937), pp. 617–622

Parsons, Sara E., *History of the Massachusetts General Hospital Training School of Nursing* (Boston: Whitcomb and Barrows, 1922)

Parvin, Theophilus, *Lectures on Obstetric Nursing* (Philadelphia: Blakiston, Son, 1889)

Patton, James Welch, and Simkins, Francis Butler, *The Women of the Confederacy* (Richmond: Garrett and Massie, 1936)

Payne, Joseph Frank, *English Medicine in the Anglo-Saxon Times* (Oxford: Clarendon Press, 1904)

Pearson, Lu Emily, *Elizabethans at Home* (Palo Alto: Stanford University, 1957)

Peters, Dorothy, "The Kewanee Story," *American Journal of Nursing* 61 (1961), pp. 74–79

Petry, Lucile, "The U.S. Cadet Nurse Corps: A Summing up," *American Journal of Nursing* 45 (1945), pp. 1027–1028

Pfeiffer, R. H., *State Letters of Assyria* (New Haven: Yale University, 1935)

Phillips, E. D., *Greek Medicine* (London: Thames and Hudson, 1973)

Phillips, "Health Planning: New Hope for a Fresh Start," *Hospitals: Journal of the American Hospital Association* 49 (March 16, 1975), pp. 35–38

Pinel, Philippe, *A Treatise on Insanity,* translated by D. D. Davis (New York: Hafner, 1962)

Plain Directions for the Care of the Sick (New York: Mutual Life Insurance Co., 1874)

Plautus, *Two Menaechmuses,* edited and translated by Paul Nixon, in vol. 2 in the Loeb, *Plautus,* 5 vols. (London: William Heinemann, 1959–1963)

Pliny, *Natural History,* edited and translated by H. Rackham, W. H. S. Jones, and E. E. Eichholza, 10 vols. (London: William Heinemann, 1947–1963)

Plutarch, *Parallel Lives,* edited and translated by B. Perrin, 11 vols. (London: William Heinemann, 1954–1962)

Poël, Emma, *Life of Amelia Wilhelmina Sieveking,* translated by Catherine Winkworth (London: Longmans, Green, 1863)

Poole, Ernest, *Nurses on Horseback* (New York: Macmillan, 1935)

Power, Sir D'Arcy, *A Short History of Surgery* (London: John Bale Sons, and Danielsson, Ltd., 1933)

Practical Thoughts on Sisterhoods (New York: T. Whittaker, 1864)

Proceedings: Issues in Family Nurse Practitioner Education at the Baccalaureate Level. Conference held at the California State College, Sonoma, June 16–17, 1975

Proceedings of the Thirty-eighth Convention of the American Nurses Association, vol. I, House of Delegates, 1952

Ramphal, Marjorie, "Peer Review," *American Journal of Nursing* 74 (1974), pp. 63–67

Rathbone, Eleanor F., *William Rathbone, A Memoir* (New York: Macmillan, 1905)

Rathbone, William, *Sketch of the History and Progress of District Nursing From Its Commencement in the Year 1859 to the Present Date* (New York: Macmillan, 1890)

Raymond Rich Associates, "Report on the Structure of Organized Nursing," *American Journal of Nursing* 46 (1946), p. 648

Recordon, G., "Le cinquantenaire de l'école des infirmières de l'assistance publique," *Revue de l'assistance publique à Paris* 8 (1957), pp. 423–428

Redmond, Juanita, *I Served on Bataan* (Philadelphia: J. B. Lippincott, 1943)

Reinkemeyer, Sister Agnes M., "It Won't Be Hospital Nursing," *American Journal of Nursing* 68 (1968), pp. 1936–1940

Reinkemeyer, Sister Mary Hubert, "An Inherited Pathology," *Nursing Outlook* 15 (November, 1967), pp. 51–53

Reissman, Leonard, *Change and Dilemma in the Nursing Profession* (New York: G. P. Putnam's Sons, 1957)

Reiter, Francis, *The Improvement of Nursing Practice* (New York: ANA Publication, 1961)

Report of the Committee Appointed to Consider the Cubic Space of Metropolitan Workhouses, Paper No. XVI, pp. 64–79

"Report of Committee on the Training of Nurses," *Transactions of the American Medical Association,* 1869, pp. 161–174

Report of the Nursing Consultant Group to the Surgeon-General, *Toward Quality in Nursing, Needs and Goals* (Washington, D.C.: U.S. Department of Health, Education, and Welfare, 1963)

Reznick, Allen E., *Lillian D. Wald: The Years at Henry Street* (unpublished PhD dissertation, University of Wisconein, 1973)

Richards, Linda, "Early Days in the First American Training School for Nurses," *American Journal of Nursing* 73 (1973), pp. 574–575

Richards, Linda, "Recollections of a Pioneer Nurs," *American Journal of Nursing* 3 (1903), pp. 245–252

Richards, Linda, *Reminiscences of Linda Richards: America's First Trained Nurse* (Boston: Whitcomb and Barrows, 1911)

Riehl, Joan P., and McVay, Joan Wilcox (Editors) *The Clinical Nurse Specialist: Interpretations* (New York: Appleton-Century-Crofts, 1973)

Riesman, David, *The Story of Medicine in the Middle Ages* (New York: Hoeber, 1935)

Robb, Isabel Hampton, "Address of the President Before the Third Annual Convention of the Associated Alumnae of Trained Nurses in the United States," *American Journal of Nursing* 1 (1900), pp. 97–104

Robb, Isabel Hampton, "The Three Years' Course of Training in Connection with the Eight Hour System," *First and Second Annual Reports of the American Society of Superintendents of Training Schools for Nurses,* 1897

Robert, Mary M., *American Nursing: History and Interpretation* (New York: Macmillan, 1954)

Roberts, Mary M., "Lavinia Lloyd Dock—Nurse, Feminist, Internationalist," *American Journal of Nursing* 56 (1956), pp. 176–179

Robinson, Victor, *White Caps: The Story of Nursing* (Philadelphia: J. B. Lippincott, 1946)

Roemer, Ruth, "The Nurse Practitioner in Family Planning Services: Law and Practice," *Family Planning Population Reporter,* 6, No. 3, (June, 1977), pp. 28–34

Roemer, Ruth, "Nursing Functions and the Law: Some Perspectives from Australia and Canada," *The Law and the Expanded Role of the Nurse,* edited by Bonnie Bullough (New York: Appleton-Century-Crofts, 1975)

Rogers, Martha E., *Educational Revolution in Nursing* (New York: Macmillan, 1961)

Rogers, Martha, *Reveille in Nursing* (Philadelphia: F. A. Davis, 1964)

Rosaria, Sister Mary, *The Nurse in Greek Life* (Boston: privately printed, 1917)

Rose, Marie L., "What About Our Own Catastrophe," *American Journal of Nursing* 32 (1932), pp. 62–63

Rosen, George, *History of Public Health* (New York: M. D. Publications, 1958)

Rosen, George, *Madness in Society* (New York: Harper Torchbooks, 1964)

Ross, Ishbel, *Angel of the Battlefield* (New York: Harper, 1956)

Ross, Ishbel, *Child of Destiny* (London: Victor Gollancz, 1950)

Ross, Margaret, *Memoirs of a Private Nurse* (Glasgow: McNaugton and Sinclair, n.d.)

Rothstein, William G., *American Physicians in the 19th Century: From Sects to Science* (Baltimore: Johns Hopkins, 1972)

Royal Australian Nursing Federation and the National Florence Nightingale Committee of Australia, *Survey Report on the Wastage of General Trained Nurses from Nursing in Australia* (Canberra: 1967)

Russell, William L., "Men Nurses in Psychiatric Hospitals," *American Journal of Nursing* 34 (1934), p. 19

Sachs, Theodore B., "The Tuberculosis Nurse," *American Journal of Nursing* 8 (1908), p. 597

Sackett, David L., "The Burlington Randomized Trial of the Nurse Practitioner: Health Outcomes of Patients," *Annals of Internal Medicine* 80 (February 1974); reprinted in Bonnie and Vern Bullough (Editors) *Expanding Horizon for Nurses* (New York: Springer, 1977)

Sadler, Alfred M., and Sadler, Blair L., "Recent Developments in the Law Relating to Physicians' Assistants," *Vanderbilt Law Review* 24 (November 1971), p. 1205

Safier, Gwendolyn, *Contemporary American Leaders in Nursing: An Oral History* (New York: McGraw-Hill, 1977)

Sarner, Harvey, *The Nurse and the Law* (Philadelphia: W. B. Saunders, 1968)

Saunders, Lyle, "The Changing Role of Nurses," *American Journal of Nursing* 54 (1954), pp. 1094–1098

Scarborough, John, *Roman Medicine* (Ithaca: Cornell, 1969)

Schoenmaker, Adrian, "Nursing's Dilemma: Male Versus Female Admissions Choice," *Nursing Forum* XV (1976), pp. 406–412

Schoenmaker, Adrian, and Radosevich, David M., "Men Nursing Students: How They Perceive their Situation," *Nursing Outlook* 24 (May, 1976), pp. 298–301

Schryver, Grace Fay, *History of the Illinois Training School for Nurses, 1880–1929* (Chicago: Board of Directors of the Illinois Training School for Nurses, 1930)

Schulman, Sam, "Basic Functional Roles in Nursing: Mother Surrogate and Healer," in *Patients, Physicians and Illness,* edited by E. Gartly Jaco (Glencoe, Illinois: The Free Press, 1958)

Schutt, Barbara G., "Frontier's Family Nurses," *American Journal of Nursing* 72 (1972), pp. 903–909

Schutt, Barbara G., "The Right to Strike," (editorial), *American Journal of Nursing* 68 (1968), p. 1455

Schwier, Mildred E.; Paskewita, Lena R.; Peterson, Frances K., and Elliot, Florence E., *Ten Thousand Nurse Faculty Members in Basic Professional Schools of Nursing* (New York: National League for Nursing, 1953), p. 48

Schwitalla, Alphonse M., "President Economic Objectives of the Nursing Profession," *American Journal of Nursing* 33 (1933), pp. 1135–1142

Scott, Jessie M., "Federal Support for Nursing Education, 1964–1972," *American Journal of Nursing* 72 (1972), pp. 1855–1861

Scott, William, "Shall Professional Nurse Associations Become Collective Bargaining Agents for Their Members?" *American Journal of Nursing* 44 (1944), pp. 231–232

Scott, William G.; Porter, Elisabeth K.; Smith, Donald W., "The Long Shadow," *American Journal of Nursing* 66 (1966), pp. 538–554

Sculco, Cynthia D., "An American Nurse at the London Hospital," *Nursing Outlook* 24 (August, 1967), pp. 504–508

Seagrave, Gordon, *Burma Surgeon* (New York: W. W. Norton, 1943)

Seneca, *De Constantia,* in vol. I *Moral Essays,* edited and translated by John W. Basore (London: William Heinemann, 1951–1958)

Seton, R., *Memoirs, Letters and Journals of Elizabeth Seton,* 2 vols. (New York: 1869)

Seymer, Lucy Ridgely, *A General History of Nursing* (New York: Macmillan, 1933)

Seymer, Lucy Ridgely, *Selected Writings of Florence Nightingale* (New York: Macmillan, 1954)

Sharp, Bonita H., "The Beginning of Nursing Education in the United States: An Analysis of the Times," *Journal of Nursing Education* 12 (April, 1973), pp. 26–32

Shoemaker, Sister M. Theophane, *History of Nurse-Midwifery in the United States* (Washington, D.C.: The Catholic University of America, 1947)

Shryock, Richard H., *The Development of Modern Medicine,* 2nd edition (New York: Alfred A. Knopf, 1947)

Shryock, Richard H., *The History of Nursing* (Philadelphia: W. B. Saunders, 1959)

Shryock, Richard H., *Medical Licensing in America* (Baltimore: Johns Hopkins, 1967)

Shryock, Richard H., *Medicine in America: Historical Essays* (Baltimore: Johns Hopkins, 1966)

Sidel, W., "Feldshers and Feldsherism: The Role and Training in the Feldsher in the U.S.S.R." Bonnie and Vern Bullough, Editors, *New Directions for Nurses* (New York: Springer, 1971)

Siegel, G. E., and Bryson, S., "Redefinition of the Role of the Public Health Nurse in Child Health Supervision," *American Journal of Public Health* 53 (1972), pp. 1015–1024

Sigerist, Henry E., *American Medicine* (New York: W. W. Norton, 1934)

Sigerist, Henry E., *The Great Doctors* (New York: W. W. Norton, 1933)

Sigerist, Henry E., *A History of Medicine,* 2 vols. (New York: Oxford University, 1951–1961)

Sills, Grayce M., "Historical Developments in Psychiatric and Mental Health Nursing," Madelene Leininger, editor, *Contemporary Issues in Mental Health Nursing* (Boston: Little, Brown, 1973)

Silver, H., and Ford, L., "The Pediatric Nurse Practitioner at Colorado," *American Journal of Nursing* 67 (1967), pp. 1143–1144

Silver, H.; Ford, L., and Stearly, S., "A Program to Increase Health Care for Children: The Pediatric Nurse Practitioner Program," *Pediatrics* 39 (1967), pp. 756–760

Sinai, Nathan; Anderson, Odin W.; Dollar, Melvin L., *Health Insurance in the United States* (New York: The Commonwealth Fund, 1946)

Singer, Charles, *Greek Biology and Medicine* (Oxford: Clarendon Press, 1922)

Singer, Charles, *A Short History of Anatomy and Physiology from the Greeks to Harvey,* (reprint of *The Evolution of Anatomy* (New York: Dover, 1957)

The Size and Shape of the Medical Care Dollar, U.S. Department of Health, Education and Welfare, Social Security Administration (Washington, D.C.: U.S. Government Printing Office, 1970)

Skardon, Alvin W., *Church Leader in the Cities: William August Muhlenberg* (Philadelphia: University of Pennsylvania, 1971)

Slaughter, Frank G., *Immortal Magyar* (New York: Henry Schuman, 1950)

Smith, Adelaide W., *Reminiscences of an Army Nurse During the Great War* (New York: 1911)

Smith, Donald W., "The Wagner-Murray-Dingel Bill, Senate Bill 1050 H.R. 3293," *American Journal of Nursing* 45 (1945), pp. 933–936

Smith, Lena Mae, "Deaconess," *Mennonite Encyclopedia* 4 vols. (Scottdale, Pennsylvania: Mennonite Publishing House, 1955–1959), II, pp. 22–25

Somers, Herman Miles, and Somers, Anne Ransay, *Doctors, Patients and Health Insurance* (Washington, D.C.: The Brookings Institution, 1961)

Soranus, *Gynecology,* translated with an introduction by Owsei Temkin (Baltimore: Johns Hopkins, 1956)

Southey, Robert, *Sir Thomas Moore; or Colloquies on the Progress and Prospects of Society* (London: Murray, 1829), II, p. 318 and appendix. *The Life and Correspondence of the Late Robert Southey,* edited by Charles Cuthbert Southey, 6 vols. (London: Longmans, Green, 1850)

Southwood, Martin, *John Howard: Prison Reformer* (London: Independent Press, 1958)

Spingarn, Natalie Davis, "Biggest of the Health Professions, Nursing is Beset with Paradoxes," *The Chronicle of Higher Education,* February 4, 1974

Standard Curriculum for Schools of Nursing (New York: NLNE, 1917)

Standlee, Mary W., *The Great Pulse: Japanese Midwifery and Obstetrics through the Ages* (Rutland, Vermont: Charles E. Tuttle, 1959)

Stanley, Mary, *Hospitals and Sisterhoods* (London: Murray, 1854)

"Statutory Status of Six Professions," *Research Bulletin of the National Educational Association* 16 (September, 1938), pp. 184–223

Staupers, Mabel K., *No Time for Prejudice* (New York: Macmillan, 1961)

Staupers, Mabel K., "Story of the National Association of Colored Graduate Nurses," *American Journal of Nursing* 51 (1951), pp. 222–223

Stead, E. A. Jr., "Training and Use of Paramedical Personnel," *New England Journal of Medicine* 277 (October 12, 1967), pp. 800–801

Stein, Leonard, "The Doctor-Nurse Game," *American Journal of Nursing* 68 (1968), pp. 101–105, also in *New Directions for Nurses,* edited by Bonnie and Vern Bullough (New York: Springer, 1971), pp. 129–137

Stern, Madeleine, "Civil War Nurses," *Americana* XXXVII (1943), pp. 296–325

Stevenson, N., "Curriculum Development in Practical Nurse Education," *American Journal of Nursing* 64 (1964), pp. 81–86

Stewart, Isabel M., *The Education of Nurses: Historical Foundations and Modern Trends* (New York: Macmillan, 1945)

Stewart, Isabel M., "The Movement for Shorter Hours in Nurses' Training Schools," *American Journal of Nursing* 19 (1919), pp. 439–443

Stewart, Isabel M., and Gelinas, Agnes, *A Century of Nursing* (New York: G. P. Putnam's Sons, 1950)

Stopes, Charlotte Carmichael, *The Life of Henry, Third Earl of Southampton* (Cambridge: Cambridge University, 1922)

Strachey, Lytton, *Eminent Victorians* (New York: G. P. Putnam's Sons, 1918)

Strauss, Anselm, "The Structure and Ideology of American Nursing," in F. Davis, edition, *The Nursing Profession: Five Sociological Essays* (New York: Wiley, 1966)

"A Study of Industrial Nursing Services," *Public Health Nursing* 32 (1940), pp. 631–636

Sturluson, Snorri, *Heimskringla,* translated from the Icelandic by William Morris and E. Magnusson, 4 vols. (London: Bernard Quaritch, 1893–1905), "The Story of Magnus the Good," chap. xxix

Sushruta Samhita, translated and edited by K. K. Bhishagratna, 2nd edition, 3 vols. (India: Chowkhamba Sanscrit Series, 1963)

Swanton, John R., *The Indians of the Southeastern United States* (Smithsonian Institute, Bureau of American Ethnology, Bulletin No. 137, Washington, D.C., 1946)

Tacitus, *Dialogus,* edited and translated by Sir William Peterson (London: William Heinemann, 1946)

Tacitus, *Germania,* edited and translated by Maurice Hutton (London: William Heinemann, 1924)

Talbot, C. H., *Medicine in Medieval England* (London: Oldbourne, 1967)

Taylor, Henry L., *Professional Education in the United States* (Albany: University of the State of New York, 1900)

Tenon, J., *Memoirs sur les hôpitaux de Paris* (Paris: Pierres, 1788)

"A Tentative Plan for One National Nursing Organization," *American Journal of Nursing* 48 (1948), p. 321

Thatcher, Virginia S., *A History of Anesthesia: With Emphasis on the Nurse Specialist* (Philadelphia: J. B. Lippincott, 1952)

Theodoretus of Cyrrhus, *Ecclasiastical History,* edited by Leon Parmentier under title of *Theodoret Kirchengeschichte* 2nd edition (Berlin: Akademie-Verlag, 1954)

Thomas de Celano, *Vite Prima* and *Vite Secundo,* 2 vols. (Florence: College of S. Bonaventura, 1926–1927)

Thompson, Campbell R., *The Devils and Evil Spirits of Babylonia* (London: Luzac, 1903)

Thomas, Adah M., *Pathfinders—A History of the Progress of Colored Graduate Nurses* (New York: Kay, 1929)

Thurston, Herbert, "Deaconesses," *Catholic Encyclopedia,* 16 vols. (New York: Appleton, 1908–1914) IV, p. 651

Tighe, B., *Review of the Training Programs and Utilization of Paraprofessionals in Medicine and Dentistry,* Institute for the Study of Health and Society (1972), pp. 34–35

Titus, Shirley, "Economic Facts of Life for Nurses," *American Journal of Nursing* 52 (1952), pp. 1109–1112

Titus, Shirley, "Factors Determining the Development of Nursing and Schools of Nursing (with Special Reference to Vanderbilt University School of Nursing)," in *Methods and Problems of Medical Education* (New York: The Rockefeller Foundation, 1932)

Todd, J., and Gask, G. E., "The Origin of Hospitals" in *Science, Medicine and History,* edited by E. A. Underwood, 2 vols. (Oxford: Oxford University, 1953)

Tooley, Sarah A., *The History of Nursing in the British Empire* (London: S. H. Bousfield, 1906)

Trail, H. D., *Social England* (New York: G. P. Putnam's Sons, 1897)

"Trained Attendants and Practical Nurses," *American Journal of Nursing* 44 (1944), pp. 7–8

Trenchard, Edward C., *The Services and Sacrifices of the Daughters of the Republic During the Civil War* (New York: 1912)

Trexler, Bernice J., "Hospital Patients in Florence," *Bulletin of the History of Medicine* 48 (1974), pp. 41–58

Two Letters on Protestant Sisterhoods, 3rd edition (New York: R. Craighead, printer, 1856)

Tyler, Alice Felt, *Freedom's Ferment: Phases of American Social History to 1860* (Minneapolis: University of Minnesota, 1944)

U.S. Army Nurse Corps, *The Army Nurse* (Washington, D.C.: 1944)

U.S. Bureau of Labor Statistics, *The Economic Status of Registered Professional Nurses* (Washington, D.C.: 1947)

U.S. Department of Health, Education, and Welfare, Division of Nursing, *Health Manpower Source Book; 2. Nursing Personnel* (Washington, D.C.: U.S. Government Printing Office, Public Health Publication No. 263, Section 2, revised 1969), p. 53

U.S. Department of Health, Education and Welfare, *Extending the Scope of Nursing Practice: A Report of the Secretary's Committee to Study Extended Roles for Nurses* (November, 1971)

U.S. Navy Nurse Corps, *White Task Force* (Washington, D.C.: 1943)

U.S. Public Health Service, *The U.S. Cadet Nurse Corps and Other Federal Nurse Training Programs, 1943–1948* (Washington, D.C.: U.S. Government Printing Office, 1950)

Vasiliev, A. A., *History of the Byzantine Empire,* 2nd edition (Madison: University of Wisconsin, 1952)

"Vassar Preparatory Course: A New Experiment in Nursing Education," *American Journal of Nursing* 18 (1918), p. 1155

Vegetius, *Military Institutions of the Romans,* translated by John Clark (Harrisburg, Pennsylvania: The Military Service Publishing Company, 1944)

Veith, Ilza, *The Yellow Emperor's Classic of Internal Medicine*, new edition (Berkeley: University of California, 1972)

Verney, Sir Harry, *Florence Nightingale at Harley Street: Her Reports to the Governors of Her Nursing Home, 1853-1854* (London: J. M. Dent & Sons, 1970)

Vreeland, Ellwynne M., "Fifty Years of Nursing in the Federal Government Nursing Services," *American Journal of Nursing* 50 (1950), pp. 626-631

Wald, Lillian D., *The House on Henry Street* (Boston: Little, Brown & Company, 1933)

Walsh, James J., *History of Medicine in New York* (New York: National American Society, 1919)

Walsh, James J., *These Splendid Sisters* (New York: J. H. Sears, 1927) and articles on various nursing orders in the *New Catholic Encyclopedia* (Washington, D.C.: The Catholic University of America, 1967)

Walsh, Mary Roth, *Doctors Wanted: No Women Need Apply* (New Haven, Connecticut: Yale University, 1977)

Walsh, Mary Roth, "Feminism: A Support System for Women Physicians," *Journal of the American Medical Women's Association* (June, 1976)

Walters, Verle; Chater, Shirley; Vivier, Mary Louise; Urres, Judith H., and Wilson, Holly Skodal, "Technical and Professional Nursing: An Exploratory Study," *Nursing Research* 21 (March/April, 1972), pp. 124-131

Walton, Harold, and Nelson, Kathryn Jensen, *Historical Sketches of the Medical Work of Seventh Day Adventists* (Washington, D.C.: Review & Herald Publishing Company, 1948)

Warrington, Joseph, *The Nurses Guide* (Philadelphia: Thomas Cowperwaite, 1893), excerpted in Anne L. Austin, *History of Nursing Source Book* (New York: G. P. Putnam's Sons, 1949)

Waters, Isabella, *Visiting Nursing in the United States* (New York: Charities Publication Committee, 1909)

Weiner, Dora B., "The French Revolution, Napoleon, and the Nursing Profession," *Bulletin of the History of Medicine* XLVI (1972), pp. 274-305

Welborn, Mary Catherine, "The Long Tradition: A Study on Fourteenth Century Medical Dentology," *Medieval and Historiographical Essays in Honor of James Westfall Thompson* (Chicago: University of Chicago, 1938)

Werminghouse, Esther H., *Annie W. Goodrich; Her Journey to Yale* (New York: Macmillan, 1950)

West, Margaret, and Hawkins, Christy, *Nursing Schools at the Mid-Century* (New York: NCINS, 1950)

West, Roberta Mayhew, *History of Nursing in Pennsylvania* (Pennsylvania State Nurses' Association, 1933)

Whitman, Walt, *Complete Writings*, 10 vols. (New York: G. P. Putnam's Sons, 1902)

Whitney, Janet, *Elizabeth Fry* (Boston: Little, Brown & Company, 1936)

Whitney, Jessamine S., "Tuberculosis Among Young Women—With Special Reference to Tuberculosis Among Nurses," *American Journal of Nursing* 28, pp. 766-768

"Who is Mrs. Nightingale?" *London Times*, October 30, 1854

Willius, F. A., and Keys, Thomas E., (eds.), *Cardiac Classics* (St. Louis: C. V. Mosby, 1941)

Winslow, C.E.A., "The Role of the Visiting Nurse in the Campaign for Public Health," *American Journal of Nursing* 11 (1911), pp. 909-920

Witte, Frances W., "Opportunities in Graduate Education for Men Nurses," *American Journal of Nursing* 34 (1934), p. 133

Wittmeyer, Annie T., *Under the Guns: A Woman's Reminiscences of the Civil War* (Boston: 1895)

Women in the Modern World, edited by Viba B. Boothe for the American Academy of Political and Social Science (1929)

Woodham-Smith, Cecil, *Florence Nightingale, 1820–1910* (New York: McGraw-Hill, 1951)

Woodward, E. D., *The Age of Reform, 1815–1870* (Oxford: Clarendon Press, 1938)

Woodward, Ella S., "Federal Aspects of Unemployment Among Professional Women," *American Journal of Nursing* 34 (1934), pp. 534–538

Woodward, Ella S., "The WPA and Nursing," and "WPA Nursing," *American Journal of Nursing* 37 (1937), pp. 994–997; 38 (1938), p. 733

Woody, T., *A History of Women's Education in the United States*, 2 vols. (Lancaster, Pennsylvania: Science Press, 1929)

Woolsey, Abby Howland, *Hospitals and Training Schools Report of the Standing Committee on Hospitals of the State Charities Aid Association* (New York: May 24, 1876); reprinted in *A Century of Nursing* (New York: G. P. Putnam's Sons, 1950), p. 129

Woolsey, Jane Stuart, *Hospital Days* (New York: 1870)

Worcester, Alfred, *Nurses and Nursing* (Cambridge: Harvard University, 1927)

Wormeley, Katharine Prescott, *The Other Side of the War with the Army of the Potomac* (Boston: Ticknor, 1889), later published as *The Cruel Side of War* (Boston: Roberts, 1898)

Worthington, C. G., *The Woman in Battle* (Hartford: 1876)

"WPA Nursing," *American Journal of Nursing* 38 (1938), p. 733

Xelainche, X., "La profession d'infirmière," *Quatre novelles années d'action hôspitalière sociale et medico-sociale, 1956 à 1960* (Paris: Imprimerie Municipale, 1960)

Xenophon, *Anabasis*, edited and translated by C. L. Brownson and O. J. Todd, 2 vols. (London: William Heinemann, 1947–1953)

Xenophon, *Oeconomicus*, edited and translated by E. C. Marchant (London: William Heinemann, 1953)

Zimmerman, Anne, "The ANA Economic Security Program in Retrospect," *Nursing Forum* 10, No. 3 (1971), pp. 313–321

Zimmermann, Anne, "Taft-Hartley Amended; Implications for Nursing: The Industrial Model," *American Journal of Nursing* 75 (1975), pp. 284–288

Index